Lung Transplantation

Guest Editor

ROBERT M. KOTLOFF, MD

CLINICS IN CHEST MEDICINE

www.chestmed.theclinics.com

June 2011 • Volume 32 • Number 2

SAUNDERS an imprint of ELSEVIER, Inc.

W.B. SAUNDERS COMPANY
A Division of Elsevier Inc.

1600 John F. Kennedy Boulevard • Suite 1800 • Philadelphia, Pennsylvania 19103

http://www.theclinics.com

CLINICS IN CHEST MEDICINE Volume 32, Number 2
June 2011 ISSN 0272-5231, ISBN-13: 978-1-4557-0430-9

Editor: Sarah E. Barth
Developmental Editor: Eva Kulig

Clinics in Chest Medicine (ISSN 0272-5231) is published quarterly by Elsevier Inc., 360 Park Avenue South, New York, NY 10010-1710. Months of issue are March, June, September, and December. Periodicals postage paid at New York, NY and additional mailing offices. Subscription prices are $293.00 per year (domestic individuals), $475.00 per year (domestic institutions), $140.00 per year (domestic students/residents), $321.00 per year (Canadian individuals), $583.00 per year (Canadian institutions), $399.00 per year (international individuals), $583.00 per year (international institutions), and $195.00 per year (international and Canadian students/residents). International air speed delivery is included in all Clinics subscription prices. All prices are subject to change without notice. **POSTMASTER:** Send address changes to Clinics in Chest Medicine, Elsevier Health Sciences Division, Subscription Customer Service, 3251 Riverport Lane, Maryland Heights, MO 63043. **Customer Service: Telephone: 1-800-654-2452** (U.S. and Canada); **1-314-447-8871** (outside U.S. and Canada). **Fax: 1-314-447-8029. E-mail: journalscustomerservice-usa@elsevier.com** (for print support); **journalsonlinesupport-usa@elsevier.com** (for online support).

Reprints. For copies of 100 or more of articles in this publication, please contact the Commercial Reprints Department, Elsevier Inc., 360 Park Avenue South, New York, NY 10010-1710. Tel.: 212-633-3812; Fax: 212-462-1935; E-mail: reprints@elsevier.com.

Clinics in Chest Medicine is covered in *MEDLINE/PubMed (Index Medicus), Current Contents/Clinical Medicine, EMBASE/ Excerpta Medica, Science Citation Index,* and *ISI/BIOMED.*

Printed and bound by CPI Group (UK) Ltd, Croydon, CR0 4YY

Transferred to Digital Print 2011

Contributors

GUEST EDITOR

ROBERT M. KOTLOFF, MD
Professor of Medicine, Chief, Section of
Advanced Lung Disease and Lung
Transplantation, Pulmonary, Allergy,
and Critical Care Division, University of
Pennsylvania Medical Center,
Philadelphia, Pennsylvania

AUTHORS

VIVEK N. AHYA, MD
Medical Director, Lung Transplantation
Program; Assistant Professor of Medicine,
Pulmonary, Allergy, and Critical Care Division,
Department of Medicine, University of
Pennsylvania School of Medicine,
Philadelphia, Pennsylvania

SELIM M. ARCASOY, MD, FCCP, FACP
Professor of Clinical Medicine, Medical
Director, Lung Transplantation Program,
Division of Pulmonary, Allergy, and Critical
Care Medicine, Columbia University Medical
Center, New York, New York

SANGEETA M. BHORADE, MD
Medical Director, Lung Transplantation
Program; Associate Professor of Medicine,
Section of Pulmonary and Critical Care
Medicine, University of Chicago Medical
Center, Chicago, Illinois

EMILY A. BLUMBERG, MD
Professor of Medicine, Division of Infectious
Diseases, University of Pennsylvania Medical
Center, University of Pennsylvania School of
Medicine, Philadelphia, Pennsylvania

DONG-FENG CHEN, PhD, Diplomate ABHI
Associate Professor, Director, Clinical
Transplantation Immunology Laboratory,
Department of Pathology, Duke University
Medical Center, Durham, North Carolina

JASON D. CHRISTIE, MD, MS
Associate Professor of Medicine and
Epidemiology, Division of Pulmonary,
Allergy and Critical Care Medicine;
Department of Biostatistics and
Epidemiology, Center for Clinical
Epidemiology and Biostatistics,
University of Pennsylvania School
of Medicine, Philadelphia, Pennsylvania

PAUL A. CORRIS, MBBS, FRCP
Professor of Thoracic Medicine, Institute of
Cellular Medicine, Newcastle University,
Newcastle upon Tyne Hospitals, NHS
Foundation Trust, Newcastle upon Tyne,
United Kingdom

GERARD J. CRINER, MD
Professor of Medicine, Florence P.
Bernheimer Distinguished Service
Chair, and Director, Division of Pulmonary
and Critical Care Medicine and
Temple Lung Center, Temple
University School of Medicine,
Philadelphia, Pennsylvania

MARCELO CYPEL, MD, MSc
Clinical Fellow, Division of Thoracic
Surgery, Toronto Lung Transplant
Program, Toronto General Hospital,
University of Toronto, Toronto,
Ontario, Canada

MICHAEL EBERLEIN, MD, PhD
Fellow, Division of Pulmonary and Critical
Care Medicine, Johns Hopkins Hospital,
Johns Hopkins University School of Medicine,
Baltimore; Staff Clinician, Critical Care
Medicine Department, Clinical Center, National
Institutes of Health, Bethesda, Maryland

MARC ESTENNE, MD, PhD
Professor, Department of Chest Medicine,
Erasme University Hospital, Université
Libre de Bruxelles, Brussels, Belgium

TIMOTHY FLORETH, MD
Fellow, Section of Pulmonary and Critical
Care Medicine, University of Chicago
Medical Center, Chicago, Illinois

EDWARD R. GARRITY, MD, MBA
Professor of Medicine, Vice Chair of
Clinical Operations, and Associate Director,
Transplantation Services, Division of
Pulmonary and Critical Care Medicine,
University of Chicago, Chicago, Illinois

DENIS HADJILIADIS, MD, MHS
Assistant Professor of Medicine,
Section of Advanced Lung Disease and
Lung Transplantation, Pulmonary,
Allergy, and Critical Care Division,
University of Pennsylvania Medical Center,
Philadelphia, Pennsylvania

STEVEN M. KAWUT, MD, MS
Associate Professor of Medicine and
Epidemiology; Director, Pulmonary Vascular
Disease Program, Pulmonary, Allergy, and
Critical Care Division, Department of Medicine
and the Center for Clinical Epidemiology and
Biostatistics, University of Pennsylvania
School of Medicine, Philadelphia, Pennsylvania

**SHAF KESHAVJEE, MD, MSc,
FRCSC, FACS**
Surgeon-in-Chief, James Wallace
McCutcheon Chair in Surgery Director, Toronto
Lung Transplant Program; Director, Latner
Thoracic Research Laboratories Scientist,
McEwen Centre for Regenerative Medicine
Program; Medical Director, Surgical Services
and Critical Care University Health Network,
Division of Thoracic Surgery, Institute of
Biomaterials and Biomedical Engineering,
University of Toronto, Toronto, Ontario,
Canada

CHRISTIANE KNOOP, MD, PhD
Professor, Department of Chest Medicine,
Erasme University Hospital, Université
Libre de Bruxelles, Brussels, Belgium

ROBERT M. KOTLOFF, MD
Professor of Medicine, Chief, Section
of Advanced Lung Disease and Lung
Transplantation, Pulmonary, Allergy,
and Critical Care Division, University of
Pennsylvania Medical Center,
Philadelphia, Pennsylvania

MARYL KREIDER, MD, MS
Assistant Professor of Medicine,
Section of Advanced Lung
Disease and Lung Transplantation,
Pulmonary, Allergy, and Critical
Care Division, University of
Pennsylvania Medical Center,
Philadelphia, Pennsylvania

HANS J. LEE, MD
Associate Director, Interventional
Pulmonology, Virginia Commonwealth
University; Director, Interventional
Pulmonology Fellowship Program,
Virginia Commonwealth University
Medical Center, Richmond, Virginia

JAMES C. LEE, MD
Assistant Professor of Medicine,
Division of Pulmonary, Allergy and
Critical Care Medicine, University of
Pennsylvania School of Medicine,
Philadelphia, Pennsylvania

TEREZA MARTINU, MD
Assistant Professor of Medicine,
Lung and Heart-Lung Transplant Program,
Division of Pulmonary and Critical Care,
Department of Medicine, Duke University
Medical Center, Durham, North Carolina

JONATHAN B. ORENS, MD
Professor of Medicine, Associate
Director and Clinical Chief, Medical
Director of Lung Transplantation,
Division of Pulmonary and Critical Care
Medicine, Johns Hopkins Hospital, Johns
Hopkins University School of Medicine,
Baltimore, Maryland

SCOTT M. PALMER, MD, MHS
Associate Professor of Medicine, Scientific
Director, Lung and Heart-Lung Transplant
Program, Division of Pulmonary and Critical
Care, Department of Medicine, Duke University
Medical Center, Durham, North Carolina

ELIZABETH N. PAVLISKO, MD
Clinical Associate, Division of Thoracic
Pathology, Department of Pathology, Duke
University Medical Center, Durham, North
Carolina

JONATHAN PUCHALSKI, MD, MEd
Assistant Professor of Medicine (Pulmonary)
and Director, Thoracic Interventional Program
(TIP), Yale School of Medicine, Yale University,
New Haven, Connecticut

HILARY Y. ROBBINS, MD
Assistant Professor of Clinical Medicine,
Lung Transplantation Program, Division of
Pulmonary, Allergy, and Critical Care
Medicine, Columbia University
Medical Center, New York, New York

KAREN D. SIMS, MD, PhD
Discovery Medicine, Virology, Bristol-Myers
Squibb, Princeton, New Jersey

GREGORY I. SNELL, MD
Professor, Lung Transplant Service,
Alfred Hospital and Monash University,
Melbourne, Australia

DANIEL H. STERMAN, MD
Chief, Section of Interventional Pulmonology
and Thoracic Oncology, University of
Pennsylvania Medical Center, Philadelphia,
Pennsylvania

GLEN P. WESTALL, MD
Lung Transplant Service, Alfred
Hospital and Monash University,
Melbourne, Australia

JONATHAN C. YEUNG, MD
General Surgery Resident, Research
Fellow - Latner Thoracic Surgery
Laboratories, University of Toronto,
Toronto, Ontario, Canada

ROGER D. YUSEN, MD, MPH
Associate Professor of Medicine,
Divisions of Pulmonary and Critical Care
Medicine and General Medical Sciences,
Washington University School of
Medicine, St Louis, Missouri

Contents

Decisions about patient selection, timing of listing, and choice of procedure are important steps in optimizing the outcome of lung transplantation. Selection of candidates for lung transplantation requires an appreciation of the effect of pretransplant patient characteristics on posttransplant outcomes. Familiarity with the natural history of the underlying disease and of disease-specific prognostic factors is essential in making decisions about when to list candidates. Decisions about transplanting 1 or 2 lungs are principally determined by the underlying disease, but in cases in which both procedures are acceptable, factors such as survival benefit, patient's age, and center-specific preferences come into play.

Lung allocation in the United States has changed significantly with the introduction of the Lung Allocation Score (LAS) system in May 2005. Since then, organ allocation is no longer based on waiting time but on a measure of transplant benefit (the difference between survival with vs without a transplant). The LAS system has met its primary goal of reducing time and mortality on the waiting list. Better understanding of pretransplant factors that influence long-term posttransplant outcomes of the individual patient will be instrumental in improving the LAS system in the future.

This article reviews recent developments in the selection, assessment, and management of the potential lung donor that aim to increase donor organ use. The scarcity of suitable donor organs results in long waiting times and significant mortality for those patients awaiting transplant. Strategies to expand the donor pool can substantially improve donor lung use rates. Although further long-term studies are required to confirm that long-term outcomes are not being compromised, the available evidence suggests that the traditional factors defining a lung as marginal or extended do not actually compromise outcomes within the framework of current donor management strategies.

Two novel approaches have been developed to potentially increase the availability of donor lungs for lung transplantation. In the first approach, lungs from donation after cardiac death (DCD) donors are used to increase the quantity of organ donors. In the second approach, a newly developed normothermic ex vivo lung perfusion

(EVLP) technique is used as a means of reassessing the adequacy of lung function from DCD and from high-risk brain death donors prior to transplantation. This EVLP technique can also act as a platform for the delivery of novel therapies to repair injured organs ex vivo.

Patients who are excellent candidates for lung transplantation often die on the waiting list because they are too sick to survive until an organ becomes available. Improvements in lung transplant outcomes, patient selection, and artificial lung device technologies have made it possible to bridge these patients to successful life-saving transplantation. Extracorporeal life support (ECLS) should be tailored to minimize morbidity and provide the appropriate mode and level of cardiopulmonary support for each patient's physiologic requirements. Novel device refinements and further development of ECLS in an ambulatory and simplified manner will help maintain these patients in better condition until transplantation.

Lung transplant offers the hope of prolonged survival and significant improvement in quality of life to patients with advanced lung disease. However, the medical literature lacks strong evidence and shows conflicting information regarding the effects of lung transplantation on these outcomes. Tools that integrate survival and quality-of-life information allow for more comprehensive evaluations of the benefits and risks of lung transplant. Higher-quality information leads to improved knowledge and more-informed decision making.

Immunosuppressive therapy has contributed significantly to improved survival after solid organ transplantation. Nevertheless, treatment-related adverse events and persistently high risk of chronic graft rejection remain major obstacles to long-term survival after lung transplantation. The development of new agents, refinements in techniques to monitor immunosuppression, and enhanced understanding of transplant immunobiology are essential for further improvements in outcome. In this article, conventional immunosuppressive regimens, novel approaches to preventing graft rejection, and investigational agents for solid organ transplantation are reviewed.

Primary graft dysfunction (PGD) is the most important cause of early morbidity and mortality following lung transplantation. PGD affects up to 25% of all lung transplant procedures and currently has no proven preventive therapy. Lung transplant recipients who recover from PGD may have impaired long-term function and an increased risk of bronchiolitis obliterans syndrome. This article aims to provide a state-of-the-art review of PGD epidemiology, outcomes, and risk factors, and to summarize current efforts at biomarker development and novel strategies for prevention and treatment.

Acute cellular rejection affects greater than one-third of lung transplant recipients. Alloreactive T-lymphocytes constitute the basis of lung allograft rejection. Recent evidence supports a more complex immune response to the allograft. Interaction between recipient genetics, immunosuppression therapies, and allograft environmental exposures likely contribute to high rejection rates after lung transplantation. A greater understanding of the heterogeneous mechanisms of lung rejection is critical to developing effective therapies that target the precise pathophysiology of the disease and ultimately improve long-term lung transplant outcomes.

Chronic, progressive, and irreversible loss of lung function is the major medium-term and long-term complication after lung transplantation and the leading cause of death. Over the past decade, progress has been made in understanding the pathogenesis of bronchiolitis obliterans. Alloimmune factors and nonalloimmune factors may contribute to its development. Understanding the precise mechanism of each type of chronic allograft dysfunction may open up the field for new preventive and therapeutic interventions. This article reviews major new insights into the clinical aspects, pathophysiology, risk factors, diagnosis, and management of chronic allograft dysfunction after lung transplantation.

Infections are a major cause of morbidity and mortality after lung transplantation. Pretransplant assessments for infection risk and immunization updates may help reduce posttransplant infections. In addition careful choice of posttransplant prophylaxis for cytomegalovirus and fungal infections is critical. Because of the potential association of infections such as respiratory viral infections and gram-negative bacterial infections with bronchiolitis obliterans syndrome, prompt attention to these pathogens is critical. Choice of antimicrobials for prophylaxis and treatment should take into consideration both adverse effects and drug interactions associated with antimicrobial choice.

Malignancy is an important complication of thoracic organ transplantation and is associated with significant morbidity and mortality. Lung transplant recipients are at greater risk for cancer than immunocompetent persons, with cancer-specific incidence rates up to 60-fold higher than the general population. The increased risk for cancer is attributed to neoplastic properties of immunosuppressive medications, oncogenic viruses, and cancer-specific risk factors. This article addresses the epidemiology, presentation, and treatment of the most common malignancies after

Clinics in Chest Medicine

ISSUES OF RELATED INTEREST

Pediatric Clinics of North America, Volume 57, Issue 2, Pages 353–634 (April 2010)
Optimization of Outcomes for Children After Solid Organ Transplantation
Vicky Lee Ng and Sandy Feng, *Guest Editors*

THE CLINICS ARE NOW AVAILABLE ONLINE!

Access your subscription at:
www.theclinics.com

Preface

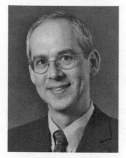

Robert M. Kotloff, MD
Guest Editor

"This patient, satisfying stringent preset technical and moral criteria for the procedure, is believed to be the first recipient of a successful lung transplant."

Hardy and colleagues, 1963[1]

"With this experimental work completed and with the use of cyclosporine eliminating the need for perioperative corticosteroids, we returned to the clinical sphere and reported the first two successful single-lung transplantations."

Grossman and colleagues, 1990 (referring to transplants performed by Joel Cooper in 1983–1984)[2]

"It depends on what the meaning of the word 'is' is."

Bill Clinton (42nd President of the United States)[3]

James Hardy is credited with performing the first human lung transplantation in 1963; the patient died 18 days later of multisystem organ failure but the allograft remained functional up to the time of death. Two decades later, Joel Cooper performed the first lung transplantation that resulted in meaningful survival; the recipient lived for 7 years before dying of renal failure. Both pioneering surgeons lay claim to the first "successful" procedure. Neither surgeon is wrong—it is simply a matter of how one defines success. Nearly 50 years and 32,000 procedures after the initial attempt, we are still debating the meaning of this word as it applies to lung transplant outcomes. Should lung transplantation be judged by the absolute longevity of its recipients, by the relative gain in survival compared to survival without the procedure, or by gains in quality of life and functional status independent of survival? Should it be judged against other vital organ transplant procedures, whose long-term outcomes continue to outpace those achieved with lung transplantation?

This issue of the *Clinics in Chest Medicine* provides readers with an overview of the current state of lung transplantation. The articles comprising this monograph, written by leading authorities in the field, cover the entire transplant process, from selection and management of transplant candidates and donors, to outcomes achieved in recipients, to management of the protean complications that constrain these outcomes. The issue concludes with discussions of evolving therapies that can serve as either an alternative or a bridge to transplantation for patients with chronic obstructive pulmonary disease or pulmonary hypertension. The ultimate goal of this compilation is to allow readers to formulate their own opinions on whether lung transplantation should be deemed a "successful" intervention. This is an essential exercise for frontline caregivers who are often responsible for initiating referrals for transplant evaluation and whose counseling can color the perspective of patients even before they arrive at the transplant center.

I would like to express my sincere gratitude to the authors who committed precious time to produce the scholarly works that comprise this monograph. I would also like to thank Sarah Barth from Elsevier for orchestrating this effort and keeping everyone on task. I owe a special debt of gratitude to Nancy Blumenthal, CRNP, who graciously shouldered extra patient care responsibilities to allow me to devote time to this project and who has set the standard for collaborative practice in the care of transplant patients.

Clin Chest Med 32 (2011) xiii–xiv
doi:10.1016/j.ccm.2011.03.002

Finally, I would like to thank my wife, Debbie, and sons, Eric, Brian, and Ethan; it is through them that I define success in my own life.

Robert M. Kotloff, MD
Pulmonary, Allergy, and Critical Care Division
838 West Gates Building
University of Pennsylvania Medical Center
3400 Spruce Street
Philadelphia, PA 19104, USA

E-mail address:
kotloffr@uphs.upenn.edu

REFERENCES

1. Hardy JD, Webb WR, Dalton ML Jr, et al. Lung homotransplantation in man. JAMA 1963;186: 1065–74.
2. Grossman RF, Frost A, Zamel N, et al. Results of single-lung transplantation for bilateral pulmonary fibrosis. The Toronto Lung Transplant Group. N Engl J Med 1990;322:727–33.
3. Testimony of William Jefferson Clinton before the Grand Jury, August 17, 1998. Available at: http://jurist.law.pitt.edu/transcr.htm. Accessed March 8, 2011.

Candidate Selection, Timing of Listing, and Choice of Procedure for Lung Transplantation

Maryl Kreider, MD, MS, Denis Hadjiliadis, MD, MHS, Robert M. Kotloff, MD*

KEYWORDS

• Lung transplantation • Selection criteria • Techniques

Lung transplant recipients face innumerable challenges posed by surgery, immunosuppression, drug toxicities, and rejection. To maximize the likelihood of a successful outcome, candidates selected to undergo this arduous procedure ideally must be free of significant medical comorbidities and sufficiently fit to handle these insults. Because of the inherent risks involved, it is also essential that patients are not listed prematurely, but only at a time when living with their underlying disease poses even greater risk. This strategy requires an appreciation of the natural history of lung disease to determine when the disease has entered an advanced and imminently life-threatening stage. Unique to lung transplantation, decisions must often be made about whether to replace 1 or both organs.

This review discusses the decision process leading up to the transplant surgery. These decisions (patient selection, timing of listing, and choice of procedure type) are critically important steps in optimizing the outcome of lung transplantation.

INDICATIONS FOR TRANSPLANTATION

The indications for lung transplantation include a diverse array of pulmonary diseases of the airways, parenchyma, and vasculature. Chronic obstructive pulmonary disease (COPD) represents the leading indication for lung transplantation worldwide, accounting for approximately one-third of all procedures performed to date.[1] The number of procedures performed for idiopathic pulmonary fibrosis (IPF) has been steadily increasing and although still second to COPD worldwide, IPF is now the leading indication in the United States.[2] Cystic fibrosis (CF) (16%), emphysema caused by α-$_1$-antitrypsin deficiency (7%), sarcoidosis (3%), non-CF bronchiectasis (3%), and lymphangioleiomyomatosis (1%) represent other less common indications.[1] Once a leading indication for transplantation, idiopathic pulmonary arterial hypertension (IPAH) now accounts for only 2% of procedures, reflecting major advances in the medical management of these patients. Transplantation of patients with lung involvement caused by scleroderma remains controversial because of concerns that esophageal dysmotility and reflux could increase the risk for aspiration and accelerated graft loss. Nonetheless, short-term functional outcomes and survival after transplantation of carefully selected patients with scleroderma are comparable with other patient populations.[3,4] Limited attempts to use lung transplantation for definitive cure of bronchoalveolar carcinoma,

Funding source: This work was supported in part by the Craig and Elaine Dobbin Pulmonary Research Fund.
Section of Advanced Lung, Disease and Lung Transplantation, Pulmonary, Allergy, and Critical Care Division, University of Pennsylvania Medical Center, 838 West Gates, 3400 Spruce Street, Philadelphia, PA 19104, USA
* Corresponding author.
E-mail address: kotloffr@uphs.upenn.edu

Clin Chest Med 32 (2011) 199–211
doi:10.1016/j.ccm.2011.02.001
0272-5231/11/$ – see front matter © 2011 Published by Elsevier Inc.

a subtype of lung cancer with a low metastatic potential, were met with an unacceptably high rate of cancer recurrence, leading most centers to view this as a contraindication.[5]

CANDIDATE SELECTION

There are few absolute contraindications to lung transplantation. There is general consensus that listing is contraindicated by: recent malignancy (other than nonmelanoma skin cancer); infection with the human immunodeficiency virus; hepatitis B or C virus with histologic evidence of significant liver damage; active or recent cigarette smoking, drug abuse, or alcohol abuse; severe psychiatric illness; documented and recurrent noncompliance with medical care; and absence of a consistent and reliable social support network.[6] The presence of significant extrapulmonary vital organ dysfunction precludes isolated lung transplantation, but multiorgan procedures such as heart-lung or lung-liver can be considered in highly select patients.[7,8] When extreme, obesity and malnutrition are commonly viewed as absolute contraindications but cutoffs vary among centers.[6] The risk posed by other medical comorbidities such as diabetes mellitus, osteoporosis, gastroesophageal reflux, and coronary artery disease must be assessed individually based on severity of disease, presence of end-organ damage, and ease of control with standard therapies.

Although the cutoff is admittedly arbitrary, most transplant centers define an upper age cutoff for transplant eligibility, commonly 65 years of age. However, there has been an increasing trend to expand the age range, based principally on the argument that suitability for transplant should be based on physiologic rather than chronologic age criteria. This trend has been most pronounced in the United States, where patients 65 years and older accounted for 19% of transplant recipients in 2008 compared with less than 5% before 2002.[2] A recent single-center study of 50 carefully selected patients 65 years or older found no difference in 1-year and 3-year posttransplant survival rates compared with a cohort less than the age of 65 years.[9] However, the Scientific Registry of Transplant Recipients (SRTR), a comprehensive database of US transplants, documents a 10-year survival rate among recipients 65 years and older of only 13% compared with 23% for those 50 to 64 years, and 38% for those younger than 50 years.[2]

Candidates for lung transplantation are functionally limited (New York Heart Association class III or IV) but, ideally, still ambulatory. Many programs screen for and exclude profoundly debilitated patients by requiring a minimum distance on a standard 6-minute walk test (6MWT).[10] An evolving area of controversy centers on the eligibility of ventilator-dependent patients in the intensive care unit (ICU), most of whom are nonambulatory. Ventilator dependence before transplantation has long been recognized as a risk factor for increased posttransplant mortality, and transplantation of these patients was typically discouraged in the past. The new lung allocation system in the United States, which prioritizes patients based on medical urgency and short-term net survival benefit, has forced transplant centers to reconsider this philosophy by assigning the highest allocation scores to ventilator-dependent patients. Many programs are now willing to maintain select ventilator-dependent patients on their active waiting list, anticipating that transplantation occurs in short order and reserving the option of delisting patients who develop intercurrent complications or progressive debility. A recent analysis of 586 ventilator-dependent patients documents inferior but not abysmal short-term outcomes; 1-year and 2-year survival rates were 62% and 57%, respectively, compared with 79% and 70% for unsupported patients.[11] Even more controversial is the transplantation of patients on extracorporeal membrane oxygenation support, for whom 1-year and 2-year posttransplant survival rates are only 50% and 45%, respectively.[11]

Previous pleurodesis is associated with an increased risk of intraoperative bleeding, particularly when cardiopulmonary bypass is used, but this is not a contraindication to transplantation in experienced surgical hands.[12,13] Previous lung volume reduction surgery (LVRS) in patients with COPD can similarly increase the risk of pleural bleeding but does not seem to adversely affect survival or functional outcomes.[14] In contrast, pleural thickening associated with mycetomas can render explantation of the native lung difficult and bloody, and there is the additional risk of soiling the pleural space with fungal organisms if the mycetoma cavity is violated. In 1 small series, the presence of a mycetoma in the native lung was associated with a perioperative mortality of 45%.[15] In light of this, it seems prudent to exclude those patients with mycetomas with either extensive pleural reaction or cavities abutting the pleural surface.

Chronic infection of the airways is a universal feature of CF and poses unique concerns in selecting patients with CF for transplantation. Most patients with CF are infected with Pseudomonas aeruginosa by the time they are considered for lung transplantation. Although these organisms are often highly resistant, the effect of the resistance pattern on survival after transplantation seems to be small. Two single-center retrospective studies found that posttransplant survival of patients with CF with panresistant *Pseudomonas aeruginosa* was similar to that of patients harboring sensitive strains.[16,17] In contrast to these studies, Hadjiliadis and colleagues[18] found that patients harboring pan-resistant organisms had lower, albeit still highly favorable, survival rates compared with patients with sensitive strains: 87% versus 97% at 1 year and 58% versus 86% at 5 years. Taken in sum, these 3 studies suggest that patients with panresistant *Pseudomonas aeruginosa* should not be excluded from consideration for lung transplantation.

The situation is more complex in relation to pretransplant infection of patients with CF with *Burkholderia cepacia*. Published series document an adverse effect on outcomes, with 1-year survival rates in the range of 50% to 67% for patients with *B cepacia* compared with 83% to 92% for those without.[19,20] Using predictive models of pretransplant and posttransplant survival, Liou and colleagues[21] have suggested that patients with CF infected with *B cepacia* do not derive a survival benefit from transplantation. These and other negative reports have led most centers in the United States to exclude candidates with *B cepacia* from consideration for lung transplantation. However, it has become clear that *B cepacia* is not a single entity but a heterogeneous collection of species (previously referred to as genomovars) with varying pathogenicity and effect on posttransplant outcomes. Recent studies have attributed the observed excessive posttransplant mortality to *B cenocepacia* (genomovar III) and possibly to *B gladioli*.[22,23] In contrast, infection with other members of the *B cepacia complex* does not seem to adversely affect posttransplant survival. Should additional epidemiologic studies corroborate these observations, transplant eligibility in the future may be dictated by the particular species that the patient harbors.

Aspergillus species are isolated from pretransplant respiratory cultures in up to 50% of patients with CF. Although this finding may increase the risk of posttransplant *Aspergillus* infections of the bronchial anastomosis, it does not represent a contraindication to transplantation.[24,25] Nontuberculous mycobacteria are isolated in up to 20% of patients with CF referred for consideration of lung transplantation. The most common mycobacterium isolated is *Mycobacterium avium* complex; its presence does not adversely affect outcomes after lung transplantation. In contrast, pretransplant recovery of *Mycobacterium abscessus* has been associated with subsequent development of serious infections after transplantation, albeit not conclusively with

reduced survival. Some centers view the presence of *Mycobacterium abscessus* as a relative contraindication[26]

DISEASE-SPECIFIC CONSIDERATIONS IN CANDIDATE LISTING

Familiarity with the natural history of the underlying disease and of disease-specific prognostic factors is essential in making decisions about the timing of listing of candidates for lung transplantation. Prognostic factors for the diseases constituting the most common indications for transplant are reviewed in the sections to follow. Many of these prognostic factors have been incorporated into guidelines published by the International Society of Heart and Lung Transplantation (ISHLT) (**Box 1**).[6] The prognostic indices that have been identified to predict the natural history of individual lung diseases are imprecise, identifying populations of patients at increased risk for death but of more limited usefulness in predicting the course of an individual patient. Thus, not every patient who fulfills the criteria set forth in the ISHLT guidelines necessarily warrants immediate listing, and such decisions should also take into account the patient's clinical trajectory, functional status, quality of life, and willingness to accept the attendant risks and uncertainties of transplantation.

COPD

COPD is associated with a highly variable and protracted natural history, typically evolving over many years in an insidious fashion. Even at an advanced stage, long-term survival is possible and as a result it is often difficult to determine the exact point at which lung transplantation should be offered. Historically, the postbronchodilator FEV_1 was touted as the best single predictor of prognosis in COPD.[27] Other risk factors that have been associated with an increased mortality risk include hypoxemia, hypercapnia, low body mass index, poor performance on a 6MWT, and magnitude of dyspnea.[28] More recently, Celli and colleagues[29] devised a multidimensional grading system referred to as the BODE index (body mass index [B], degree of airflow obstruction [O], dyspnea [D], and exercise capacity [E], measured by the 6MWT). The investigators prospectively validated the index and showed that it was a better predictor of risk of death than FEV_1 alone. The BODE index score ranges from 0 to 10, with the higher scores indicating higher risk of death. In the study, the highest quartile (BODE score of 7–10) was associated with a mortality of 80% at 4 years.

Box 1
Disease-specific guidelines for listing for lung transplantation

COPD

- BODE index of 7 to 10 or at least 1 of the following:
- History of hospitalization for exacerbation associated with acute hypercapnia (Pco_2 exceeding 50 mm Hg)
- Pulmonary hypertension or cor pulmonale, or both, despite oxygen therapy
- Forced expiratory volume after 1 second (FEV_1) of less than 20% and either carbon monoxide diffusion in the lung (DL_{CO}) of less than 20% or homogeneous distribution of emphysema.

IPF

- Histologic or radiographic evidence of usual interstitial pneumonia (UIP) and any of the following:
- A DL_{CO} of less than 39% predicted
- A 10% or greater decrement in forced vital capacity (FVC) during 6 months of follow-up
- A decrease in pulse oximetry less than 88% during a 6MWT
- Honeycombing on high-resolution computed tomography (HRCT) (fibrosis score of >2)

CF

- FEV_1 <30% of predicted, or rapidly declining lung function if FEV_1 >30% (females and patients <18 years of age have a poorer prognosis; consider earlier listing) and/or any of the following:
- Increasing oxygen requirements
- Hypercapnia
- Pulmonary hypertension

IPAH

- Persistent New York Heart Association (NYHA) class III or IV on maximal medical therapy
- Low (350 m) or declining 6MWT
- Failing therapy with intravenous epoprostenol, or equivalent
- Cardiac index of less than 2 L/min/m^2
- Right atrial pressure exceeding 15 mm Hg

Sarcoidosis

- NYHA functional class III or IV and any of the following:
- Hypoxemia at rest
- Pulmonary hypertension
- Increased right atrial pressure exceeding 15 mm Hg

Data from Orens JB, Estenne M, Arcasoy S, et al. International guidelines for the selection of lung transplant candidates: 2006 update–a consensus report from the pulmonary scientific council of the International Society for Heart and Lung Transplantation. J Heart Lung Transplant 2006;25:745–55.

A subsequent study by Martinez and colleagues[30] examined the predictive usefulness of serial measurements of the BODE index. The study examined patients who had participated in the National Emphysema Treatment Trial and who were therefore characterized by the presence of advanced airflow obstruction (mean FEV_1 predicted of 27%) and an average baseline BODE score of approximately 5. The investigators found that an increase in BODE score of greater than 1 point over a 6-month to 24-month period of observation was associated with a 2-fold increase in death among medically treated patients and a 3-fold increase among the group that had undergone LVRS.

The ISHLT guidelines have adopted the BODE score as the principle but not exclusive parameter to be used in determining the appropriate timing of listing patients with COPD.[6] Specifically, listing is recommended for patients with a BODE score of 7 to 10 or at least 1 of the following: (1) history of hospitalization for exacerbation associated with acute hypercapnia (Pco_2 >50 mmHg); (2) pulmonary hypertension and/or cor pulmonale, despite oxygen therapy; or (3) FEV_1 less than 20% and either DL_{CO} less than 20% or homogeneous distribution of emphysema.

Assuming that listing criteria for patients with COPD accurately identify candidates with a poor prognosis, lung transplantation would be expected to confer a survival advantage but this has been difficult to show. Studies that have compared survival of patients with COPD on the waiting list with posttransplantation survival have yielded conflicting results, with 1 study from the United States[31] suggesting that transplantation does not confer a survival advantage whereas 2 European studies came to the opposite conclusion.[32,33] Recently, Thabut and colleagues[34] developed multivariate parametric models to simulate the survival of patients with COPD while on the waiting list and after transplantation to assess whether there were particular factors that portend a survival benefit from transplantation in this patient population. In building their models, the investigators used the SRTR database containing 8182 patients with COPD listed for lung transplantation between 1986 and 2004. A major determinant of survival benefit proved to be the type of transplant procedure used: approximately 45% of the patients with COPD in the United Network for Organ Sharing database were predicted to derive a survival benefit of at least 1 year by undergoing bilateral lung transplantation (BLT) compared with only 22% who would derive such a benefit if single lung transplantation (SLT) was used. In addition to the type of transplant procedure chosen, survival benefit was heavily influenced by FEV_1 and several other functional and physiologic parameters. As an example, nearly 80% of patients with an FEV_1 less than 16% but only 11% of those with an FEV_1 greater than 25% were predicted to gain at least a year of life with BLT. A calculator that generates an estimate of survival benefit for an individual patient with a particular set of parameters is available at http://www.copdtransplant.fr/ and, if validated in future studies, could serve an important role in patient selection.

A final issue specific to the COPD population is the potential effect of LVRS on listing for lung transplantation. For those patients with an FEV_1 less than 25% who meet criteria for both surgical procedures, there is the option of offering LVRS first, reserving transplantation for failure to respond to LVRS or to subsequent functional decline after a period of sustained improvement. Successful LVRS can postpone the need for transplantation for up to several years, and the associated improvement in functional and nutritional status can optimize the patient's suitability as a transplant candidate.[14,35–37]

IPF

IPF is a debilitating disorder with no proven treatment and a median survival from the time of diagnosis of 3 to 4 years. The decision to list a patient with advanced and progressive IPF for lung transplantation is usually straightforward but can be problematic for patients with early or more indolent disease. Many studies have attempted to define the factors that distinguish those who die quickly from those with a more chronic course; these factors are discussed in detail later.

Underlying pathology
The presence of UIP on pathology, the histologic sine qua non of IPF, generally portends a poor prognosis. In contrast, nonspecific interstitial pneumonitis (NSIP) is typically associated with slower progression and longer survival; within this histologic group, the cellular subset follows a more indolent course than the fibrotic subset.[38–40] Among patients with suspected IPF, surgical lung biopsies obtained from multiple sites show concurrent presence of UIP and NSIP in approximately 25% of cases.[41] In these cases of discordant UIP, the prognosis is identical to that of patients who exclusively show a pattern of UIP. The presence of a greater number of fibroblast foci within a pattern of UIP also has been associated with a poorer prognosis.[42,43]

Radiology
Several scoring systems have been developed to quantify the degree of fibrosis on HRCT scans in patients with IPF. Higher scores generally reflect a greater degree of reticulation and honeycombing, and a paucity of ground glass opacities. Although minor differences exist in the mechanics of the scoring systems, all have shown a direct correlation between higher fibrosis scores and mortality.[44–46] Among patients with biopsy-proven UIP, those who have the classic radiographic features of the disease may have a worse survival than those who have atypical features.[45–47] For example, Flaherty and colleagues[47] documented a median survival of 2.1 years for patients deemed to have definite or probable UIP by 2 expert radiologists compared with a median survival of 5.8 years for those with indeterminate features or features more suggestive of NSIP. Similarly, Sumikawa and colleagues[46] reported mean survival rates of 3.8 years, 4.8 years, and 6.4 years for patients with HRCT patterns interpreted as definite UIP, consistent with UIP, and suggestive of alternative diagnosis, respectively.

Pulmonary function testing
Mugolkuk and colleagues[48] found that baseline diffusing capacity measurement, in conjunction with HRCT fibrotic score, offered the best prediction of 2-year survival for patients with IPF. Using receiver operator character analysis, a 39% predicted diffusing capacity was the optimal cutoff

for distinguishing survivors from nonsurvivors. However, other studies have failed to consistently define which baseline parameters, if any, are best at predicting outcomes.[44,48–51] In contrast, multiple studies have reported that longitudinal changes in pulmonary function parameters over a 6-month to 12-month period from time of diagnosis are a more powerful predictor of outcome than are baseline values.[49,52,53] For example, in 1 study a decline in FVC of 10% or greater in the first 6 months was associated with a 2-fold increase in the risk of death compared with patients whose FVC was unchanged during this period.[52] A recent study found that even marginal declines in FVC (5%–10%) over 6 months were associated with an increased mortality compared with those with stable disease.[54]

6MWT

Both the lowest saturation achieved during a 6MWT and the absolute distance walked are independently associated with prognosis. In 1 study of patients with biopsy-proven UIP, those whose oxygen saturation decreased to 88% or less during a 6MWT performed on room air had a 4-year survival rate of only 35%, whereas those who maintained higher levels had a survival rate of 69%.[50] In another study, patients with IPF who were awaiting lung transplantation and who walked less than 207 m (679 feet) had a 4-fold increase in mortality compared with those who had a longer walk distance.[51] The persistence of significant tachycardia 1 minute after completion of the 6MWT (decrease in heart rate from last minute of test of less than 13 beats per minute) was recently documented to be a strong predictor of mortality, performing better than either distance walked or saturation.[55]

Pulmonary hypertension

Secondary pulmonary hypertension is encountered in 30% to 60% of patients with advanced IPF.[56,57] There is an emerging consensus in the literature that pulmonary hypertension is associated with significantly worse mortality.[57–59] For example, a study that relied on echocardiographic estimates of pulmonary artery pressures found median survival rates of 4.8 years, 4.1 years, and 0.7 years for patients with IPF with estimated pulmonary artery systolic pressures of less than 35 mm Hg, 35 to 50 mm Hg, and greater than 50 mm Hg, respectively.[59]

Acute exacerbations

Although IPF typically progresses in a stuttering fashion, seemingly stable patients may experience sudden and precipitous decline. These so-called acute exacerbations are characterized by unexplained worsening or development of dyspnea within 30 days, new bilateral ground glass opacities or consolidation superimposed on the background of UIP changes, and no evidence of infection, heart failure, pulmonary embolus, or other cause of acute lung injury.[60] In 1 study examining the natural history of patients with mild to moderate IPF, 21% of patients died during a 76-month period of observation, and half of these deaths were caused by acute exacerbations. Pulmonary function parameters before these acute events were generally stable and provided no signal of impending decompensation. Other studies have suggested rates of acute exacerbations in the range of 5% to 61%, with short-term mortality approaching 100% for those requiring admission to an ICU for respiratory failure.[60–62]

Combination of IPF and emphysema

There is increasing recognition of the unique features of a subgroup of patients with IPF who have concomitant emphysema.[63,64] Because of the counterbalancing effects of IPF and emphysema on elastic recoil, spirometric and lung volume parameters are typically well preserved in these patients and often belie the severity of the underlying condition. Characteristically, these patients are at greater risk of developing pulmonary hypertension than patients with IPF alone. When present, pulmonary hypertension portends an extremely poor prognosis in this group, with a 1-year survival of only 60% and 5-year survival of 25%.[63,64]

Guidelines for listing

In light of the generally poor prognosis and the possibility of rapid and unexpected decompensation, the ISHLT guidelines recommend that patients with histologic or radiographic evidence of UIP should be referred to a lung transplant center for evaluation at the time of diagnosis, independent of the degree of functional impairment. The intention is not to immediately list all patients, but to initiate the process of patient education and allow sufficient time to address potential barriers to transplantation (eg, obesity, deconditioning, high-dose corticosteroid use). In addition, the testing and consultations necessary for listing can be completed to facilitate expedited listing in the event of sudden decline in the future. The ISHLT guidelines for active listing incorporate many of the negative prognostic factors identified earlier: (1) diffusing capacity less than 39% predicted; (2) a 10% or greater decrease in FVC over a 6-month period; (3) desaturation less than 88% on a 6MWT; and/or (4) honeycombing on an HRCT. Although not stated in the ISHLT guidelines, patients with combined IPF and emphysema are a special case; listing should be based on presence of pulmonary hypertension rather than standard pulmonary function parameters.

CF

Kerem and colleagues[65] published a landmark study in 1992 that identified FEV_1 as the single most significant predictor of mortality in patients with CF. These investigators found that an FEV_1 less than 30% predicted was associated with a 2-year mortality of 50%. For a given FEV_1, females and patients less than the age of 18 years had a higher 2-year mortality than their counterparts. Based on this study, the recommendation that patients with CF with an FEV_1 less than 30% be listed for transplantation became widespread, with consideration given to earlier referral of females and younger patients. Subsequent studies from several other CF centers documenting more favorable median survival rates of 3.9 to 4.6 years associated with an FEV_1 less than 30% challenged but did not alter this recommendation.[66,67]

More recent studies have attempted to assess the risk of death in patients with CF using models incorporating multiple patient characteristics. In 2001, Liou and colleagues[68] published a 5-year survivorship model that was derived from data on 5800 patients in the CF Foundation Patient Registry and validated using data from an additional 5800 Registry patients. In addition to FEV_1, age, gender, weight, presence of diabetes, pancreatic insufficiency, number of acute exacerbations per year, and infection with *Staphylococcus aureus* and *Burkholderia cepacia* were identified as independent predictors of prognosis by multivariate analysis and were incorporated into the model. When applied to the validation cohort, this complex model predicted survival in superior fashion to the simpler model proposed by Kerem and colleagues using FEV_1 alone.

Mayer-Hamblett and colleagues[69] developed and validated a 2-year mortality model using methods identical to those of Liou and a more current and larger cohort of patients (n = 14,572) from the CF Foundation Patient Registry. In contrast to the findings of Liou and colleagues, their multivariate model showed no greater ability to predict short-term mortality than the simpler FEV_1 criterion proposed by Kerem and colleagues. Both the multivariate model and the FEV_1 alone showed a positive predictive value for 2-year mortality in the range of only 50% (ie, half of the patients predicted to die within 2 years would actually survive). Because the Mayer-Hamblett model chose a different outcome than the Liou model (2-year vs 5-year mortality), it cannot be firmly concluded that the findings of the 2 studies are necessarily contradictory but these contrasting studies do serve to raise a degree of uncertainty about overreliance on predictive models to guide transplant decisions.

A potential limitation of both of these models is that they included all patients with CF, independent of disease severity and transplant eligibility. These models might not be applicable to the specific population of potential CF transplant candidates, a more homogenous population of patients with many shared clinical characteristics and a narrower spectrum of physiologic abnormalities. Addressing this concern, Vizza and colleagues[70] examined 146 patients with CF awaiting lung transplantation at Washington University. Shorter 6-minute walk distance, presence of diabetes mellitus, and higher pulmonary artery systolic pressure were predictive of mortality on the waiting list. However, the investigators noted that there was no threshold for any of these factors that reliably separated the patients who died from those still alive. In a larger analysis of 343 patients with CF listed at 4 transplant centers, Belkin and colleagues[71] identified FEV_1 less than 30%, hypercapnia, and need for nutritional intervention (appetite stimulant, placement of a gastrojejunostomy tube, or parenteral nutrition) as predictors of an increased risk of mortality.

Two studies have focused on the prognosis of patients with CF admitted to the ICU with severe pulmonary exacerbation. Sood and colleagues documented a 76% in-hospital mortality among 25 patients with CF with hypercapnic respiratory failure, most of whom required intubation and mechanical ventilatory support. Of the 6 patients successfully discharged, only 3 (12% of the original group) survived to 1 year after discharge. In contrast, 1-year survival was 82% for the subset of patients with respiratory failure who underwent lung transplantation while in the ICU. Ellaffi and colleagues[72] reported a 48% 1-year survival rate among 21 patients with CF admitted to the ICU with severe pulmonary exacerbations (excluding 2 patients who received lung transplants). This more favorable prognosis may relate to differences in the severity of exacerbations; most patients in the study by Ellaffi and colleagues were managed with noninvasive ventilation. All 4 of the patients reported by Ellaffi and colleagues who required intubation and conventional ventilation died.

Failure of these various studies to define a common set of reliable prognostic factors has limited the ability to make definitive recommendations on timing of listing for patients with CF. The

ISHLT guidelines state that an FEV_1 less than 30% predicted should prompt referral of the patient to a transplant center but not necessarily immediate listing. The decision to proceed with transplantation should be based on "a comprehensive evaluation that must take into account several indicators of disease severity such as FEV_1, increases in oxygen need, hypercapnia, need for noninvasive ventilation, functional status, and pulmonary hypertension".[6] Given the low expectation of survival for patients with CF who require intubation for CF exacerbations, these patients should be considered for emergent listing and transplantation.

IPAH

In 1991, the Patient Registry for Characterization of Primary Pulmonary Hypertension reported a median survival of 2.8 years for patients with IPAH.[73] Survival was shown to correlate with NYHA functional class and with hemodynamic indices of right ventricular function. Based on these data, an equation to predict mortality was developed, incorporating mean pulmonary arterial pressure, right atrial pressure, and cardiac index. This equation was used for many years in determining when to list patients with IPAH for lung transplantation.

The subsequent development of effective vasodilator therapy has markedly improved the prognosis of patients with IPAH and has undermined the usefulness of the previously described equation. Intravenous epoprostenol, the oldest and most extensively studied agent, is associated with a 5-year survival of 55%, compared with 28% for historical controls.[74] Long-term follow-up of patients taking the newer agents is more limited, but available data suggest a favorable effect on survival.[75] However, not all patients respond to vasodilator therapy and, for those who do show initial improvement, subsequent deterioration may ensue, often precipitously. Factors that portend a poor prognosis among patients receiving epoprostenol include pretreatment NYHA class IV functional status or history of right heart failure, persistence of class III to IV functional status after 3 months of treatment, and failure of pulmonary vascular resistance to decrease by 30% from pretreatment baseline.[74] For example, 3-year survival of those with persistent class III to IV functional status is only 33% compared with 88% for those who improve to class I to II.

Other factors associated with a poor prognosis in patients with IPAH include hyponatremia,[76] echocardiographic evidence of severe right ventricular dysfunction as assessed by the degree of tricuspid annular displacement,[77] and 6MWT distance of less than 332 m.[78]

Given the availability of potentially effective treatment, it is appropriate to delay evaluation for lung transplantation until response to maximum medical therapy can be assessed. Listing for transplantation is appropriate for those patients with persistent NYHA class III or IV despite a minimum of 3 months of maximum therapy. The ISHLT guidelines suggest several other parameters for listing, although not all of these are necessarily independent prognostic variables: (1) low (350 m) or declining 6MWT; (2) failing therapy with intravenous epoprostenol or equivalent; (3) cardiac index less than 2 L/min/m²; or (4) right atrial pressure exceeding 15 mm Hg. Although patients with IPAH generally receive lower priority than patients with IPF and CF under the new allocation system in the United States., an exception is granted to increase the lung allocation score of a patient with IPAH to the 90th percentile of all scores nationally when (1) a patient is deteriorating on optimal therapy, (2) right atrial pressure is greater than 15 mm Hg, and (3) cardiac index is less than 1.8 L/min/m².[79]

Sarcoidosis

Sarcoidosis is associated with a highly variable but generally favorable natural history; only a few patients progress to a stage of advanced and irreversible pulmonary disease that prompts consideration of lung transplantation. Arcasoy and colleagues[80] studied a cohort of 43 patients with sarcoidosis listed for lung transplantation in an effort to identify factors predictive of a high risk of death. In univariate analysis, hypoxemia, increased pulmonary artery pressure, low cardiac output, and increased right atrial pressure all portended an increased short-term risk of death. Survivors and nonsurvivors did not differ with respect to standard pulmonary function parameters. In multivariate analysis, only a right atrial pressure exceeding 15 mm Hg proved to be independently predictive of death. In a subsequent study of 405 sarcoid patients entered into the SRTR database, increased pulmonary artery pressure and hypoxemia were again identified as strongly predictive of short-term mortality whereas pulmonary function parameters were not.[81] Right atrial pressure was not analyzed in this study. The ISHLT guidelines incorporate the findings of these 2 studies into their recommendation that sarcoid patients with the following characteristics be considered for listing for lung transplantation: NYHA functional class III to IV with hypoxemia, pulmonary hypertension, and/or right atrial pressure exceeding 15 mm Hg.[6]

CHOICE OF PROCEDURE

At the time a patient is placed on the active waiting list, the transplant team must also identify the specific procedure for which the patient is listed. Three surgical options are available: heart-lung transplantation (HLT), SLT, and BLT. Indications for each are shown in **Box 2** and described in the sections to follow.

Historically, HLT was the first procedure to be successfully performed but it has been largely supplanted by lung transplantation alone. Fewer than 80 procedures are performed worldwide on an annual basis.[1] The principle indication is Eisenmenger syndrome with surgically irreparable cardiac lesions. HLT is still occasionally performed on patients with IPAH. However, experience with lung transplantation alone has shown that the right ventricle has a remarkable ability to recover once pulmonary artery pressures have normalized, obviating concurrent cardiac replacement in all but the most severely decompensated patients. HLT is also occasionally offered for patients with advanced lung disease and concurrent severe left ventricular dysfunction or extensive coronary artery disease. The small number of patients

---

Box 2
Major indications for lung transplant procedures

HLT

- Eisenmenger syndrome with unrepairable cardiac defects
- IPAH (with right ventricular decompensation)
- Advanced lung disease with concurrent severe left ventricular dysfunction or extensive coronary artery disease

BLT

- IPAH
- Eisenmenger syndrome with surgically correctable cardiac defects
- Advanced lung disease with significant secondary pulmonary hypertension
- CF
- Non-CF bronchiectasis
- COPD
- IPF

SLT

- COPD (particularly older patients)
- IPF

---

requiring HLT in the United States face potentially protracted waiting times because of the preferential allocation of hearts to status 1A cardiac transplant candidates.

For most candidates, the choice is between SLT and BLT. This decision is dictated chiefly by the underlying disease but in cases in which both procedures are acceptable, additional factors such as the patient's age and functional status and center-specific preferences come into play. For patients with CF and other forms of suppurative lung disease, BLT is the exclusive procedure used, because leaving a chronically infected native lung behind runs the risk of infecting the allograft. BLT is also the procedure of choice for IPAH and for patients with severe, secondary pulmonary hypertension. This approach ensures that cardiac output is evenly distributed between 2 allografts as opposed to SLT, in which a single allograft must bear the burden of nearly the entire cardiac output (and the attendant risk of exaggerated pulmonary edema) because of exceedingly high vascular resistance in the native lung.

The situation with COPD and IPF, the 2 leading indications for transplantation, is more complex, because both SLT and BLT have been shown to be suitable. Historically, SLT was the predominant procedure for both diseases. However, over the past decade there has been a steady increase in the proportion of BLTs performed, and BLT now accounts for two-thirds of all procedures for COPD and just more than half of procedures performed for IPF.[1] Driving this preference in the population with COPD are studies that have suggested superior survival with BLT compared with SLT. In a cohort of 2260 adult lung transplant recipients with COPD entered into the ISHLT registry, a multivariate analysis performed by Meyer and colleagues[82] revealed that procedure type was an independent predictor of survival, with an overall risk ratio for mortality of 0.57 for BLT compared with SLT. Analysis of the interaction of age with procedure type showed that the survival benefit of BLT was apparent until approximately age 60 years, after which SLT was associated with a lower mortality, albeit not statistically significant. A subsequent analysis of more than 9000 COPD lung transplant recipients in the ISHLT registry by Thabut and associates[34] yielded similar findings. Median survival after BLT was superior to that after SLT (6.41 years vs 4.51 years) and the survival benefit of BLT was consistently shown for patients younger than 60 years across a variety of statistical methods to account for confounding factors. Again, a survival advantage to BLT could not be confirmed in recipients older than 60 years. In addition to a survival benefit, use of BLT for patients with COPD avoids the serious, albeit uncommon, complications associated with leaving an emphysematous lung in place: lung cancer and native lung hyperinflation.

It is more difficult to identify a compelling rationale for the increased use of BLT in patients with IPF, in the absence of secondary pulmonary hypertension. Meyer and colleagues[83] assessed the effect of procedure type on outcomes in 821 patients with pulmonary fibrosis registered in the SRTR database. For patients younger than 60 years, survival was better after SLT compared with BLT. When posttransplant survival was reanalyzed contingent on survival beyond the first posttransplant month, there was no difference in outcomes between the 2 procedures. This finding suggests that the inferior survival associated with BLT was likely because of increased perioperative mortality. For patients older than 60 years, survival was similar after SLT and BLT but the analysis was limited by the small number of patients in the BLT group. Recently, Thabut and colleagues[84] published a larger multivariate analysis of the SRTR database, involving 3327 patients with IPF (2146 SLT and 1181 BLT recipients). After adjustment for baseline characteristics, survival associated with the 2 procedures was similar. Analysis of hazard ratio for death as a function of time after transplant showed an increased risk of death associated with BLT in the perioperative period that was offset by a lower mortality risk subsequently.

A recent analysis by Nathan and colleagues[85] of patients with IPF listed for transplantation exposes a hidden risk of BLT in this population. These investigators reported that listing for BLT was associated with longer waiting times and an increased risk of dying on the waiting list compared with listing for SLT. In the absence of an offsetting posttransplant survival advantage to BLT, the potential net effect is increased loss of life for the population with IPF.

SUMMARY

Decisions about patient selection, timing of listing, and choice of procedure are critically important steps in optimizing the outcome of lung transplantation. Selection of candidates for lung transplantation requires an appreciation of the effect of pretransplant patient characteristics on posttransplant outcomes. Familiarity with the natural history of the underlying disease and of disease-specific prognostic factors is essential in making decisions about when to list candidates. Decisions about transplanting 1 or 2 lungs are principally determined by the underlying disease, but in cases in which both procedures

are acceptable, factors such as survival benefit, patient's age, and center-specific preferences come into play.

REFERENCES

1. Christie JD, Edwards LB, Kucheryavaya AY, et al. The registry of the International Society for Heart and Lung Transplantation: twenty-seventh official adult lung and heart-lung transplant report–2010. J Heart Lung Transplant 2010;29:1104–18.
2. Yusen RD, Shearon TH, Qian Y, et al. Lung transplantation in the United States, 1999–2008. Am J Transplant 2010;10:1047–68.
3. Schachna L, Medsger TA Jr, Dauber JH, et al. Lung transplantation in scleroderma compared with idiopathic pulmonary fibrosis and idiopathic pulmonary arterial hypertension. Arthritis Rheum 2006;54:3954–61.
4. Shitrit D, Amital A, Peled N, et al. Lung transplantation in patients with scleroderma: case series, review of the literature, and criteria for transplantation. Clin Transplant 2009;23:178–83.
5. de Perrot M, Chernenko S, Waddell TK, et al. Role of lung transplantation in the treatment of bronchogenic carcinomas for patients with end-stage pulmonary disease. J Clin Oncol 2004;22:4351–6.
6. Orens JB, Estenne M, Arcasoy S, et al. International guidelines for the selection of lung transplant candidates: 2006 update–a consensus report from the pulmonary scientific council of the International Society for Heart and Lung Transplantation. J Heart Lung Transplant 2006;25:745–55.
7. Harringer W, Haverich A. Heart and heart-lung transplantation: standards and improvements. World J Surg 2002;26:218–25.
8. Grannas G, Neipp M, Hoeper MM, et al. Indications for and outcomes after combined lung and liver transplantation: a single-center experience on 13 consecutive cases. Transplantation 2008;85:524–31.
9. Mahidhara R, Bastani S, Ross DJ, et al. Lung transplantation in older patients? J Thorac Cardiovasc Surg 2008;135:412–20.
10. Levine SM. A survey of clinical practice of lung transplantation in North America. Chest 2004;125:1224–38.
11. Mason DP, Thuita L, Nowicki ER, et al. Should lung transplantation be performed for patients on mechanical respiratory support? The US experience. J Thorac Cardiovasc Surg 2010;139:765–73, e761.
12. Dusmet M, Winton TL, Kesten S, et al. Previous intrapleural procedures do not adversely affect lung transplantation. J Heart Lung Transplant 1996;15:249–54.
13. Detterbeck FC, Egan TM, Mill MR. Lung transplantation after previous thoracic surgical procedures. Ann Thorac Surg 1995;60:139–43.

14. Burns KE, Keenan RJ, Grgurich WF, et al. Outcomes of lung volume reduction surgery followed by lung transplantation: a matched cohort study. Ann Thorac Surg 2002;73:1587–93.

15. Hadjiliadis D, Sporn TA, Perfect JR, et al. Outcome of lung transplantation in patients with mycetomas. Chest 2002;121:128–34.

16. Aris RM, Gilligan PH, Neuringer IP, et al. The effects of panresistant bacteria in cystic fibrosis patients on lung transplant outcome. Am J Respir Crit Care Med 1997;155:1699–704.

17. Dobbin C, Maley M, Harkness J, et al. The impact of pan-resistant bacterial pathogens on survival after lung transplantation in cystic fibrosis: results from a single large referral centre. J Hosp Infect 2004;56:277–82.

18. Hadjiliadis D, Steele MP, Chaparro C, et al. Survival of lung transplant patients with cystic fibrosis harboring panresistant bacteria other than *Burkholderia cepacia*, compared with patients harboring sensitive bacteria. J Heart Lung Transplant 2007;26:834–8.

19. Aris RM, Routh JC, LiPuma JJ, et al. Lung transplantation for cystic fibrosis patients with *Burkholderia cepacia* complex. Survival linked to genomovar type. Am J Respir Crit Care Med 2001;164:2102–6.

20. Chaparro C, Maurer J, Gutierrez C, et al. Infection with *Burkholderia cepacia* in cystic fibrosis: outcome following lung transplantation. Am J Respir Crit Care Med 2001;163:43–8.

21. Liou TG, Adler FR, Huang D. Use of lung transplantation survival models to refine patient selection in cystic fibrosis. Am J Respir Crit Care Med 2005; 171:1053–9.

22. Alexander BD, Petzold EW, Reller LB, et al. Survival after lung transplantation of cystic fibrosis patients infected with *Burkholderia cepacia* complex. Am J Transplant 2008;8:1025–30.

23. Murray S, Charbeneau J, Marshall BC, et al. Impact of *Burkholderia* infection on lung transplantation in cystic fibrosis. Am J Respir Crit Care Med 2008; 178:363–71.

24. Helmi M, Love RB, Welter D, et al. *Aspergillus* infection in lung transplant recipients with cystic fibrosis: risk factors and outcomes comparison to other types of transplant recipients. Chest 2003;123:800–8.

25. Nunley DR, Ohori P, Grgurich WF, et al. Pulmonary aspergillosis in cystic fibrosis lung transplant recipients. Chest 1998;114:1321–9.

26. Chalermskulrat W, Sood N, Neuringer IP, et al. Non-tuberculous mycobacteria in end stage cystic fibrosis: implications for lung transplantation. Thorax 2006;61:507–13.

27. Traver GA, Cline MG, Burrows B. Predictors of mortality in chronic obstructive pulmonary disease. A 15-year follow-up study. Am Rev Respir Dis 1979;119:895–902.

28. Martinez FJ, Kotloff R. Prognostication in chronic obstructive pulmonary disease: implications for lung transplantation. Semin Respir Crit Care Med 2001;22:489–98.

29. Celli BR, Cote CG, Marin JM, et al. The body-mass index, airflow obstruction, dyspnea, and exercise capacity index in chronic obstructive pulmonary disease. N Engl J Med 2004;350:1005–12.

30. Martinez FJ, Han MK, Andrei AC, et al. Longitudinal change in the BODE index predicts mortality in severe emphysema. Am J Respir Crit Care Med 2008;178:491–9.

31. Hosenpud JD, Bennett LE, Keck BM, et al. Effect of diagnosis on survival benefit of lung transplantation for end-stage lung disease. Lancet 1998;351:24–7.

32. De Meester J, Smits JM, Persijn GG, et al. Listing for lung transplantation: life expectancy and transplant effect, stratified by type of end-stage lung disease, the Eurotransplant experience. J Heart Lung Transplant 2001;20:518–24.

33. Charman SC, Sharples LD, McNeil KD, et al. Assessment of survival benefit after lung transplantation by patient diagnosis. J Heart Lung Transplant 2002;21:226–32.

34. Thabut G, Christie JD, Ravaud P, et al. Survival after bilateral versus single lung transplantation for patients with chronic obstructive pulmonary disease: a retrospective analysis of registry data. Lancet 2008;371:744–51.

35. Meyers BF, Yusen RD, Guthrie TJ, et al. Outcome of bilateral lung volume reduction in patients with emphysema potentially eligible for lung transplantation. J Thorac Cardiovasc Surg 2001;122:10–7.

36. Senbaklavaci O, Wisser W, Ozpeker C, et al. Successful lung volume reduction surgery brings patients into better condition for later lung transplantation. Eur J Cardiothorac Surg 2002;22:363–7.

37. Bavaria JE, Pochettino A, Kotloff RM, et al. Effect of volume reduction on lung transplant timing and selection for chronic obstructive pulmonary disease. J Thorac Cardiovasc Surg 1998;115:9–17.

38. Travis WD, Matsui K, Moss J, et al. Idiopathic nonspecific interstitial pneumonia: prognostic significance of cellular and fibrosing patterns: survival comparison with usual interstitial pneumonia and desquamative interstitial pneumonia. Am J Surg Pathol 2000;24:19–33.

39. Bjoraker JA, Ryu JH, Edwin MK, et al. Prognostic significance of histopathologic subsets in idiopathic pulmonary fibrosis. Am J Respir Crit Care Med 1998; 157:199–203.

40. Daniil ZD, Gilchrist FC, Nicholson AG, et al. A histologic pattern of nonspecific interstitial pneumonia is associated with a better prognosis than usual interstitial pneumonia in patients with cryptogenic fibrosing alveolitis. Am J Respir Crit Care Med 1999;160:899–905.

41. Flaherty KR, Travis WD, Colby TV, et al. Histopathologic variability in usual and nonspecific

interstitial pneumonias. Am J Respir Crit Care Med 2001;164:1722–7.

42. King TE Jr, Schwarz MI, Brown K, et al. Idiopathic pulmonary fibrosis: relationship between histopathologic features and mortality. Am J Respir Crit Care Med 2001;164:1025–32.

43. Nicholson AG, Fulford LG, Colby TV, et al. The relationship between individual histologic features and disease progression in idiopathic pulmonary fibrosis. Am J Respir Crit Care Med 2002;166:173–7.

44. Gay SE, Kazerooni EA, Toews GB, et al. Idiopathic pulmonary fibrosis: predicting response to therapy and survival. Am J Respir Crit Care Med 1998;157: 1063–72.

45. Lynch DA, David Godwin J, Safrin S, et al. High-resolution computed tomography in idiopathic pulmonary fibrosis: diagnosis and prognosis. Am J Respir Crit Care Med 2005;172:488–93.

46. Sumikawa H, Johkoh T, Colby TV, et al. Computed tomography findings in pathological usual interstitial pneumonia: relationship to survival. Am J Respir Crit Care Med 2008;177:433–9.

47. Flaherty KR, Thwaite EL, Kazerooni EA, et al. Radiological versus histological diagnosis in UIP and NSIP: survival implications. Thorax 2003;58:143–8.

48. Mogulkoc N, Brutsche MH, Bishop PW, et al. Pulmonary function in idiopathic pulmonary fibrosis and referral for lung transplantation. Am J Respir Crit Care Med 2001;164:103–8.

49. Collard HR, King TE Jr, Bartelson BB, et al. Changes in clinical and physiologic variables predict survival in idiopathic pulmonary fibrosis. Am J Respir Crit Care Med 2003;168:538–42.

50. Lama VN, Flaherty KR, Toews GB, et al. Prognostic value of desaturation during a 6-minute walk test in idiopathic interstitial pneumonia. Am J Respir Crit Care Med 2003;168:1084–90.

51. Lederer DJ, Arcasoy SM, Wilt JS, et al. Six-minute-walk distance predicts waiting list survival in idiopathic pulmonary fibrosis. Am J Respir Crit Care Med 2006;174:659–64.

52. Flaherty KR, Mumford JA, Murray S, et al. Prognostic implications of physiologic and radiographic changes in idiopathic interstitial pneumonia. Am J Respir Crit Care Med 2003;168:543–8.

53. Latsi PI, du Bois RM, Nicholson AG, et al. Fibrotic idiopathic interstitial pneumonia: the prognostic value of longitudinal functional trends. Am J Respir Crit Care Med 2003;168:531–7.

54. Zappala CJ, Latsi PI, Nicholson AG, et al. Marginal decline in forced vital capacity is associated with a poor outcome in idiopathic pulmonary fibrosis. Eur Respir J 2010;35:830–6.

55. Swigris JJ, Swick J, Wamboldt FS, et al. Heart rate recovery after 6-min walk test predicts survival in patients with idiopathic pulmonary fibrosis. Chest 2009;136:841–8.

56. Arcasoy SM, Christie JD, Ferrari VA, et al. Echocardiographic assessment of pulmonary hypertension in patients with advanced lung disease. Am J Respir Crit Care Med 2003;167:735–40.

57. Lettieri CJ, Nathan SD, Barnett SD, et al. Prevalence and outcomes of pulmonary arterial hypertension in advanced idiopathic pulmonary fibrosis. Chest 2006;129:746–52.

58. Hamada K, Nagai S, Tanaka S, et al. Significance of pulmonary arterial pressure and diffusion capacity of the lung as prognosticator in patients with idiopathic pulmonary fibrosis. Chest 2007; 131:650–6.

59. Nadrous HF, Pellikka PA, Krowka MJ, et al. Pulmonary hypertension in patients with idiopathic pulmonary fibrosis. Chest 2005;128:2393–9.

60. Collard HR, Moore BB, Flaherty KR, et al. Acute exacerbations of idiopathic pulmonary fibrosis. Am J Respir Crit Care Med 2007;176:636–43.

61. Blivet S, Philit F, Sab JM, et al. Outcome of patients with idiopathic pulmonary fibrosis admitted to the ICU for respiratory failure. Chest 2001;120:209–12.

62. Saydain G, Islam A, Afessa B, et al. Outcome of patients with idiopathic pulmonary fibrosis admitted to the intensive care unit. Am J Respir Crit Care Med 2002;166:839–42.

63. Cottin V, Le Pavec J, Prevot G, et al. Pulmonary hypertension in patients with combined pulmonary fibrosis and emphysema syndrome. Eur Respir J 2010;35:105–11.

64. Cottin V, Nunes H, Brillet PY, et al. Combined pulmonary fibrosis and emphysema: a distinct underrecognised entity. Eur Respir J 2005;26:586–93.

65. Kerem E, Reisman J, Corey M, et al. Prediction of mortality in patients with cystic fibrosis. N Engl J Med 1992;326:1187–91.

66. Doershuk CF, Stern RC. Timing of referral for lung transplantation for cystic fibrosis: overemphasis on FEV1 may adversely affect overall survival. Chest 1999;115:782–7.

67. Milla CE, Warwick WJ. Risk of death in cystic fibrosis patients with severely compromised lung function. Chest 1998;113:1230–4.

68. Liou TG, Adler FR, Fitzsimmons SC, et al. Predictive 5-year survivorship model of cystic fibrosis. Am J Epidemiol 2001;153:345–52.

69. Mayer-Hamblett N, Rosenfeld M, Emerson J, et al. Developing cystic fibrosis lung transplant referral criteria using predictors of 2-year mortality. Am J Respir Crit Care Med 2002;166:1550–5.

70. Vizza CD, Yusen RD, Lynch JP, et al. Outcome of patients with cystic fibrosis awaiting lung transplantation. Am J Respir Crit Care Med 2000;162:819–25.

71. Belkin RA, Henig NR, Singer LG, et al. Risk factors for death of patients with cystic fibrosis awaiting lung transplantation. Am J Respir Crit Care Med 2006;173:659–66.

72. Ellaffi M, Vinsonneau C, Coste J, et al. One-year outcome after severe pulmonary exacerbation in adults with cystic fibrosis. Am J Respir Crit Care Med 2005;171:158–64.

73. D'Alonzo GE, Barst RJ, Ayres SM, et al. Survival in patients with primary pulmonary hypertension. Results from a national prospective registry. Ann Intern Med 1991;115:343–9.

74. Sitbon O, Humbert M, Nunes H, et al. Long-term intravenous epoprostenol infusion in primary pulmonary hypertension: prognostic factors and survival. J Am Coll Cardiol 2002;40:780–8.

75. Galie N, Manes A, Negro L, et al. A meta-analysis of randomized controlled trials in pulmonary arterial hypertension. Eur Heart J 2009;30:394–403.

76. Forfia PR, Mathai SC, Fisher MR, et al. Hyponatremia predicts right heart failure and poor survival in pulmonary arterial hypertension. Am J Respir Crit Care Med 2008;177:1364–9.

77. Forfia PR, Fisher MR, Mathai SC, et al. Tricuspid annular displacement predicts survival in pulmonary hypertension. Am J Respir Crit Care Med 2006;174:1034–41.

78. Miyamoto S, Nagaya N, Satoh T, et al. Clinical correlates and prognostic significance of six-minute walk test in patients with primary pulmonary hypertension. Comparison with cardiopulmonary exercise testing. Am J Respir Crit Care Med 2000;161:487–92.

79. Chan KM. Idiopathic pulmonary arterial hypertension and equity of donor lung allocation in the era of the lung allocation score: are we there yet? Am J Respir Crit Care Med 2009;180:385–7.

80. Arcasoy SM, Christie JD, Pochettino A, et al. Characteristics and outcomes of patients with sarcoidosis listed for lung transplantation. Chest 2001;120:873–80.

81. Shorr AF, Davies DB, Nathan SD. Predicting mortality in patients with sarcoidosis awaiting lung transplantation. Chest 2003;124:922–8.

82. Meyer DM, Bennett LE, Novick RJ, et al. Single vs bilateral, sequential lung transplantation for end-stage emphysema: influence of recipient age on survival and secondary end-points. J Heart Lung Transplant 2001;20:935–41.

83. Meyer DM, Edwards LB, Torres F, et al. Impact of recipient age and procedure type on survival after lung transplantation for pulmonary fibrosis. Ann Thorac Surg 2005;79:950–7 [discussion: 957–8].

84. Thabut G, Christie JD, Ravaud P, et al. Survival after bilateral versus single-lung transplantation for idiopathic pulmonary fibrosis. Ann Intern Med 2009;151:767–74.

85. Nathan SD, Shlobin OA, Ahmad S, et al. Comparison of wait times and mortality for idiopathic pulmonary fibrosis patients listed for single or bilateral lung transplantation. J Heart Lung Transplant 2010;29:1165–71.

Lung Allocation in the United States

Michael Eberlein, MD, PhD[a,b,]*,
Edward R. Garrity, MD, MBA[c], Jonathan B. Orens, MD[a]

KEYWORDS
- Lung transplantation • Lung allocation
- Lung allocation score

After Bruce Reitz and Norman Shumway performed the first successful combined heart-lung transplant in 1981 and Joel Cooper the first successful human single-lung transplant in 1983, there was exponential growth in the number of cadaveric donor lung transplants performed worldwide through the 1990s.[1,2] This growth was paralleled by an increase in the number of centers with lung transplant programs. However, the volume of transplants performed started to plateau in the mid 1990s, primarily due to the limited number of available donor lungs (**Fig. 1**). Before 2005, lungs were allocated to potential recipients based on accumulated time on the lung transplant waiting list after matching for ABO blood type. As wait times grew to as long as 2 or more years, many patients with rapidly progressive lung diseases did not survive the prolonged wait time to transplantation. In May of 2005 the Lung Allocation Score (LAS) system was implemented specifically to provide a fairer method of allocating donor lungs. The goal was to decrease wait-list mortality, provide transplants to those most in need while avoiding futile transplants, and to deemphasize wait time and geography as factors in allocation. While achieving these goals, the introduction of the system also coincided with the greatest annual increase in the volume of lung transplantations, which occurred in the period 2004 to 2005 when

transplants increased by 21%.[3] This article reviews the history of lung donor allocation in the United States, the development of the LAS, and the impact of this system on the outcomes of lung transplantation.

HISTORY OF LUNG ALLOCATION IN THE UNITED STATES

In 1984 the US Congress enacted the National Organ Transplant Act (NOTA), which established the Organ Procurement and Transplantation Network (OPTN) to operate and monitor a national system for allocating organs. Although lung transplant candidates were registered with the OPTN by transplant programs, the OPTN initially provided a thoracic organ allocation provision only for heart and heart-lung transplantation, but not for isolated single or double lung transplantation. In 1990 OPTN thoracic organ allocation policies were amended to include provisions for the allocation of donor lungs to isolated lung transplant candidates. From 1990 to 1995 donor lungs were allocated purely on the basis of the recipient's time on the waiting list. The average waiting time was approximately 2 years, which resulted in a large number of recipients being put on the list earlier than would have been predicted based on disease severity, so that they could accrue

The authors have nothing to disclose.
a Division of Pulmonary and Critical Care Medicine, Johns Hopkins Hospital, Johns Hopkins University School of Medicine, 1830 East Monument Street, 5th floor, Baltimore, MD 21205, USA
b Critical Care Medicine Department, Clinical Center, National Institutes of Health, 10 Center Drive, Bethesda, MD 20892, USA
c Division of Pulmonary and Critical Care Medicine, University of Chicago Medical Center, University of Chicago, 5841 South Maryland Avenue, MC 0999, Chicago, IL 60637, USA
* Corresponding author. Division of Pulmonary and Critical Care Medicine, Johns Hopkins Hospital, Johns Hopkins University School of Medicine, 1830 East Monument Street, 5th floor, Baltimore, MD 21205.
E-mail address: meberle3@jhmi.edu

Clin Chest Med 32 (2011) 213–222
doi:10.1016/j.ccm.2011.02.004
0272-5231/11/$ – see front matter. Published by Elsevier Inc.

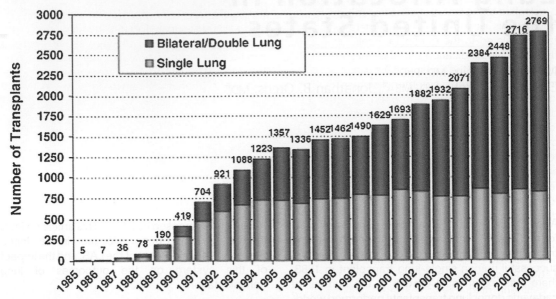

Fig. 1. Number of lung transplant procedures reported by year and procedure type. These data include transplants reported to the Registry of the International Society for Heart and Lung Transplantation from organ exchange organizations in countries with a data-sharing agreement as well as transplants reported voluntarily from centers in countries without a specific data-sharing agreement. Therefore, this graph may not fully represent the total number of procedures worldwide or the trend in activity. (*Reproduced from* Christie JD, Edwards LB, Kucheryavaya AY, et al. The Registry of the International Society for Heart and Lung Transplantation: twenty-seventh official adult lung and heart-lung transplant report—2010. J Heart Lung Transplant 2010;29(10):1105; with permission.)

time. An unintended consequence was that there was often no association between location on the waiting list and severity of disease. As there are variations in disease progression between patients with the same diagnosis and even more so between patients with different diagnosis, wait time was a poor surrogate for disease progression.[4] Often when a donor organ was allocated the organs were refused, as the candidate's disease had not progressed as quickly as anticipated and transplantation would have been premature. On the other hand, those patients with advanced or rapidly deteriorating disease who could not withstand the long waiting period were not accommodated by this allocation system. Because of the disproportionately high mortality rate for patients with idiopathic pulmonary fibrosis (IPF) on the waiting list, the United Network for Organ Sharing (UNOS) implemented the first change to the lung allocation system in 1995 by taking this diagnosis into account. Specifically, patients with IPF listed for transplantation were granted an additional 90 days at the time of listing, ostensibly to expedite transplantation.

On December 20, 1999, the US Department of Health and Human Services issued its Final Rule regarding organ allocation, which mandated the development of allocation systems based on

medical need rather than waiting time.[5] Subsequently the OPTN created what would become to be known as the Lung Allocation Subcommittee, composed of members of the UNOS Thoracic Organ Transplantation Committee. This subcommittee, charged with devising a new allocation policy, ultimately created the LAS system.

THE DERIVATION AND MECHANICS OF THE LAS SYSTEM

The lung allocation subcommittee had as goal to design an allocation score system that would lead to: (a) a reduction of mortality on the waiting list; (b) a prioritization of candidates based on urgency while avoiding futile transplants; and (c) a decreased emphasis on the role of waiting time and geography in lung allocation within the limits of ischemic time.[6] To achieve the second goal, the subcommittee chose to consider not simply medical urgency but also "net transplant benefit"; that is, the increase in survival anticipated with transplantation. The process to reach these goals is described in detail by Egan and colleagues[6] and is briefly summarized here.

As a first step, risk factors associated with mortality while on the waiting list and for the first posttransplant year were identified. The analysis was limited to the first year after transplantation, as beyond this period survival is dictated more by factors related to the transplant itself and less to the underlying indication and the patient's condition at the time of the transplant. This initial analysis focused on the 4 most common diseases for which lung transplantation is performed (emphysema/chronic obstructive pulmonary disease [COPD], idiopathic pulmonary arterial hypertension [IPAH], cystic fibrosis, and IPF). These diseases account for approximately 80% of lung transplants. The subcommittee then restricted the analysis of risk factors to objective criteria that would be difficult to manipulate. Subsequently, less common diseases comprising the other 20% of transplants were analyzed and eventually grouped with the original 4 diagnoses based on clinical characteristics or similar patterns of risk factors for mortality. **Table 1** shows the diagnosis groups and their constituent diagnoses. The next step was to generate multivariate models for estimated 1-year wait-list survival (wait-list urgency measure) and 1-year posttransplant survival. The factors used in making these survival calculations are summarized in **Table 2**. Several predictors are included for both measures: age, functional status, forced vital capacity percentage of predicted, continuous mechanical ventilation, and diagnosis. Wait-list and posttransplant survival, expressed as number of days alive in the ensuing year, were obtained from the areas under the respective 1-year survival curves (**Fig. 2**). The raw LAS is calculated as the net

transplant benefit measure (posttransplant survival minus wait-list survival) minus the medical urgency measure (wait-list survival). By counting wait-list survival twice in the calculation, the LAS gives relatively more weight to transplant urgency than to net transplant benefit. Because the raw allocation score can take values from −730 to +365, it is then normalized to a 0 to 100 scale as follows: normalized LAS = 100 × [(raw LAS + 2)/365]/3 × 365. Patients with the highest LAS have the highest priority for receiving a donor lung offer. In addition, the LAS system continues to use geographic proximity to the donor hospital (geographic zones) and ABO match as allocation factors. Size matching, donor/recipient cytomegalovirus serology, and other additional factors are considerations for the transplant center receiving the donor organ offer.

The LAS applies to candidates older than 12 years. Because the number of pediatric candidates younger than 12 years is small, there were insufficient data to create reliable regression models, and waiting time remains the primary determinant of allocation.

An appeal process was included with the implementation of the LAS system. Should a transplant center believe that a candidate's LAS does not adequately reflect the urgency of a patient's clinical status, an appeal may be filed with the UNOS Lung Review Board. After review, the Lung Review Board may assign a different score than the one calculated.

Table 1
Diagnosis groups and their constituent diagnoses

LAS Group A	LAS Group B	LAS Group C	LAS Group D
Obstructive Lung Disease	Pulmonary Vascular Disease	Cystic Fibrosis or Immunodeficiency Disorders	Restrictive Lung Disease
Chronic obstructive pulmonary disease	Primary pulmonary hypertension	Cystic fibrosis	Idiopathic pulmonary fibrosis
Emphysema	Eisenmenger syndrome	Common variable immune deficiency	Bronchiolitis obliterans and organizing pneumonia
α1-Antitrypsin deficiency	All specific pulmonary vascular diseases including pulmonary venous obstructive disease, chronic thromboembolic disease, and secondary pulmonary hypertension	Hypogamma-globulinemia	Hypersensitivity pneumonitis
Lymphangioleio-myomatosis			Acute respiratory distress syndrome/pneumonia
Bronchiectasis			Bronchoalveolar carcinoma
Sarcoidosis with mean pulmonary artery pressure ≤30 mm Hg			Lung retransplant/graft failure

Table 2
Factors used to calculate LAS when the allocation system was implemented

Factors Used to Predict Waiting List Survival	Factors Used to Predict Posttransplant Survival
Forced vital capacity (FVC) (% predicted)	FVC (% predicted)
Pulmonary artery systolic pressure	Mean pulmonary capillary wedge pressure ≥20 mm Hg
O_2 required at rest (L/min)	Continuous mechanical ventilation
Age at offer	Age at transplant
Body mass index	Serum creatinine (mg/dL)
New York Heart Association (NYHA) functional status	NYHA functional status
Diagnosis	Diagnosis
Six-minute walk distance <150 feet	
Continuous mechanical ventilation	
Diabetes	

IMPACT OF THE LAS SYSTEM ON WAIT-LIST POPULATION

Since its implementation in May 2005, the LAS system has had a major effect on the population of patients awaiting lung transplantation in the United States. The most profound change was observed in waiting time to transplant. For many years before LAS implementation, waiting time averaged well over 2 years. In 2004, for example, the median time to transplant was 792 days. The time to transplant in 2006, the first year with complete data after initiation of the LAS system, had dropped to 134 days (95% confidence interval, 114–151 days). The time to transplant has remained less than 200 days in each year after implementation of the LAS system. In general, higher LAS at listing results in shorter median time to transplant (**Fig. 3**).[3] For example, those candidates with a LAS of 50 or higher waited a median of 38 days to receive a transplant in 2008. Although the lung allocation system favors patients with higher LAS, the distribution of LAS

among patients receiving transplants indicates that candidates with scores of at least 30 have had good access to organs. Because there is no longer any advantage to accruing time, the new allocation system has led to a dramatic reduction in the number of patients actively waiting for a lung transplant; the active wait-list population dropped from 2163 patients in 2004 to 1005 patients in 2007, a 54% decrease.

The primary diagnoses of lung transplant recipients have changed gradually over the last decade. The percentage of patients with COPD undergoing transplantation declined over this period and reached a nadir at 29% in 2008.[3] By contrast, the percentage of patients with IPF has been on the increase, and in 2007 IPF overtook COPD as the leading indication for transplantation. Although these trends began prior to the implementation of the LAS system (**Fig. 4**), adoption of the LAS system likely influenced these trends, as its mechanism of preferentially allocating organs to those with greatest medical urgency and net transplant benefit favors IPF patients over those

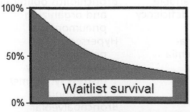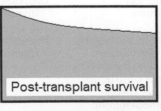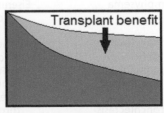

Fig. 2. Transplant benefit. The area under the curve (*left panel*) depicts wait-list survival, a measure of transplant urgency. The area under the curve (*middle panel*) depicts posttransplant survival, a measure of projected posttransplant survival. The difference between the two curves (*right panel*) is the transplant benefit. (*Adapted from* Egan TM, Murray S, Bustami RT, et al. Development of the new Lung Allocation System in the United States. Am J Transplant 2006;6:1220; with permission.)

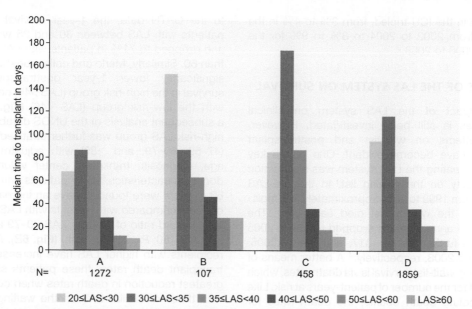

Fig. 3. Median time to transplant by diagnosis group (A–D) and LAS group at listing for patients who received lung transplants for the period 2006 to 2008. (*Reproduced from* Yusen RD, Shearon TH, Qian Y, et al. Lung transplantation in the United States, 1999–2008. Am J Transplant 2010;10(4 Pt 2):1047–68; with permission.)

with COPD. Analyzing a cohort of more than 4000 patients, Merlo and colleagues[7] showed that 53% of patients with LAS greater than 46 had IPF versus only 24% with LAS less than 46. The ability to expeditiously transplant critically ill patients under the LAS system led to an increase in recipients who came from the intensive care unit (ICU) at the time of transplant. The percentage of

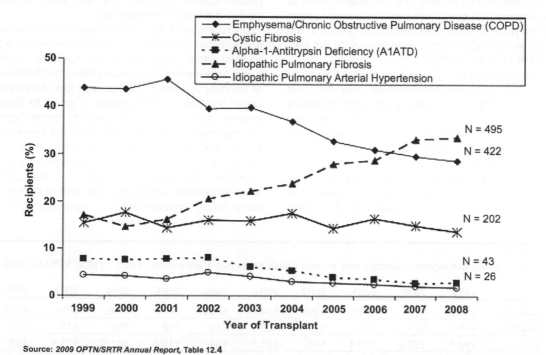

Source: *2009 OPTN/SRTR Annual Report,* Table 12.4

Fig. 4. Primary diagnosis of deceased donor lung transplant recipients, 1999 to 2008. (*Reproduced from* Yusen RD, Shearon TH, Qian Y, et al. Lung transplantation in the United States, 1999–2008. Am J Transplant 2010;10 (4 Pt 2):1047–68; with permission.)

patients in the ICU tripled, from 3% to 4% in the period from 2002 to 2004 to 8% to 9% for the period 2006 to 2008.[3]

IMPACT OF THE LAS SYSTEM ON SURVIVAL

The impact of the LAS system on clinical outcomes is still being investigated. However, initial effects on wait-list and posttransplant survival have become evident. One of the key aims in creating the LAS system was a reduction in mortality on the waiting list. In the pre-LAS period from 1999 to 2004 approximately 500 registrants on the waiting list died each year. The number of annual deaths dropped to 398 in 2005 and then further to 300, 317, and 266 in 2006, 2007, and 2008, respectively.[3] A better means of estimating wait-list survival is via death rates, which account for the number of patient-years at risk. Like the absolute death counts, the death rates for patients on the lung transplant waiting list dropped from a peak of 190.5 deaths per 1000 patient-years in 1999 to a low of 101.7 in 2006 (a 46% decline). Wait-list death rates dropped following implementation of the LAS system but did not decrease as dramatically as the absolute number of deaths (Table 3). LAS group D (restrictive lung disease) had the highest annual number of deaths pre-LAS, and it had the largest decrease in the number of deaths in the LAS era. The absolute number of deaths and the death rate also decreased in each of the other primary lung diagnostic groups in the LAS era of 2006 to 2008 compared with the pre-LAS era of 2002 to 2004.

Survival rates at 1, 3, and 5 years post transplant have shown some improvement over the past 10 years (Fig. 5). Of note, 1-year posttransplant survival rates have not significantly changed following implementation of the LAS system, but longer-term survival data for recipients in the LAS era do not yet exist. Although overall 1-year survival rates have not changed, multiple studies have demonstrated an association between higher LAS scores and lower 1-year survival rates. According to the OPTN data, the 1-year survival rate for patients with LAS between 30 and 35 was 86%, and dropped to 71% in patients with LAS greater than 60. Similarly, Merlo and colleagues[7] reported significantly lower 1-year posttransplantation survival in the high-risk group (LAS >46) compared with the low-risk group (LAS <46) (Fig. 6A). In a subsequent analysis of the UNOS database, the high-risk LAS group was further stratified by LAS (47–59, 60–79, and ≥80) with adjustments for age, diagnosis, transplant center volume, and donor characteristics.[8] Only patients with LAS of 60 or more were found to have an increased risk of death compared with patients with LAS of 46 or less (hazard ratio of 1.52 for LAS 60–79 and 2.02 for LAS ≥80; P <.001 for both) (Fig. 6B). Although recipients with higher LAS have increased posttransplant death rates, these patients show the greatest reduction in death rates when compared with those of similar LAS on the waiting list (ie, they appear to derive the greatest net transplant survival benefit).[3]

THE "HIGH LAS" PATIENT POPULATION: IS THIS A REASONABLE POPULATION TO PRIORITIZE?

The LAS system is more heavily weighted toward the risk of mortality on the waiting list than risk of posttransplant mortality, as the LAS system counts the former measure twice.

Under the pre-LAS system, rapidly deteriorating and critically ill candidates with limited expected survival often were not listed because under a wait time–based allocation system the likelihood of survival to transplantation was low. However, under the LAS system priority is given to these acutely and critically ill patient populations. Iribarne and colleagues[9] analyzed LAS scores at listing and at transplant from May 2005 to November 2007. Their study demonstrated that over time, LAS scores at listing and at transplant were increasing, supporting the proposition that since implementation of LAS, more acutely and

Table 3
Lung waiting list reported deaths and annual death rates per 1000 patient-years at risk, 1999 to 2008

	1999	2000	2001	2002	2003	2004	2005	2006	2007	2008
Patients	4868	5141	5374	5399	5549	5650	5269	4798	4676	4119
Deaths	599	519	532	529	489	512	398	300	317	266
Rate	190.5	152.6	149.1	145	131.5	135	115.5	101.7	125.9	128

Includes patients alive on the waiting list at any time during the year. Period at risk begins on the later of January 1 or waiting list registration, and ends on the earlier of December 31, date of death, or date of removal for other reasons.
Data from OPTN/SRTR Data as of May 4, 2009.

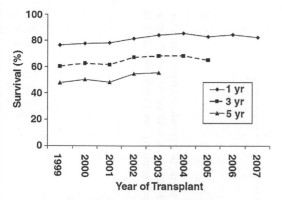

Source: *2009 OPTN/SRTR Annual Report,* Table 12.15

Fig. 5. Unadjusted patient survival for recipients of deceased donor lung transplants, by year of transplant, 1999 to 2007. (*Reproduced from* Yusen RD, Shearon TH, Qian Y, et al. Lung transplantation in the United States, 1999–2008. Am J Transplant 2010;10(4 Pt 2):1047–68; with permission.)

critically ill candidates were being listed and transplanted.

In addition to the association with increased posttransplant mortality discussed earlier, higher LAS is also associated with higher rates of primary graft dysfunction and longer lengths of stay in ICU.[10] Russo and colleagues[11] reported on post-transplant complications and survival in patients with a LAS greater than 75 at time of transplant (197 patients, 5.23% of the 3769 patients analyzed). Patients with a LAS greater than 75 had longer transplant hospitalizations (mean of 38 days vs 22 days, P<.005), greater frequency of infections (28% vs 9%, P<.001), need for dialysis (14 vs 5 per 100 patients, P<.001), and decreased 1-year survival (64% vs 83%, P<.001) compared with patients with LAS less than 50. When the investigators further subdivided the high-risk LAS group into recipients with LAS of 80 to 89 and 90 to 100, median survival of 2.28 and 1.56 years, respectively, was documented. An analysis of the impact of LAS on resource use provides an additional perspective. Arnaoutakis and colleagues[12] stratified patients by LAS quartiles and reported on total hospital charges for all admissions within 1 year following transplant. In the LAS quartile 4 (LAS 44.9–94.3), the mean total hospital charges were significantly greater than in the LAS quartiles 1 to 3 ($292,247 vs $188,342, P<.002). Thus, the principle that guided the creation the LAS system—to allow allocation of organs to patients who are more urgently in need of a transplant—comes with the burden of higher resource use, morbidity, and mortality in the subgroup of patients with very high LAS.

LIMITATIONS OF THE LAS SYSTEM

An important integrity check of the LAS is the comparison of LAS survival projections against prospectively observed survival of patients transplanted under the LAS system. For those receiving transplants from May 4, 2005 to December 31, 2007, the LAS posttransplant model predicted 317 days of life in the first posttransplant year, and 324 days were actually observed.[3] Although the average values were very similar, for individual recipients LAS did not make consistently accurate predictions for days of life in the first posttransplant year. In this regard, 10% of transplanted patients had an overestimate of their first year of survival by 180 days or more and 10% had an underestimate of their survival of 60 days or more. Gries and colleagues[13] reported on the predictive potential of the LAS for posttransplant survival at 1 and 5 years by reviewing the UNOS database, and found that overall prediction of long-term survival was poor. Specifically, receiver operator characteristics analysis demonstrated an area under the curve of 0.580 for 1-year survival prediction and 0.566 for 5-year survival prediction.

Another concern that has been raised about the LAS system is that it does not accurately predict wait-list survival in patients with IPAH. It has previously been demonstrated that the best predictors of mortality in this patient population are right atrial pressure and cardiac index, hemodynamic parameters that reflect the status of the right ventricle. Of note, however, the current LAS system does not include these parameters in its calculations. Failure to include these parameters may be responsible for underestimation of the risk of death for IPAH patients on the waiting list. Supporting this contention, Chen and colleagues[14] analyzed 7952 registrants in the UNOS database between 2002 and 2008, and found that wait-list mortality following LAS implementation decreased for all diagnostic groups except IPAH. Although the IPAH population experienced the highest wait-list mortality of all the major diagnostic groups under the LAS system (20% at 1 year), they were the least likely to undergo transplantation. A recently added exception to the LAS system (see below) will potentially address this shortcoming.

NEW AND ANTICIPATED CHANGES TO THE LAS SYSTEM

The LAS system was designed to include a structured process to allow evolution and improvement of the allocation mechanism based on prospective data collection. The OPTN Thoracic Committee periodically audits the performance of the LAS

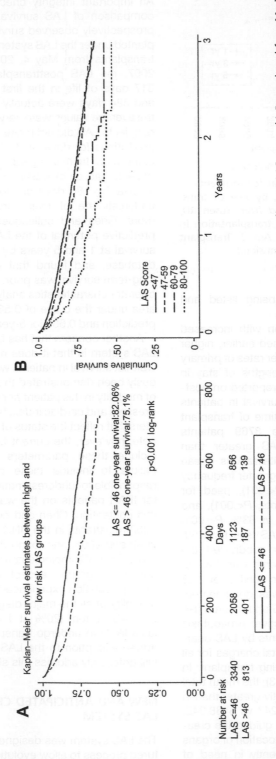

Fig. 6. (A) Kaplan-Meier survival estimates between high-risk and low-risk LAS groups. (B) Cumulative survival according to LAS score. (A Reproduced from Merlo CA, Weiss ES, Orens JB, et al. Impact of U.S. Lung Allocation Score on survival after lung transplantation. J Heart Lung Transplant 2009;28:769–75, with permission; B Reproduced from Liu V, Zamora MR, Dhillon GS, et al. Increasing lung allocation scores predict worsened survival among lung transplant recipients. Am J Transplant 2010;10(4):915–20, with permission.)

system, and proposed updates are reviewed. The frequent reevaluation of the LAS allows for refinement to the algorithm by adjusting hazard ratios or variable weights when appropriate, but also allows for the potential inclusion of new variables. If proposed revisions receive a favorable review by the Committee they undergo a period of public comment and ultimately are presented to the OPTN Board of Directors for approval. An example of this process was the response of Thoracic Committee to evidence demonstrating increased wait-list mortality in candidates with IPAH who experienced (a) deterioration on optimal therapy, (b) right atrial pressure greater than 15 mm Hg, and (c) cardiac index less than 1.8 L/min/m^2. A transplant physician caring for such a candidate can request an LAS modification by sending an appeal to the Lung Review Board. If approved, the candidate's LAS will be increased to the 90th percentile of all lung allocation scores.

The first substantive change in the parameters used to calculate LAS was the inclusion of Pco_2 data in the algorithm in 2008. This modification of the LAS system was in response to information generated from auditing Pco_2 data, which demonstrated that inclusion of current Pco_2 and change in Pco_2 over time improved the LAS estimates of wait-list survival.[15] Similarly, recent analysis indicated improved prediction of wait-list survival by including current and serial total bilirubin values. This improvement was particularly true for primary lung diagnostic group B (pulmonary vascular disease) patients with a peak total bilirubin greater than 1.0 mg/dL who experienced a 50% increase in total bilirubin within a 6-month period.[15] Following positive feedback during the public comment phase, the OPTN Board of Directors approved the inclusion of bilirubin data to the LAS system in July 2009. However, to date the LAS system has not incorporated bilirubin values, as concerns remain about additional expenses for collection of bilirubin data and programming this change into the OPTN computer systems. In the interim, consideration is being given to incorporating the bilirubin modifications into the online LAS calculator,[16] thus providing transplant centers with the necessary data to make exception requests to the Lung Review Board in cases where bilirubin data significantly affect LAS.

SUMMARY

Lung allocation in the United States has changed significantly following the introduction of the LAS system in May 2005. Organ allocation is no longer based on waiting time, but balances a measure of wait-list urgency and a measure of net transplant benefit. The LAS system has met its primary goals of reducing wait-list time and mortality and of prioritizing patients based on need. Since implementation of the LAS system, changes in transplant diagnosis and severity of disease at time of transplant have occurred, but thus far no changes in short-term posttransplant mortality have been observed. The association between higher LAS and increased posttransplant morbidity and mortality highlights the tension between prioritizing sicker patients and optimizing posttransplant outcomes. Better understanding of pretransplant factors that influence long-term posttransplant outcomes of the individual patient will be instrumental in improving the LAS system in the future.

REFERENCES

1. Reitz BA, Wallwork JL, Hunt SA, et al. Heart-lung transplantation: successful therapy for patients with pulmonary vascular disease. N Engl J Med 1982; 306:557–64.
2. Toronto Lung Transplant Group. Unilateral lung transplantation for pulmonary fibrosis. N Engl J Med 1986;314:1140–5.
3. Yusen RD, Shearon TH, Qian Y, et al. Lung Transplantation in the United States, 1999–2008. Am J Transplant 2010;10(4 Pt 2):1047–68.
4. Davis SQ, Garrity ER. Organ allocation in lung transplant. Chest 2007;132:1646–51.
5. U.S. Department of Health and Human Services. Health Resources and Services Administration. The final rule for transplantation. Available at: http://ecfr.gpoaccess.gov/cgi/t/text/text-idx?c_ecfr&tpl_/ecfrbrowse/Title42/42cfr121_main_02.tpl. Accessed September 27, 2010.
6. Egan TM, Murray S, Bustami RT, et al. Development of the new lung allocation system in the United States. Am J Transplant 2006;6(5 Pt 2):1212–27.
7. Merlo CA, Weiss ES, Orens JB, et al. Impact of U.S. Lung Allocation Score on Survival After Lung Transplantation. J Heart Lung Transplant 2009;28:769–75.
8. Liu V, Zamora MR, Dhillon GS, et al. Increasing lung allocation scores predict worsened survival among lung transplant recipients. Am J Transplant 2010; 10(4):915–20.
9. Iribarne A, Russo MJ, Davies RR, et al. Despite decreased wait-list times for lung transplantation, lung allocation scores continue to increase. Chest 2009;135(4):923–8.
10. Kozower BD, Meyers BF, Smith MA, et al. The impact of the lung allocation score on short-term transplantation outcomes: a multicenter study. J Thorac Cardiovasc Surg 2008;135:166–71.
11. Russo MJ, Iribarne A, Hong KN, et al. High lung allocation score is associated with increased morbidity

and mortality following transplantation. Chest 2010; 137(3):651–7.

12. Arnaoutakis GJ, Allen JG, Merlo CA, et al. Impact of the lung allocation score on resource utilization after lung transplantation in the United States. J Heart Lung Transplant 2010. DOI:10.1016/j.healun.2010.06.018.

13. Gries CJ, Rue TC, Heagerty PJ, et al. Development of a predictive model for long-term survival after lung transplantation and implications for the lung allocation score. J Heart Lung Transplant 2010; 29(7):731–8.

14. Chen H, Shiboski SC, Golden JA, et al. Impact of the lung allocation score on lung transplantation for pulmonary arterial hypertension. Am J Respir Crit Care Med 2009;180(5):468–74.

15. Organ Procurement and Transplantation Network. Policies. Revision to policy 3.7.6.1. Available at: http://optn.transplant.hrsa.gov/policiesAndBylaws/policies.asp. Accessed September 27, 2010.

16. Lung allocation score calculator. Available at: http://optn.transplant.hrsa.gov/resources/professionalResources.asp?index=88. Accessed September 27, 2010.

Selection and Management of the Lung Donor

Gregory I. Snell, MD*, Glen P. Westall, MD

KEYWORDS

- Lung transplant • Donor • Management
- Donor lung assessment

The sources of donor organs for use in lung transplant (LTx) and the selection criteria used have taken a quantum leap forward in the last few years. Novel sources of lungs are being used, and there is now overwhelming evidence that all LTx programs need to be routinely considering the use of a broad range of donor lungs and not just those previously described as ideal.[1,2] The authors provide evidence and expert consensus that it is no longer scientifically correct to claim that less than 25% of offered donor lungs can be successfully transplanted.[3,4] As part of the overall strategy to maximize the number of transplantable lungs, donor lung optimization and novel lung donor assessment strategies are discussed. Put together, these changes in the concept of the lung donor pool are arguably producing the biggest revolution in LTx in the last 20 years.

NOVEL SOURCES OF TRANSPLANTABLE DONOR LUNGS

Traditionally, cadaveric ABO blood-group–matched donation-after-brain death (DBD) double and single LTxs have been almost exclusively used for clinical LTx; however, other organ sources are evolving.

Living-Related Lobar Donors

In the setting of an ongoing shortage of cadaveric donors, living-related lobar LTx continues to be routinely performed in Japan. Enterprising Japanese surgeons have used such lungs in increasingly innovative configurations,[5] with outcomes following living-related lobar LTx that are superior, or at least comparable, to standard cadaveric LTx.[6]

Cadaveric Lobar Donors

There have been several reports of successful early and intermediate term outcomes from cadaveric lobar LTx or cut-down LTx.[7,8] This procedure may be a particular strategy to enable pediatric LTx, where waiting list mortality has traditionally been high in the setting of a limited donor pool.[9]

Cadaveric Donation-after-Cardiac Death Donors

In recent times, clinical donation-after-cardiac death (DCD) LTx has expanded dramatically, accounting for up to 20% of some national lung donor pools.[10] A variety of techniques have been used depending on the exact nature of the organ source (the so-called Maastricht category) and the local political-legal-ethical system.[11] Several centers report excellent early and intermediate term results, potentially superior to traditional DBD lungs.[10,12,13] The techniques and results are detailed in another article elsewhere in this issue.

Cadaveric ABO Blood Group Incompatible Donors

Although there is an established and blossoming literature to support ABO blood group incompatible (ABOi) renal transplant (primarily elective

Support for this work comes from the Margaret Pratt Foundation.
Lung Transplant Service, Alfred Hospital and Monash University, 5th Floor, Commercial Road, Melbourne 3004, Australia
* Corresponding author.
E-mail address: g.snell@alfred.org.au

Clin Chest Med 32 (2011) 223–232
doi:10.1016/j.ccm.2011.02.002

living-related),[14,15] until recently, the only published experience with ABOi LTx had come from inadvertent clerical errors.[16,17] Struber and colleagues[18] describe the first intentional ABOi cadaveric LTx, where, using a complex protocol of perioperative antibody depletion, blood group AB lungs were successfully transplanted into a blood group O recipient. The previous LTx cases[16,17] actually describe reasonable outcomes, and we are aware of an unpublished case of LTx of blood group B lungs into blood group O recipient who survived 9 years with intact graft function. Given these anecdotes, ABOi LTx focusing on lungs of blood group A2 and A2B donors into blood group B and even O recipients with low anti-A titers warrants further consideration,[19] particularly in the African American and Asian populations, in which B blood group exceeds 20% of the recipient pool.[15]

EXTENDING THE SPECTRUM OF TRANSPLANTABLE DONOR LUNGS

The potential pool of donor lungs available for transplant has traditionally been reduced by concerns regarding perceived poor function in the donor and the perception of a high risk of failure postoperatively.[4] Although available donor lungs can be conceived as an iceberg with only the tip useable (Fig. 1), we contend the situation is quite different.

Ideal and Extended Donors

The ideal donor is a young donor with no prior lung disease, no current medical problems, and excellent pulmonary function (Box 1). Aiming for optimal clinical results, and in the absence of data, the early transplant physicians and surgeons chose

> **Box 1**
> **Ideal donor lung selection criteria**
>
> 1. Age less than 55 years
> 2. ABO blood group compatible, DBD donor
> 3. Appropriate size match
> 4. Clear chest radiograph
> 5. Pao$_2$/fraction of inspired oxygen (Fio$_2$) >300 on 5 cm H$_2$O positive end-expiratory pressure (PEEP)
> 6. Tobacco history of less than 20 pack years
> 7. Absence of chest trauma
> 8. No evidence of aspiration or sepsis
> 9. Absence of purulent secretions at bronchoscopy
> 10. Absence of organisms on sputum Gram stain
> 11. No history of primary pulmonary disease or active pulmonary infection
>
> *Data from* Refs.[3,4,20]

such donors as the starting point for LTx.[4] However, the reality of the donor pool is that ideal donors represent only a fraction of the pool, and many units long ago moved to considering and transplanting organs that were not perfect, so-called extended donors.[3,4,20] The extended group actually has 2 subgroups: (1) general medical concerns in the donor, such as older age, history of prior cancer, or positive hepatitis serology and (2) specific lung issues, such as prior smoking history, asthma, recent aspiration, fluid overload, or infection. The former potentially leads to late graft/recipient problems in a graft that works well to start with, whereas the latter is

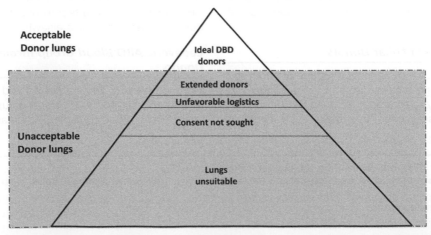

Fig. 1. An iceberg schema of the historical view of the total pool of donor lungs available for transplant.

more likely to lead to acute dysfunction. Of course, some factors, like smoking history, might have the potential to actually impact both short- and long-term outcomes.

The evidence supporting the view that the lung donor pool should routinely consider many organs traditionally regarded as extended includes the pooled analyses of several single-center studies and expert consensus.[2,21,22] In a 2009 review, Van Raemdonck and colleagues[21] noted that the percentage of marginal donors transplanted ranged between 24% and 77% in the 10 LTx units analyzed. Seven studies cited in the meta-analysis reported equivalent outcomes to traditional ideal DBD donors, with 2 studies showing inferior early outcomes.[23,24] Van Raemdonck's team has taken this review to heart by recently reporting a doubling of transplant numbers by using extended donors.[25] The 2 studies with negative outcomes (a higher 30-day mortality) tended to have an older donor population with a higher cigarette intake than the other studies.[23,24] This result highlights the challenge with all single-center studies, as there are variations between centers in how extended organs are defined and into what recipients they are transplanted.

In our Alfred Hospital cohort of 151 patients who underwent transplant between 2000 and 2005, we attempted to characterize donor and recipient matching.[26] We have a system where extended donors have been used for many years, and we choose recipients based on need and logistics.[3,27,28] We were able to calculate the lung donor score (a marker of apparent donor quality)[29] and the lung allocation score (a marker of apparent recipient risk of mortality)[30] and show that there was no statistical difference in the subsequent 5-year survival for the 4 different combinations of donors and recipients split around median values (better or worse donors, healthier or sicker recipients).

Two studies have analyzed the use of lungs across larger donor pools. Reyes and colleagues[31] have recently completed important analyses of the United Network for Organ Sharing Registry, quantifying the degree of compliance with current US ideal donor guidelines and the impact of the guideline variables and novel variables on survival. They studied more than 10,000 primary LTxs since 1999 and noted that 56% varied from the guidelines (41% chest radiograph abnormality, 21% smoked >20 pack years, and 18% had a PaO_2/FiO_2 <300). The common variances within the guidelines (eg, PaO_2/FiO_2 down to 230, abnormal chest radiograph, purulent secretions) were not associated with an increased mortality. Novel donor factors including donor diabetes, donor positive cytomegalovirus serology, a recent smoking history, an African American donor, blood type A, death other than from head trauma, and gender, race, and size mismatches were associated with poorer survival. The investigators conclude that the "donor PaO_2 range can be widened and a suspicious chest radiograph, evidence of airway sepsis and purulent secretions ignored".[31] Although this study describes the fate of lungs actually accepted and transplanted, it represents only less than 20% of all lungs offered for transplant during the same period.[20,32]

We have recently published Australian data on the fate of all lungs offered for transplant.[3] Our Alfred Hospital experience in 2006 showed that our team was able to successfully use 66% of local donors, with the remaining 18% functionally unusable and 16% logistically unusable (**Fig. 2**). Of interstate (rest of Australia = 500–3000 miles) donors, we used 50% of lung offers from states where there was no LTx program and 32% of offers from where a program was present but had rejected these organs. The survival rate was 100% at 6 months and 96% at 12 months, with no attributable effect of donor quality. Overall, 54% of all Australian donor lungs were actually transplanted in the study year, despite the tyranny of distance. We concluded that a "strategy of perioperative lung donor evaluation and intervention suggests the number of truly unusable donor lungs is actually only a small fraction of the donor pool."

The Impact of Specific Donor Factors on LTx Outcomes

Donor age
Review of mortality statistics and potential donor audits suggests that donor organ availability could be significantly increased by expanding the acceptable age limit. The Australian Bureau of Statistics data for 2008[33] notes a death rate per 1000 population that increases exponentially with age. The death rate is 14.5 for those aged 10 to 55 years (our ideal donor pool), 12.5 for those aged 55 to 65 years (extended donor pool), and 22.1 for those aged 65 to 75 years, per 1000 population. The current ideal donor pool represents only 29% and the extended donor pool only 54% of the total deaths of those younger than 75 years. An Australian donor audit[34] noted that, although many of these older deaths would not occur in a traditional scenario that would allow organ donation (eg, sepsis, cancer, death at home), there was still a significant potential of donors (particularly DCD) from emergency departments that were currently not being used. On reviewing these data and applying conservative acceptance criteria (ie, otherwise ideal donors), we recognize

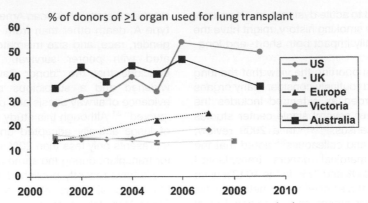

% of donors of ≥1 organ used for lung transplant

- US
- UK
- Europe
- Victoria
- Australia

Fig. 2. Percentage of donors from whom at least 1 organ was recovered who were successfully used as lung donors. Data is shown for the United States,[32] United Kingdom,[75] Europe,[76] Victoria, and Australia.[77]

that this represents a significant potential supply of donor lungs.[3,4]

The proportion of cadaveric donors older than 60 years has increased during the past decade and now represents more than 10% of the total cadaveric donor pool.[35] Although LTx has been successfully performed using organs from older donors, some investigators have suggested that the combination of older donor age and long ischemic times (ie, beyond 8 hours) is associated with increased mortality.[36] However, a recent study evaluating LTx outcomes using lungs from donors older than 60 years (median, 65 years; range, 60–77 years) reported a lower 10-year survival but outcomes that were otherwise not dissimilar to those observed with lungs from younger donors.[37] These investigators suggest that older donor lungs should be avoided in higher-risk recipients (patients with pulmonary fibrosis or pulmonary hypertension) and those with expected longer ischemic time.

Donor history of malignancy
LTx conveys the risk of direct transmission of cancer cells present in the donor at the time of implantation. Since the Cincinnati Transplant Tumor Registry first reported an unacceptably high rate of tumor transmission in patients receiving organs from donors with malignancies,[38] the use of donors with a history of recent and active malignancy has been contraindicated. Exceptions include cases in which the risk of tumor transmission is low (eg, basal cell skin cancer, in situ cervical carcinoma of the cervix). In the specific case of primary brain tumors and LTx, there have only been 2 cases of transmission of tumors to recipients,[39–41] both with glioblastoma multiforme.

Difficulties arise when the donor history of cancer is distant and the cancer is presumed cured. Transmission of breast cancer[42] and melanoma[43] to transplant recipients aged 8 and 32 years, respectively, after apparent cure of the same malignancy in the donor has been reported. In the melanoma cases, the past history of skin cancer was not available at the time of organ donor assessment and lung acceptance, a situation we have anecdotally seen at The Alfred Hospital. In both melanoma transmission cases,[43] death followed within 2 years of LTx. On balance, the risk of donor-to-recipient cancer transmission is based on histology and stage of tumor, type of therapies and interventions, and length of cancer-free survival.[44,45] At present, the incidence of donor-related malignancy remains rare, but as noted earlier, might be expected to increase given the trend to using lungs from older, smoking organ donors.

Donor history of infection
Infection in the donor lung is common, especially if the donor is ventilated for more than 48 hours.[46] Bronchial secretions in the donor are commonly observed at bronchoscopy, and a positive result on Gram stain on donor bronchial wash does not preclude subsequent organ donation,[31] although not all support this view.[47] Despite 2 large studies demonstrating that the lung is the most common site of infection in organ donors, the subsequent transmission of pulmonary infection from donor to recipient remains low (<10%).[48,49]

Screening of transplant donors for infection is limited by the available diagnostic tests, with serologic testing being routinely performed for the more common chronic viral infections. In the absence of more sensitive, rapid, and comprehensive molecular diagnostic tools, donor-to-recipient transmission of rarer infections, including human immunodeficiency virus, West Nile virus, lymphocytic choriomeningitis virus, and rabies, have been reported.[50–53]

The use of organs from donors infected with either hepatitis B virus (HBV) or hepatitis C virus (HCV) remains controversial and anecdotal. LTx recipients receiving organs from HBV core antibody–positive donors should be vaccinated peritransplant, if not already vaccinated. One- and 5-year survivals are not detrimentally affected when lung and heart-lung transplantation is performed using lungs from HBV core antibody–positive donors.[54] Lungs from HBV surface antigen (sAg)–positive donors may be considered for HBV sAg–positive recipients who have access to lamivudine treatment.[55] Likewise, lungs from HCV-infected donors should only be reserved for HCV-infected recipients.

The Present Status of Acceptable Lung Donors

The current position on the selection of lungs for LTx is summarized in **Fig. 3**. Based on the up-to-date literature describing recent practices, most donor lungs are usable with an appropriate plan of resuscitation. It is apparent that the best term is acceptable lung donor rather than ideal and extended or marginal. This term becomes particularly relevant when Reyes and colleagues'[31] recent data are considered, which show that new factors such as donor diabetes and race, gender, and size mismatch actually have more relevance to outcomes than PaO_2/FiO_2 and radiology results. **Box 2** summarizes the current evidence defining a currently acceptable lung donor.

The weighting and potential adverse additive interactions of multiple traditional and novel donor factors that define a poor outcome from LTx remain to be clarified by future lung donor scoring studies,[29] as is discussed later. The clinical judgment of proceeding into transplant with a set of potentially suboptimal lungs needs to consider 30-day and 5-year survival with and without

transplant, with the potential recipient's particular characteristics in mind. As noted by Van Raemdonck and colleagues,[21] "the impact of less perfect donor lungs may be lessened with competent post-operative care, and the majority of recipients will still have better outcomes than not receiving a transplant."

NEW TECHNIQUES OF DONOR EVALUATION

Oto and colleagues[56] describe a high incidence of macroscopic pulmonary emboli (40 of 130 donor lungs) in the pulmonary vein effluent following flushing of donor lungs on the back-table preimplantation. The presence of these emboli (80% thrombi and 20% fat) was associated with a 4.8- and 20.6-fold increase, respectively, in the incidence of primary graft dysfunction (PGD). In this study, the incidence of subsequent PGD was decreased if therapeutic attempts were made to flush out all venous clots using larger perfusate volumes. In contrast, a recent study failed to show a routine benefit of a preimplantation retrograde flush on immediate postoperative graft function.[57] Further studies are clearly needed, but a routine retrograde venous flush is a simple tool with a potential to diagnose pulmonary emboli and prevent PGD.

A more sophisticated ex vivo perfusion technique to evaluate the quality of donor lungs has been described by Steen and colleagues.[58] Recently, this Swedish team used this ex vivo system to recondition previously rejected human DBD lungs and evaluate their function by measuring the oxygen content of the perfusate leaving the lung circulation under varying inspired oxygen fractions.[59] Cypel and colleagues[60] modified the ex vivo technique slightly to show stable donor lung function (oxygenation, resistance, and

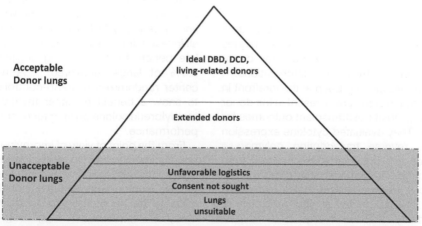

Fig. 3. A schema of the current view of the total pool of donor lungs available for transplant.

Box 2
Acceptable donor lung selection criteria in 2010

1. Age less than 70 years

2. ABO blood group compatible DBD or DCD donor

3. Approximate size match, with minor surgical trimming or lobectomy as need

4. Minor diffuse and moderate focal chest radiograph changes acceptable if good, stable/improving function

5. PaO_2/FiO_2 more than 250 on 5 cm H_2O PEEP

6. Tobacco history less than 40 pack years

7. Chest trauma not relevant if good function

8. Aspiration or minor sepsis acceptable if good, stable/improving function

9. Purulent secretions not relevant if good, stable/improving function

10. Organisms on Gram stain and ventilation time not relevant

11. Primary pulmonary disease not acceptable, unless asthma

Future acceptability considerations

1. Age acceptance up to 75 years

2. ABO incompatible transplant theoretically acceptable if low-titer recipient and antibody removal and monitoring plan

3. Lobar cut downs of larger donor lungs acceptable

4. Moderate and/or 1-sided chest radiograph changes acceptable with good, stable/improving function

5. Novel predictive donor factor recognition, eg, donor diabetes, recent smoking history

Adapted from Refs.[3,4,20]

histology) for 12 hours at physiologic temperatures using an acellular perfusate. These techniques potentially provide a useful window for donor lung assessment and therapeutic interventions.

The Toronto group[61] has been at the forefront in identifying immune signatures present in the donor lung that may predict posttransplant outcomes for the recipient. They evaluated cytokine expression by real-time reverse transcription polymerase chain reaction in biopsy samples collected from 169 donor lungs and demonstrated using a stepwise logistic regression model that a high interleukin (IL)-6 to IL-10 ratio was most predictive of 30-day mortality.[61] These assays can be performed rapidly and may in the future provide

a useful adjuvant to the assessment of donor lungs. The same group has gone on to perform gene expression profiling to identify signatures associated with PGD.[62] Microarray analysis identified 4 genes (ATP11B, FGFR2, EGLN1, and MCPH1) that were significantly overexpressed in donor lungs that developed PGD after implantation. Using different methods, the St Louis group[63] has also identified several genes involved in signaling, apoptosis, and stress-activated pathways that are upregulated in donor lungs that subsequently develop PGD.

RESUSCITATION AND OPTIMIZATION OF DONOR LUNGS

The low use rate of potential donor lungs, in part, is related to the inherent instability of the lungs following brain death. Donor lung injury may arise from direct trauma, aspiration, neurogenic edema, ventilator-associated barotrauma, or ventilator-associated pneumonia.[64] However, there are several strategies that can be implemented to aim to reverse the current low procurement rate.

Hormone Resuscitation

The autonomic storm accompanying brain death leads to neurogenic pulmonary edema and triggers the development of pulmonary and systemic inflammatory responses. Animal models have demonstrated that the presence of neurogenic edema in the donor lung predicts PGD following LTx.[65] Oto and colleagues[66] have shown a significant and clinically relevant association among PGD in the lung, heart, and kidneys from the same donor, suggesting that the systemic inflammatory response typical of brain death results in multiorgan dysfunction.

Hormone resuscitation with thyroid hormone, methylprednisolone, and vasopressin aims to ameliorate the effects associated with brain death and is generally still advocated.[2,67] However, not all investigators are convinced,[68,69] with the absolute benefit for lungs being negligible (an extra 2.8% of lungs recovered).[70] A recent single-center randomized placebo-controlled trial failed to show a benefit of either thyroid hormone or methylprednisolone on lung recovery rates or graft performance.[69]

From the point of view of improving lung function and mechanics, recent animal work by Rostron and colleagues[71] confirms a role for arginine, vasopressin, and norepinephrine as equally effective in treating the hypotensive pulmonary donor. This study refutes prior work suggesting that systemic catecholamines administered to the donor were predictive of inferior blood gases in the lung recipient.[2]

Ex vivo Resuscitation

The ex vivo perfusion technique described by Steen and colleagues[58,59] and Cypel and colleagues[60] to assess donor quality has also proved to have therapeutic properties (see chapter 3 for further discussion). Common to both ex vivo perfusion techniques is the use of hyperoncotic Steen Solution (Vitrolife AB, Sweden) that potentially dehydrates edematous lung tissue. Ingemansson and colleagues[59] report successful transplantation of 6 of 9 initially rejected pairs of donor lungs. Cypel and his Toronto colleagues have also performed several human transplants using resuscitated lungs.[72] These investigators, who previously modified donor animal immunologic responses via transfected gene therapy, are setting the stage for more sophisticated molecular and cellular repair techniques to further improve human transplant outcomes.

Donor Management Strategies

Two excellent recent reviews support the strategy of aggressive donor management coupled with the liberalization of the traditional, but actually nonevidenced, donor criteria.[2,21] Using such a strategy, in combination with a flexible collaborative approach with donor intensive care units (ICUs), it now seems possible to retrieve up to 60% of donor lungs offered up for transplant.[3] Following certification of brain death, active donor management in the ICU should include an initial bronchoscopy and repeated suctioning, physiotherapy, revision of antibiotic therapy, and fluid management. Lung recruitment strategies should be used if atelectasis is suspected. A repeat assessment, including chest radiography and serial determination of blood gas levels, may need to be undertaken before a final decision can be made.[22] This message has been adopted by ICU staff and donor transplant coordinators across Australia.

Recipient Management Strategies

One concern of broadening the definition of what is called an acceptable donor lung and transplanting lungs that were previously considered marginal is that LTx recipients may be receiving suboptimal grafts, predisposing them to early PGD and its associated complications. It thus becomes increasingly important that the immediate posttransplant care focuses on identification and appropriate management of evolving graft dysfunction. Early bronchoscopy and universal use of appropriately targeted antibiotics helps minimize the deleterious effects of donor-derived infections. Rapid and effective pain relief via either epidural or intravenously administered analgesics facilitates early extubation, thereby lessening the effect of ventilator-associated pneumonia.

Hemodynamic management early posttransplant is challenging, and previous studies have suggested that a central venous pressure (CVP) of greater than 7 mm Hg is associated with a longer duration of intubation and mortality following LTx.[73] Based on this information, we recently developed an ICU guideline that aims to optimize early posttransplant respiratory and hemodynamic management (CVP <7 mm Hg) and were able to show that its implementation resulted in less use of vasopressors and a reduced incidence of PGD.[74]

SUMMARY

The gap between the number of available donor lungs and patients waiting for transplant continues to be problematic. Notwithstanding, novel sources of donor lungs, a much broader definition of acceptability criteria, and aggressive management of the lung donor can clearly increase the number of donor lungs available. Prospective studies of novel donor factors and novel assessment techniques are now required to further expand and define acceptability limits. The ultimate aim must be the creation of strategies and tools that will allow us to consider the use of 90% of the lung donor pool.

REFERENCES

1. Williams TJ, Snell GI. Organ procurement–strategies to optimize donor availability. Semin Respir Crit Care Med 2001;22(5):541–50.
2. Botha P, Rostron AJ, Fisher AJ, et al. Current strategies in donor selection and management. Semin Thorac Cardiovasc Surg 2008;20(2):143–51.
3. Snell GI, Griffiths A, Levvey BJ, et al. Availability of lungs for transplantation: exploring the real potential of the donor pool. J Heart Lung Transplant 2008; 27(6):662–7.
4. Sundaresan S, Trachiotis GD, Aoe M, et al. Donor lung procurement: assessment and operative technique. Ann Thorac Surg 1993;56(6):1409–13.
5. Yamane M, Sano Y, Toyooka S, et al. Living-donor lobar lung transplantation for pulmonary complications after hematopoietic stem cell transplantation. Transplantation 2008;86(12):1767–70.
6. Bando T, Date H, Minami M, et al. First registry report: lung transplantation in Japan: the Japanese

Society of Lung and Heart-Lung Transplantation. Gen Thorac Cardiovasc Surg 2008;56(1):17–21.

7. Stamenkovic S, Van Raemdonck D, Verleden G, et al. Bilateral lobar lung transplantation–the first two cases in Belgium. Acta Chir Belg 2007;107(2):201–4.

8. Keating DT, Westall GP, Marasco SF, et al. Paediatric lobar lung transplantation: addressing the paucity of donor organs. Med J Aust 2008;189(3):173–5.

9. Sweet SC, Wong HH, Webber SA, et al. Pediatric transplantation in the United States, 1995–2004. Am J Transplant 2006;6(5 Pt 2):1132–52.

10. Levvey B. Excellent early results of Australian DCD lung transplantation. J Heart Lung Transplant 2010; 31(2):S63–4.

11. Kootstra G, Daemen JH, Oomen AP. Categories of non-heart-beating donors. Transplant Proc 1995; 27(5):2893–4.

12. Snell GI, Levvey BJ, Oto T, et al. Early lung transplantation success utilizing controlled donation after cardiac death donors. Am J Transplant 2008;8(6): 1282–9.

13. Mason DP, Thuita L, Alster JM, et al. Should lung transplantation be performed using donation after cardiac death? The United States experience. J Thorac Cardiovasc Surg 2008;136(4):1061–6.

14. Tyden G, Kumlien G, Genberg H, et al. ABO incompatible kidney transplantations without splenectomy, using antigen-specific immunoadsorption and rituximab. Am J Transplant 2005;5(1):145–8.

15. Nelson PW, Bryan CF. When will real benefits for minority patients be realized with A2–>B transplants? Transplantation 2010;89(11):1310–1.

16. Banner NR, Rose ML, Cummins D, et al. Management of an ABO-incompatible lung transplant. Am J Transplant 2004;4(7):1192–6.

17. Pierson RN 3rd, Loyd JE, Goodwin A, et al. Successful management of an ABO-mismatched lung allograft using antigen-specific immunoadsorption, complement inhibition, and immunomodulatory therapy. Transplantation 2002;74(1):79–84.

18. Struber M, Warnecke G, Hafer C, et al. Intentional ABO-incompatible lung transplantation. Am J Transplant 2008;8(11):2476–8.

19. Sano Y, Aoe M, Date H, et al. Minor ABO-incompatible living-related lung transplantation. Transplant Proc 2002;34(7):2807–9.

20. Orens JB, Boehler A, de Perrot M, et al. A review of lung transplant donor acceptability criteria. J Heart Lung Transplant 2003;22(11):1183–200.

21. Van Raemdonck D, Neyrinck A, Verleden GM, et al. Lung donor selection and management. Proc Am Thorac Soc 2009;6(1):28–38.

22. Snell GI, Westall GP. Donor selection and management. Curr Opin Organ Transplant 2009;14(5):471–6.

23. Pierre AF, Sekine Y, Hutcheon MA, et al. Marginal donor lungs: a reassessment. J Thorac Cardiovasc Surg 2002;123(3):421–7 [discussion: 7–8].

24. Botha P, Trivedi D, Weir CJ, et al. Extended donor criteria in lung transplantation: impact on organ allocation. J Thorac Cardiovasc Surg 2006;131(5): 1154–60.

25. Meers C, Van Raemdonck D, Verleden GM, et al. The number of lung transplants can be safely doubled using extended criteria donors; a single-center review. Transpl Int 2010;23(6):628–35.

26. Levvey B. The lung allocation score in a non-US lung transplant program. J Heart Lung Transplant 2009; 29(2):S135.

27. Gabbay E, Williams TJ, Griffiths AP, et al. Maximizing the utilization of donor organs offered for lung transplantation. Am J Respir Crit Care Med 1999;160(1): 265–71.

28. Snell GI, Griffiths A, Macfarlane L, et al. Maximizing thoracic organ transplant opportunities: the importance of efficient coordination. J Heart Lung Transplant 2000;19(4):401–7.

29. Oto T, Levvey BJ, Whitford H, et al. Feasibility and utility of a lung donor score: correlation with early post-transplant outcomes. Ann Thorac Surg 2007; 83(1):257–63.

30. Iribarne A, Russo MJ, Davies RR, et al. Despite decreased wait-list times for lung transplantation, lung allocation scores continue to increase. Chest 2009;135(4):923–8.

31. Reyes KG, Mason DP, Thuita L, et al. Guidelines for donor lung selection: time for revision? Ann Thorac Surg 2010;89(6):1756–64 [discussion: 64–5].

32. Organ Procurement and Transplant Network 2006 Annual Report. Available at: http://www.optn.org/ AR2006. Accessed December 9, 2007.

33. Deaths in Australia. Government House, Canberra Australia: Australian Bureau of Statistics Annual Report; 2008. p. 9–10.

34. Opdam HI, Silvester W. Potential for organ donation in Victoria: an audit of hospital deaths. Med J Aust 2006;185(5):250–4.

35. Ojo AO, Wolfe RA, Leichtman AB, et al. A practical approach to evaluate the potential donor pool and trends in cadaveric kidney donation. Transplantation 1999;67(4):548–56.

36. Meyers BF, Patterson GA. Current status of lung transplantation. Adv Surg 2000;34:301–18.

37. De Perrot M, Waddell TK, Shargall Y, et al. Impact of donors aged 60 years or more on outcome after lung transplantation: results of an 11-year single-center experience. J Thorac Cardiovasc Surg 2007; 133(2):525–31.

38. Penn I, Halgrimson CG, Starzl TE. De novo malignant tumors in organ transplant recipients. Transplant Proc 1971;3(1):773–8.

39. Chen F, Karolak W, Cypel M, et al. Intermediate-term outcome in lung transplantation from a donor with glioblastoma multiforme. J Heart Lung Transplant 2009;28(10):1116–8.

40. Armanios MY, Grossman SA, Yang SC, et al. Transmission of glioblastoma multiforme following bilateral lung transplantation from an affected donor: case study and review of the literature. Neuro Oncol 2004;6(3):259–63.

41. Chen H, Shah AS, Girgis RE, et al. Transmission of glioblastoma multiforme after bilateral lung transplantation. J Clin Oncol 2008;26(19):3284–5.

42. Penn I. Donor transmitted disease: cancer. Transplant Proc 1991;23(5):2629–31.

43. Bajaj NS, Watt C, Hadjiliadis D, et al. Donor transmission of malignant melanoma in a lung transplant recipient 32 years after curative resection. Transpl Int 2010;23(7):e26–31.

44. Gandhi MJ, Strong DM. Donor derived malignancy following transplantation: a review. Cell Tissue Bank 2007;8(4):267–86.

45. Kauffman HM, Cherikh WS, McBride MA, et al. Deceased donors with a past history of malignancy: an organ procurement and transplantation network/united network for organ sharing update. Transplantation 2007;84(2):272–4.

46. Bonde PN, Patel ND, Borja MC, et al. Impact of donor lung organisms on post-lung transplant pneumonia. J Heart Lung Transplant 2006;25(1):99–105.

47. Avlonitis VS, Krause A, Luzzi L, et al. Bacterial colonization of the donor lower airways is a predictor of poor outcome in lung transplantation. Eur J Cardiothorac Surg 2003;24(4):601–7.

48. Mattner F, Kola A, Fischer S, et al. Impact of bacterial and fungal donor organ contamination in lung, heart-lung, heart and liver transplantation. Infection 2008;36(3):207–12.

49. Len O, Gavalda J, Blanes M, et al. Donor infection and transmission to the recipient of a solid allograft. Am J Transplant 2008;8(11):2420–5.

50. Palacios G, Druce J, Du L, et al. A new arenavirus in a cluster of fatal transplant-associated diseases. N Engl J Med 2008;358(10):991–8.

51. Iwamoto M, Jernigan DB, Guasch A, et al. Transmission of West Nile virus from an organ donor to four transplant recipients. N Engl J Med 2003;348(22):2196–203.

52. Srinivasan A, Burton EC, Kuehnert MJ, et al. Transmission of rabies virus from an organ donor to four transplant recipients. N Engl J Med 2005;352(11):1103–11.

53. Halpern SD, Shaked A, Hasz RD, et al. Informing candidates for solid-organ transplantation about donor risk factors. N Engl J Med 2008;358(26):2832–7.

54. Dhillon GS, Levitt J, Mallidi H, et al. Impact of hepatitis B core antibody positive donors in lung and heart-lung transplantation: an analysis of the United Network For Organ Sharing Database. Transplantation 2009;88(6):842–6.

55. Shitrit AB, Kramer MR, Bakal I, et al. Lamivudine prophylaxis for hepatitis B virus infection after lung transplantation. Ann Thorac Surg 2006;81(5):1851–2.

56. Oto T, Excell L, Griffiths AP, et al. The implications of pulmonary embolism in a multiorgan donor for subsequent pulmonary, renal, and cardiac transplantation. J Heart Lung Transplant 2008;27(1):78–85.

57. Ferraro P, Martin J, Dery J, et al. Late retrograde perfusion of donor lungs does not decrease the severity of primary graft dysfunction. Ann Thorac Surg 2008;86(4):1123–9.

58. Steen S, Sjoberg T, Pierre L, et al. Transplantation of lungs from a non-heart-beating donor. Lancet 2001;357(9259):825–9.

59. Ingemansson R, Eyjolfsson A, Mared L, et al. Clinical transplantation of initially rejected donor lungs after reconditioning ex vivo. Ann Thorac Surg 2009;87(1):255–60.

60. Cypel M, Yeung JC, Hirayama S, et al. Technique for prolonged normothermic ex vivo lung perfusion. J Heart Lung Transplant 2008;27(12):1319–25.

61. Kaneda H, Waddell TK, de Perrot M, et al. Pre-implantation multiple cytokine mRNA expression analysis of donor lung grafts predicts survival after lung transplantation in humans. Am J Transplant 2006;6(3):544–51.

62. Anraku M, Cameron MJ, Waddell TK, et al. Impact of human donor lung gene expression profiles on survival after lung transplantation: a case-control study. Am J Transplant 2008;8(10):2140–8.

63. Ray M, Dharmarajan S, Freudenberg J, et al. Expression profiling of human donor lungs to understand primary graft dysfunction after lung transplantation. Am J Transplant 2007;7(10):2396–405.

64. Avlonitis VS, Fisher AJ, Kirby JA, et al. Pulmonary transplantation: the role of brain death in donor lung injury. Transplantation 2003;75(12):1928–33.

65. Avlonitis VS, Wigfield CH, Golledge HD, et al. Early hemodynamic injury during donor brain death determines the severity of primary graft dysfunction after lung transplantation. Am J Transplant 2007;7(1):83–90.

66. Oto T, Excell L, Griffiths AP, et al. Association between primary graft dysfunction among lung, kidney and heart recipients from the same multiorgan donor. Am J Transplant 2008;8(10):2132–9.

67. Cooper DK. Hormonal resuscitation therapy in the management of the brain-dead potential organ donor. Int J Surg 2008;6(1):3–4.

68. Shah VR. Aggressive management of multiorgan donor. Transplant Proc 2008;40(4):1087–90.

69. Venkateswaran RV, Patchell VB, Wilson IC, et al. Early donor management increases the retrieval rate of lungs for transplantation. Ann Thorac Surg 2008;85(1):278–86 [discussion: 86].

70. Rosendale JD, Kauffman HM, McBride MA, et al. Aggressive pharmacologic donor management

results in more transplanted organs. Transplantation 2003;75(4):482–7.

71. Rostron AJ, Avlonitis VS, Cork DM, et al. Hemodynamic resuscitation with arginine vasopressin reduces lung injury after brain death in the transplant donor. Transplantation 2008;85(4):597–606.

72. Breathing life into injured lungs: world-first technique will expand lung donor organ pool. 2008. Available at: http://insciences.org/article.php?article_id=944. Accessed October 4, 2009.

73. Pilcher DV, Scheinkestel CD, Snell GI, et al. High central venous pressure is associated with prolonged mechanical ventilation and increased mortality after lung transplantation. J Thorac Cardiovasc Surg 2005;129(4):912–8.

74. Currey J, Pilcher DV, Davies A, et al. Implementation of a management guideline aimed at minimizing the severity of primary graft dysfunction after lung transplant. J Thorac Cardiovasc Surg 2010;139(1): 154–61.

75. UK transplant annual report 2006. Available at: http://www.uktransplant.org. Accessed December 9, 2007.

76. Eurotransplant International Foundation Annual Report 2009. Available at: http://wwweurotransplantorg/files/annual_report/ar_2009pdf. Accessed June 3, 2010.

77. Australian and New Zealand Dialysis and Transplant Registry 2009 report. Available at: http://wwwanzdataorgau/v1/report_2009html. Accessed June 3, 2010.

Novel Approaches to Expanding the Lung Donor Pool: Donation After Cardiac Death and Ex Vivo Conditioning

Marcelo Cypel, MD, MSc[a], Jonathan C. Yeung, MD[b],
Shaf Keshavjee, MD, MSc, FRCSC[c],*

KEYWORDS

- Lung transplantation • Lung donation after cardiac death
- Ex vivo lung perfusion
- Pharmacologic/molecular intervention

Lung transplantation (LTx) represents a unique life-saving therapy for patients suffering from end-stage lung disease. Ever since the world's first successful lung transplant was performed in Toronto 27 years ago,[1] listing of patients in need of LTx has been constantly increasing, but the number of organ donors has remained mostly static. This donor shortage is further aggravated by very low use rates of donor lungs (~15%) from multiorgan donors due to the conservative practices of many transplant groups. Recently, two novel approaches have been developed to potentially increase the availability of donor lungs. In the first approach, lungs from donation after cardiac death (DCD) donors are used to increase the quantity of organ donors. In the second approach, a newly developed normothermic ex vivo lung perfusion (EVLP) technique is used as a means of reassessing the adequacy of lung function from DCD and brain death donors, and potentially optimizing function of injured donor lungs

initially unsuitable for transplantation. This review discusses both of these novel approaches in detail.

LUNG DONATION AFTER CARDIAC DEATH

Organs have traditionally been harvested only from individuals who have died after meeting criteria for brain death (ie, donation after brain death [DBD] donors).[2] However, to help overcome the organ donor shortage, some programs have initiated the use of DCD donors. At the First International Workshop on DCD held in Maastricht in the Netherlands in 1995, 4 types of donors were defined: Categories I (dead on arrival) and II (unsuccessful resuscitation) comprise the *uncontrolled* donors. Categories III (awaiting cardiac arrest) and IV (cardiac arrest in brain-dead donors) include the *controlled* donors (**Table 1**). The principal steps in the sequence of care in controlled and uncontrolled DCD donation are shown in

a Division Thoracic Surgery, Toronto Lung Transplant Program, Toronto General Hospital, University of Toronto, 200 Elizabeth Street, 9n969, Toronto, M5G 2C4, Canada
b Latner Thoracic Surgery Laboratories, University of Toronto, 101 College Street, 2-815, Toronto, ON M5G 1L7, Canada
c Division of Thoracic Surgery and Institute of Biomaterials and Biomedical Engineering, Toronto Lung Transplant Program, Latner Thoracic Research Laboratories, University of Toronto, 190 Elizabeth Street, RFE1-408, Toronto, M5G 2C4, Canada
* Corresponding author.
E-mail address: shaf.keshavjee@uhn.on.ca

Clin Chest Med 32 (2011) 233–244
doi:10.1016/j.ccm.2011.02.003
0272-5231/11/$ – see front matter © 2011 Elsevier Inc. All rights reserved.

Table 1
Maastricht classification of donation after cardiac death

Maastricht Categories	DCD Definition
Category I (uncontrolled)	Dead on arrival
Category II (uncontrolled)	Unsuccessful resuscitation
Category III (controlled)	Awaiting cardiac arrest
Category IV (controlled)	Cardiac arrest in a brain death donor

Fig. 1. Controlled DCD donation is the most accepted type of DCD donation to date for lungs, liver, and kidneys. Controlled DCD includes patients who have a dismal prognosis, but whose condition does not fulfill the strict definition of brain death. Supportive care that is thought to be futile is usually withdrawn from these patients at a planned time; this subsequently leads to patient death, at which time organ retrieval can proceed. The DCD donor pool is becoming substantial; from 2006 to 2008, there was an increase of 24% in the DCD category compared with a 2% decrease in the number of consented DBD donors.[3] By far the largest percentage increase in multiorgan donors in recent years has been in the DCD category, and this will significantly affect organ use in the future.

Experimental Research with Lung DCD

The lung is a unique organ in that it is not dependent on blood perfusion for aerobic metabolism but instead can use a mechanism of passive diffusion through the alveoli for oxygen delivery. The initial experimental studies performed in dogs by Egan and colleagues[4] demonstrated the feasibility of transplanting donor lungs after cardiocirculatory arrest. Lungs that were retrieved 1 hour after arrest could sustain life after transplantation; however, most recipient animals died when lungs that were retrieved 4 hours after arrest were transplanted. This group further demonstrated the importance of lung inflation and intra-alveolar oxygen concentration in a DCD setting. In unventilated animals, 77% of lung cells were nonviable 12 hours after death, which was comparable to results from nitrogen-ventilated cadaver lungs. Oxygen-ventilated cadaver rats, however, had only 26% nonviable lung cells.[5] Moreover, the degree of ultrastructural damage observed in the oxygen ventilated group at 2 and 4 hours postmortem was not significantly different from that of normal controls.[6] Thus, mechanical ventilation with oxygen after death preserved the lung ultrastructure and delayed cell death. Additional studies by Van Raemdonck and colleagues[7] demonstrated that lung inflation post mortem was critical to the preservation of lung barrier functions and that inflation with room air (Fio_2 21%) was equivalent to inflation with 100% Fio_2.

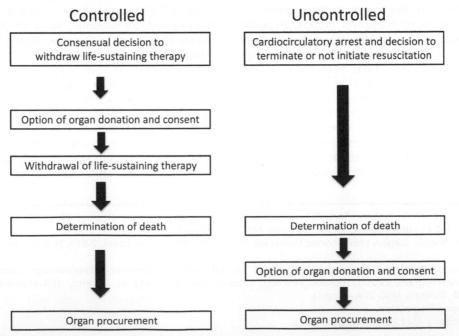

Fig. 1. Overview of sequence of care in controlled and uncontrolled donation after cardiocirculatory death.

Buchanan and colleagues[8] showed excellent gas exchange 1 week after the transplantation of lungs that were retrieved by DCD protocol 30 minutes after death in a porcine model. Greco and colleagues[9] showed similar gas-exchange characteristics of lungs from ventilated DCD pigs retrieved 30, 60, or 90 minutes after circulatory arrest compared with lungs retrieved from conventional donors. These studies supported the hypothesis that LTx from DCD donors may be feasible. Other studies were performed to determine the maximum tolerable warm ischemic time (WIT; time from arrest to cold flush) in DCD models, and 60 to 90 minutes seemed to be the acceptable limit for WIT.[7,10,11] Topical cooling by circulating cold preservation solution in the pleural cavity through large-bore chest tubes has also been proposed as a method to better preserve lungs in an uncontrolled DCD situation during transportation of the donor to the hospital and the period of time required to obtain consent for donation.[12,13]

Most of the experimental DCD studies have been performed using sudden cardiac arrest by drug administration or myocardial fibrillation. Therefore, this may not well represent the clinical scenario where a period of cardiopulmonary instability (also called the "agonal period") occurs before circulatory arrest. Concerns have been raised about the injury that may occur to the pulmonary allograft during this phase. This injury might in fact be more crucial than the postmortem insult that occurs during the warm ischemic interval and preservation process. Neutrophils can be activated and sequestrated into the lung during this time, and release proinflammatory mediators that can injure the lungs before retrieval. Tremblay and coworkers[14] investigated the impact of premortem hypotension and cardiac instability in the setting of uncontrolled DCD (traumatic blood loss, myocardial infarction). In an isolated rat lung reperfusion model, graft function was severely impaired in rats that underwent 1 hour of hemorrhagic shock by exsanguination followed by 2 to 3 hours of in situ ischemia. Another recent study demonstrated that the premortem agonal phase in DCD induces a sympathetic storm leading to capillary leak with pulmonary edema and reduced oxygenation on reperfusion. Graft quality was inferior in DCD lungs when recovered from a hypoxic cardiac arrest model in comparison with uncontrolled exsanguination or fibrillation setting.[15] Because the airway is unprotected, aspiration of gastric contents can occur during the agonal phase in a DCD donor, adding additional lung injury.

There are, however, theoretical advantages of DCD lung donation. The use of DCD organs can avoid brain death–induced lung injury. Given the low use rates of lungs today, the lung appears to be vulnerable to the effects of brain death. Neurogenic pulmonary edema is a common injury in brain-dead donors and although the mechanism is not completely clear, it is thought that the sudden and profound increase in systemic vascular resistance generated by the catecholamine storm leads to a decrease in left ventricular output and an increase in left atrial (LA) and pulmonary capillary pressure. This increased pressure can cause injury to the pulmonary epithelium and, as a result, pulmonary edema forms by both hydrostatic and increased permeability mechanisms.[16] Lung injury can also occur as a result of systemic inflammation following brain death. Increased circulating proinflammatory cytokines can result in the induction of cell adhesion molecules on pulmonary endothelial and epithelial surfaces.[17] This process leads to the recruitment of neutrophils and monocytes to the lung, causing inflammatory lung injury. The authors have previously shown that interleukin (IL)-8 levels in donor lung tissue before and after transplantation increased with time after reperfusion, and that patients who developed severe primary graft dysfunction had significantly higher IL-8 levels during ischemia and after reperfusion.[18,19] Similarly, Fisher and colleagues[20] studied the levels of IL-8 in bronchoalveolar lavage (BAL) fluid from 26 donor lungs used for transplantation, and showed that a high concentration of IL-8 in donor BAL fluid was correlated with severe graft dysfunction and with early postoperative deaths. To further study the role of proinflammatory cytokines, the authors used real-time polymerase chain reaction (RT-PCR) to study the levels of IL-6, IL-1β, IL-8, IL-10, interferon-γ, and tumor necrosis factor α in the donor lung at the end of cold ischemia, and found that the IL-6/IL-10 ratio was predictive of recipient 30-day mortality.[21]

The authors' group in Toronto recently compared inflammatory mediators in DCD and DBD donors using lung tissue biopsies from human donor lungs used for transplantation. Lungs from DCD donors showed decreased proinflammatory cytokine profiles compared with DBD lungs. In particular, levels of IL-6 and IL-8 were significantly lower in DCD lungs.[22] Moreover, in unsupervised clustering analysis of microarray data, DCD and DBD lungs generated distinct transcriptomic signatures and the two lung types differed most in pathways related to inflammation, such as nuclear factor κB. The gene sets enriched in DBD mapped to innate immunity, intracellular signaling, cytokine interaction, cell communication, and apoptosis pathways.[22] These observations support the concept that brain death results in the development of a systemic inflammatory response that can damage organs, with a deleterious impact on their function after transplantation.[23–25]

Clinical Experience with Lung DCD

The first LTx in humans was performed by James Hardy in 1963 using a lung from a DCD donor who died of a myocardial infarction. At that time, use of DCD was a necessity, as the concept of brain death was not yet legally established. Once brain death had reached general acceptance in the 1970s, all organs were harvested from DBD donors.

Uncontrolled donation

Apart from a case reported by Steen and colleagues[26] in 2001 of a DCD LTx using a donor who died of myocardial infarct in hospital (Category I), the only experience with uncontrolled DCD LTx is from the group in Madrid, who described 17 cases.[27,28] Lungs were retrieved from donors who suddenly collapsed outside the hospital (Category II). Cardiopulmonary resuscitation was started in the patient if sudden death from cardiac, neurologic, or traumatic origin occurred no longer than 15 minutes after arrival of the medical team. If these resuscitation maneuvers were not successful after more than 30 minutes, the potential donor was transported to the hospital where death was certified after cardiac massage was interrupted. Judicial and family permission for organ donation were then obtained. The cadaver was transported to the operating room and connected via the femoral vessels to an extracorporeal bypass machine with deep hypothermia and oxygenation for preservation of the abdominal organs. Both lungs were further cooled topically with 4 L of Perfadex solution at 4°C via 2 chest drains on each side. Oxygenation capacity was assessed in situ after sternotomy with a single pulmonary flush of 300 mL of venous donor blood mixed with Perfadex. An additional retrograde flush was administered on the back table after lung extraction with 250 mL Perfadex in each vein. Grade 2 or 3 primary graft dysfunction (PGD)[29] occurred in 53% of the cases. Hospital mortality rate was 17%. The survival rates were 82% at 3 months, 69%, at 1 year, and 58% at 3 years. Although PGD and mortality rates were higher than expected after conventional LTx, the investigators argued that this source of organs is valid and justifiable in the context of severe organ shortage.

Controlled donation

Controlled (Categories III and IV) DCD LTx is by far the most accepted and used DCD type for donation. In 1995, Love and colleagues[30] reported the first successful experience using a DCD lung donor. Since then, other groups slowly started to incorporate DCD transplantation into their programs, but it was not until the current decade that LTx from DCD became more widely accepted. Uncertainty about outcomes using DCD donor lungs has led transplant teams to be very conservative in organ selection when using this donor group. Whereas an average of 3.6 organs is transplanted from DBD donors, in DCD the average is 2.0.[3] About 100 cases of DCD LTx have been reported to date. **Table 2** summarizes the outcomes of DCD LTx from series where 10 or more cases have been reported. In contrast to

Table 2
Outcomes reported to date for lung transplantation using DCD donation[a]

Study	N	Category	PGD 2 or 3	BOS	Survival (Discharge, 1 y, 3 y)
de Antonio et al,[28] 2007	17	II	53%	7% 1 y, 11% 2 y, 50% 3 y	82%, 69%, 58%
Snell et al,[37] 2008	11	III	18%	9%	100%, NR, NR
Mason et al (UNOS),[35,36] 2008	36	III	NR	NR	NR, 94%, NR
Cypel et al,[33,68] 2009	10	III–IV	40%	None	100%, NR, NR
Puri et al,[34] 2009	11	III	36%	27%	82%, 82%, NR
De Oliveira et al,[31] 2010	18	III	33.3%	19.6% 1 y, 19.6% 3 y, 27.7% 5 y	94%, 88.1%, 81.9%
Erasmus et al,[38] 2010	21	III	23.8%	14.2%	95.2%, 95.2%, 90.4%

Abbreviations: BOS, bronchiolitis obliterans syndrome; NR, not recorded; PGD, primary graft dysfunction grade; UNOS, United Network for Organ Sharing.
[a] Series reporting 10 or more cases are included in this table.

uncontrolled DCD, early and intermediate outcomes of transplantation of Category III DCDs have been comparable to LTx using DBD.[31–38] Only one recent report has shown increased rates of severe PGD (36%) and higher 30-day (18%) and 18-month (36%) mortality.[34] A recent review of the United States experience using data retrospectively collected from the UNOS (United Network for Organ Sharing) database demonstrated an overall survival after LTx at 1, 12, and 24 months of 94%, 94%, and 87%, respectively, for recipients receiving lungs from DCD donors, compared with 92%, 78%, and 69%, respectively, from DBD donors. The largest single-center experience comprising 21 cases of controlled DCD LTx was reported by Erasmus and colleagues,[38] with an excellent 1-year survival of 95%. Although the DCD statistics are highly favorable, the small sample size in these studies does not allow for a definitive conclusion as to whether DCD provides better early and intermediate outcomes compared with DBD. Transplant teams have been highly selective in donor and recipient selection for DCD procedures, which may have favorably influenced the outcomes.

A better understanding of how the DCD process affects donor lungs will have a major impact in expanding the use of DCD organs and alleviating the organ shortage. The time between withdrawal of life support therapies (WLST) and cold flush in DCD lungs is a period of risk for lung injury. Once WLST is initiated, the lung is at increased risk from events such as hypotension, warm ischemia (once systolic blood pressure is <50 mm Hg or after cardiac arrest), and aspiration. Two small series have shown an inverse relationship between this "agonal" time and Pao_2/Fio_2 ratios after transplantation, but firm conclusions await performance of larger studies.[33,37]

DCD Donor Lung Evaluation and Procedure

DCD donor lung evaluation is in general similar to DBD and includes medical history, arterial blood gases, chest radiograph findings, bronchoscopy findings, and direct examination of the lungs in the operating room. Of importance, decisions about WLST, management of the dying process, and the determination of death by cardiocirculatory criteria must be independent of the donation/transplant processes. Whether WLST should occur in the intensive care unit (ICU) or in the operating room should be based on family preferences, institutional logistics, resources, and facilities.

In most protocols, the donor receives heparin (30,000 IU) 30 minutes before WLST,[33] although successful clinical DCD transplantation has been performed without donor heparinization.[38] When cardiac arrest occurs, death is certified by 2 physicians from the donor hospital ICU team after a 5- to 10-minute period of absent palpable pulses, blood pressure, and respiration. The donor is then quickly reintubated, generally by one of the LTx team members. A flexible bronchoscopy is then performed to rule out aspiration of gastric contents during cardiac arrest, presence of mucopurulent secretions, or anatomic abnormalities. Concurrent with the bronchoscopy, another member of the team performs a median sternotomy and cannulation of the pulmonary artery (PA), followed by the standard procurement technique.[39] Because there is insufficient time for careful examination of the lungs before cold flush perfusion, the decision to use the lungs for LTx and initiate recipient anesthesia is in general made only after the lungs are explanted and careful macroscopic evaluation is performed. Functional reassessment of these organs using EVLP is very useful and has become routine in some centers (see section on EVLP).

Ethical Considerations

DCD organ donation raises several very important ethical considerations.[40] Although it is generally seen as appropriate to use the human body as a source of tissues and organs to serve the well-being of other individuals, the donor's body should always be treated with great care and respect. The care of the dying patient must never be compromised by the desire to protect organs for donation or to expedite death to allow timely organ retrieval. The first responsibility of health care providers, regardless of the potential for donation, is to advance the well-being of the dying patient, including psychological, emotional, and spiritual well-being in addition to physical well-being. Decisions about care at the end of life should be based on the known values and beliefs of the patient. These decisions should be consistent with what each patient understands to be a meaningful life and death, including the ability or desire to provide organs to others. Support for families and loved ones should continue through all phases of dying: before, during, and after WLST.

It is important to recognize and minimize conflicts of interest that might occur in the setting of DCD. Conflicts of interest occur when those involved in providing health care have relationships with people or organizations outside the healing relationship that may influence their actions, regardless of whether they believe these relationships actually affect their judgment. Failure to identify and disclose such conflicts may undermine the integrity of a program and jeopardize public and professional trust.

EX VIVO LUNG PERFUSION
Rationale and Experimental Work to Date

Another novel strategy to help overcome the shortage of donor lungs is the reassessment and conditioning of injured donor lungs using normothermic EVLP. The current clinical practice of lung preservation is that of cold static preservation (CSP). During retrieval, a cold pulmonary flush using low potassium dextran preservation solution (Perfadex; Virolife, Göteborg, Sweden) is coupled with topical cooling and lung ventilation.[39,41] Thereafter, the lungs are transported at 4°C in an inflated state. Hypothermia reduces metabolic activity to the point that cell viability can be maintained in the face of ischemia (5% of metabolic rate at 37°C).[42] Cold temperature preservation continues to be an important component of lung preservation.[43,44]

Physiologic normothermic (37°C) or near-normothermic (25–34°C) ex vivo perfusion has become a popular research tool as a preservation alternative in experimental models of lung, liver, and kidney transplantation.[45–50] One important advantage of normothermic perfusion is the allowance of functional reassessment during the ex vivo phase of organ preservation. EVLP likely provides a more accurate assessment of lung function compared with in vivo assessment because: (1) it provides an excellent environment for recruitment and reexpansion of atelectatic lung areas; (2) it allows for effective clearance of bronchial secretions; (3) it allows for removal of clots in the pulmonary circulation through the use of transient retrograde perfusion at the beginning of the procedure; (4) it allows for all ventilator volumes and pressures to be transferred directly to the lungs without interference of the chest wall and diaphragm; and (5) the dextran in the perfusate solution facilitates perfusion of the pulmonary microvasculature.

Another theoretical advantage of normothermic perfusion is the maintenance of normal metabolism, permitting restoration of normal functions (using organ innate reparative mechanisms or through active therapeutic interventions). Maintenance of organs under physiologic temperatures is not a novel concept. Carrel and Lindbergh[51] described the concept of the "culture of whole organs" in 1935. However, until recently, isolated lung perfusion has been used only to study basic lung physiology, usually in small animal lungs.[52–56] In general, experimental work in isolated lung perfusion systems has shown that this leads to progressive deterioration of lung function.[57,58] The resurgence of EVLP as a potentially important tool in lung transplantation started with the work of Steen and colleagues.[59] Envisioning the use of EVLP as a method to reassess lungs from uncontrolled DCD donors (since these organs cannot be evaluated in vivo), this group described an ex vivo perfusion system and made an important contribution by developing a specific solution (Steen solution) that allows for ex vivo perfusion of the lungs without development of pulmonary edema. After a short period (60–90 minutes) of ex vivo evaluation, they demonstrated that the lung could be successfully transplanted in large animals and described its use in a case report of human LTx.[26,59]

Following these publications, other groups demonstrated the feasibility of short-term EVLP using the technique described by Steen to evaluate lung function in animal models of DCD and experimentally using injured human lungs rejected for transplantation.[13,60–65] Erasmus and colleagues[66] extended the EVLP duration to 6 hours. Although feasible, circuit-induced impairment of lung function, as evidenced by increased pulmonary vascular resistance and increased airway pressures, became apparent toward the end of the procedure.

The Toronto group modified the EVLP system and strategy in order to be able to maintain lungs in the EVLP system for at least 12 hours without additional injury. The use of an acellular perfusate, a closed circuit with protective low perfusion pressure and stable positive LA pressure (5 mm Hg), and a protective mode of mechanical ventilation (tidal volume of 7 mL/kg, rate of 7 breaths per minute, with a positive end-expiratory airway pressure of 5 cm H_2O) were critical modifications to achieve 12 hours of perfusion stability. In the authors' initial studies using normal pig lungs, stable lung function during 12 hours of EVLP was demonstrated.[67] This stability during prolonged normothermic EVLP translated into excellent posttransplant lung function ($Pao_2/Fio_2 = 527 \pm 22$ mm Hg), low edema formation, and preserved lung histology after transplantation. The acellular perfusion assessment of lung function accurately correlated with posttransplant graft function and the addition of red blood cells did not provide additional functional information compared with acellular perfusate.[67] This study provided the proof of concept that EVLP is able to maintain donor lungs for a prolonged period of time without damaging the organ. The authors further examined the impact of prolonged EVLP on ischemic injury.[68] Pig donor lungs were cold-preserved for 12 hours and subsequently divided into two groups: CSP or normothermic EVLP for an additional 12 hours (total 24 hours preservation). EVLP preservation resulted in significantly better lung oxygenation and lower edema formation rates after transplantation when compared with CSP. Alveolar epithelial cell tight junction integrity, evaluated by zona occludens–1 protein staining, was disrupted in the cell membranes after prolonged CSP but not after EVLP. Integrity of functional metabolic pathways during normothermic perfusion was confirmed by effective adenoviral GFP gene transfer and transgene expression by lung alveolar cells.[68]

Technique for EVLP

The authors have previously described the details for their acellular lung protective EVLP technique, including a detailed discussion about the rationale for the chosen ventilatory and perfusion strategies.[67] The components of the circuit are shown in **Fig. 2** and the EVLP strategy is shown in **Table 3**. The lungs are transferred from the back table to the XVIVO chamber (Vitrolife) placed

on a second draped sterile operating room back table. First, the LA cannula is connected to the circuit and a slow retrograde flow (using the circuit bridge) is performed to de-air the PA cannula. Once de-airing is complete, the PA cannula is connected to the circuit and anterograde flow is initiated at 150 mL/min with the perfusate at room temperature. The temperature of the perfusate is then gradually increased to 37°C over the next 30 minutes. Before increasing flow beyond this level, a careful check of the system is made. The PA and LA pressure readings are double checked. When a temperature of 32°C is reached (usually over 20 minutes), ventilation is started and the perfusate flow rate is gradually increased to the target flow (40% of estimated donor cardiac output) within 60 minutes. Once ventilation is started, the flow of gas (86% N_2, 6% O_2, 8% CO_2, Praxair) that will deoxygenate and provide carbon dioxide to the inflow perfusate via the gas exchange membrane is initiated (started at 0.8 L/min) and titrated to maintain inflow perfusate P_{CO_2} between 35 and 45 mm Hg.

Ex vivo Lung Perfusion Equipment

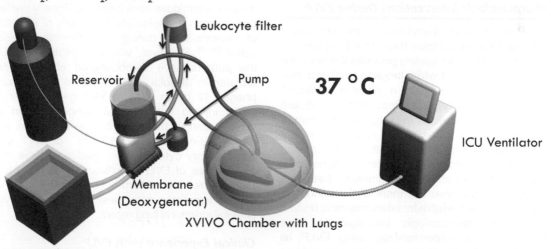

Gas for deoxygenation
86% N_2, 8% CO_2, 6% O_2

Red: Venous (Oxygenated) perfusate
Blue: Arterial (Deoxygenated) perfusate
Perfusate: Acellular Steen

Leukocyte filter

Reservoir

Pump

37 °C

ICU Ventilator

Membrane
(Deoxygenator)

XVIVO Chamber with Lungs

Heater/Cooler

Fig. 2. Components of ex vivo lung perfusion circuit. The perfusate is circulated by a centrifugal pump passing through a membrane gas exchanger and a leukocyte-depletion filter before entering the lung block through the pulmonary artery. A filtered gas line for the gas-exchange membrane is connected to an H-size tank with a specialty gas mixture of oxygen (6%), carbon dioxide (8%), and nitrogen (86%). A heat exchanger is connected to the membrane gas exchanger to maintain the perfusate at temperature. Pulmonary artery flow is controlled by the centrifugal pump and measured using an electromagnetic flow meter. The outflow oxygenated perfusate returns through the left atrial cannula to a hard-shell reservoir. Lungs are ventilated with a standard ICU-type ventilator. The lungs are contained in a specifically designed lung enclosure (XVIVO; Vitrolife, Göteborg, Sweden).

Table 3
Ventilatory and perfusion strategy for EVLP

Ventilation	
Tidal volume	7 mL/kg
PEEP	5 cm H_2O
Frequency	7 breaths/min
I/E ratio	1/2
Recruitment	1 every hour to PawP 20 cm H_2O
Perfusion	
Pump flow	40% estimated donor cardiac output
Pulmonary artery pressure	7–13 mm Hg[a]
Left atrial pressure	3–5 mm Hg[b]
Perfusate exchange	250 mL every hour
Perfusate composition	Steen solution, heparin, antibiotics, solumedrol
Perfusate pH	6.8–7.4
Perfusate Pco_2	35–45 mm Hg

Abbreviations: I/E, inspiration/expiration; PawP, pulmonary artery wedge pressure; PEEP, positive end-expiratory airway pressure.
[a] Pulmonary artery pressure is a reflection of lung quality.
[b] Left atrial pressure can be controlled by adjusting the height of the reservoir.

Pharmacologic Interventions During EVLP

EVLP offers an ideal environment for therapeutic interventions to optimize the donor lung prior to transplantation. The system provides the opportunity to better select which lungs to treat and then to reevaluate to confirm a positive treatment effect. Furthermore, side effects of the treatment are greatly minimized by the targeted treatment of the organ, and inflammatory responses in the repair process can theoretically be decreased, due to the absence of circulating immune cells. Lastly, EVLP provides flexible timing for treatment in contrast to in vivo treatment of the donor, for which the time available for interventions is limited.

Several pharmacologic investigations have been explored experimentally using EVLP as a platform. Agents to remove pulmonary edema by enhancing alveolar fluid clearance have been studied. Sakuma and colleagues[69] demonstrated the role of epinephrine in enhancing alveolar fluid clearance and removing pulmonary edema. Treated lungs demonstrated an alveolar fluid clearance of 84% above control clearance. The same group demonstrated the role of β-adrenergic stimulation in clearance of pulmonary edema

using a human EVLP model.[70] Because many donor lungs rejected for transplantation because of poor function have unrecognized pulmonary embolism,[71] Inci and colleagues[72] proposed the use of fibrinolytics during EVLP. This strategy might be especially important in DCD donors in whom donor heparinization might not be possible. Adding urokinase to the perfusate during EVLP resulted in improved graft function by reducing pulmonary vascular resistance and increasing oxygenation after 3 hours of warm ischemia. The same group demonstrated that intra-airway surfactant administration during EVLP improved donor lungs injured with acid aspiration.[73] A large number of donor lungs are declined because of infection acquired during critical illness and brain death. EVLP provides a very attractive platform for administration of high doses of antimicrobials without the risk of injuring other organs. In addition, the half-life of these drugs is significantly prolonged in the system. One recent study showed that antibiotics decreased the bacterial load,[74] but further investigations are required to prove this very promising concept.

Molecular Interventions During EVLP

Another exciting method of lung repair is gene therapy. Gene therapy in LTx is attractive because transtracheal delivery of gene vectors can localize the effect to the lung graft. Although ex vivo vector delivery is an attractive concept,[75] ex vivo gene transfer techniques have been traditionally ineffective in organ transplantation because of inhibition of metabolism during hypothermic preservation.[76–78] However, with normothermic EVLP, the authors have demonstrated efficient gene transfer in alveolar epithelial cells and macrophages 12 hours after ex vivo gene delivery.[68] Using injured human donor lungs rejected for transplantation, the authors showed that ex vivo adenoviral-mediated IL-10 (a potent anti-inflammatory cytokine) gene delivery at the start of 12 hours of EVLP significantly improved lung function, reduced inflammation (down-regulation of proinflammatory cytokines), and promoted cytoskeletal structural lung repair.

Clinical Experience with EVLP

The first clinical use of an EVLP system was described by Steen and colleagues[26] in 2001 to briefly assess lung function in an organ harvested from a DCD donor. The same group reported their experience with 60 to 90 minutes of blood-based perfusion to assess 6 high-risk donor lungs before transplantation. Although outcomes were considered acceptable, the postoperative length of stay in the ICU was longer in recipients of perfused lungs as compared with conventional transplantation (13 vs 7 days).[79,80]

The first prospective clinical trial using EVLP was recently completed at the University of Toronto, and the results have been presented at the annual meeting of the International Society of Heart and Lung Transplantation.[81] In this study, 23 lung transplants were performed after 4 hours of EVLP using the acellular protective ventilation/perfusion strategy developed by the authors' group.[67,68] This trial demonstrated that extended normothermic EVLP is safe for the assessment of high-risk donor lungs, and similar early outcomes were obtained in a comparison with conventionally selected and transplanted donor lungs.

SUMMARY

Lung transplantation using DCD donors is now a clinical reality, and outcomes from controlled donation have been comparable to brain death donors. Although the hemodynamic instability prior to death can injure the lung in DCD, the avoidance of the cytokine storm associated with brain death is a potential advantage in these organs, and some preliminary clinical studies have shown that inflammatory profiles are more favorable in lungs from DCDs when compared with DBDs.

By mimicking the lung's natural physiologic environment and by providing oxygen and other substrates necessary for active metabolism, normothermic EVLP may offer the next step in lung assessment and preservation. Treatment of donor lungs prior to transplantation, such as with pharmacologic agents to reduce pulmonary edema and inflammation or gene therapy to better prepare the organ to deal with the reperfusion and subsequent immunologic insults, will be the major goals of the future.

REFERENCES

1. Unilateral lung transplantation for pulmonary fibrosis. Toronto lung transplant group. N Engl J Med 1986;314:1140–5.
2. Barnieh L, Baxter D, Boiteau P, et al. Benchmarking performance in organ donation programs: dependence on demographics and mortality rates. Can J Anaesth 2006;53:727–31.
3. Tuttle-Newhall JE, Krishnan SM, Levy MF, et al. Organ donation and utilization in the United States: 1998-2007. Am J Transplant 2009;9:879–93.
4. Egan TM, Lambert CJ Jr, Reddick R, et al. A strategy to increase the donor pool: use of cadaver lungs for transplantation. Ann Thorac Surg 1991;52:1113–20 [discussion: 1120–1].
5. D'Armini AM, Roberts CS, Griffith PK, et al. When does the lung die? I. Histochemical evidence of pulmonary viability after "death". J Heart Lung Transplant 1994;13:741–7.
6. Alessandrini F, D'Armini AM, Roberts CS, et al. When does the lung die? II. Ultrastructural evidence of pulmonary viability after "death". J Heart Lung Transplant 1994;13:748–57.
7. Van Raemdonck DE, Jannis NC, Rega FR, et al. Extended preservation of ischemic pulmonary graft by postmortem alveolar expansion. Ann Thorac Surg 1997;64:801–8.
8. Buchanan SA, DeLima NF, Binns OA, et al. Pulmonary function after non-heart-beating lung donation in a survival model. Ann Thorac Surg 1995;60:38–44 [discussion: 44–6].
9. Greco R, Cordovilla G, Sanz E, et al. Warm ischemic time tolerance after ventilated non-heart-beating lung donation in piglets. Eur J Cardiothorac Surg 1998;14:319–25.
10. Van Raemdonck DE, Jannis NC, De Leyn PR, et al. Warm ischemic tolerance in collapsed pulmonary grafts is limited to 1 hour. Ann Surg 1998;228:788–96.
11. Kuang JQ, Van Raemdonck DE, Jannis NC, et al. Pulmonary cell death in warm ischemic rabbit lung is related to the alveolar oxygen reserve. J Heart Lung Transplant 1998;17:406–14.
12. Rega FR, Jannis NC, Verleden GM, et al. Should we ventilate or cool the pulmonary graft inside the non-heart-beating donor? J Heart Lung Transplant 2003;22:1226–33.
13. Neyrinck AP, Van De Wauwer C, Geudens N, et al. Comparative study of donor lung injury in heart-beating versus non-heart-beating donors. Eur J Cardiothorac Surg 2006;30:628–36.
14. Tremblay LN, Yamashiro T, DeCampos KN, et al. Effect of hypotension preceding death on the function of lungs from donors with nonbeating hearts. J Heart Lung Transplant 1996;15:260–8.
15. Van de Wauwer C, Neyrinck AP, Geudens N, et al. The mode of death in the non-heart-beating donor has an impact on lung graft quality. Eur J Cardiothorac Surg 2009;36:919–26.
16. Novitzky D, Wicomb WN, Rose AG, et al. Pathophysiology of pulmonary edema following experimental brain death in the chacma baboon. Ann Thorac Surg 1987;43:288–94.
17. Avlonitis VS, Fisher AJ, Kirby JA, et al. Pulmonary transplantation: the role of brain death in donor lung injury. Transplantation 2003;75:1928–33.
18. De Perrot M, Sekine Y, Fischer S, et al. Interleukin-8 release during ischemia-reperfusion correlates with early graft function in human lung transplantation. J Heart Lung Transplant 2001;20:175–6.
19. De Perrot M, Sekine Y, Fischer S, et al. Interleukin-8 release during early reperfusion predicts graft

function in human lung transplantation. Am J Respir Crit Care Med 2002;165:211–5.

20. Fisher AJ, Donnelly SC, Hirani N, et al. Elevated levels of interleukin-8 in donor lungs is associated with early graft failure after lung transplantation. Am J Respir Crit Care Med 2001;163:259–65.

21. Kaneda H, Waddell TK, de Perrot M, et al. Pre-implantation multiple cytokine mRNA expression analysis of donor lung grafts predicts survival after lung transplantation in humans. Am J Transplant 2006;6:544–51.

22. Kang CH, Anraku M, Cypel M, et al. Transcriptional signatures in donor lungs from donation after cardiac death vs after brain death: a functional pathway analysis. J Heart Lung Transplant 2010; 30(3):289–98.

23. Novitzky D. Detrimental effects of brain death on the potential organ donor. Transplant Proc 1997;29: 3770–2.

24. Takada M, Nadeau KC, Hancock WW, et al. Effects of explosive brain death on cytokine activation of peripheral organs in the rat. Transplantation 1998; 65:1533–42.

25. Kusaka M, Pratschke J, Wilhelm MJ, et al. Activation of inflammatory mediators in rat renal isografts by donor brain death. Transplantation 2000;69:405–10.

26. Steen S, Sjoberg T, Pierre L, et al. Transplantation of lungs from a non-heart-beating donor. Lancet 2001; 357:825–9.

27. Gamez P, Cordoba M, Ussetti P, et al. Lung transplantation from out-of-hospital non-heart-beating lung donors. one-year experience and results. J Heart Lung Transplant 2005;24:1098–102.

28. de Antonio DG, Marcos R, Laporta R, et al. Results of clinical lung transplant from uncontrolled non-heart-beating donors. J Heart Lung Transplant 2007;26:529–34.

29. Christie JD, Carby M, Bag R, et al. Report of the ISHLT Working Group on Primary Lung Graft Dysfunction part II: definition. A consensus statement of the International Society for Heart and Lung Transplantation. J Heart Lung Transplant 2005;24:1454–9.

30. Love RB, Stringham JC, Chomiak PN, et al. Successful lung transplantation using a non-heart-beating donor. J Heart Lung Transplant 1995;14: s88 [abstract].

31. De Oliveira NC, Osaki S, Maloney JD, et al. Lung transplantation with donation after cardiac death donors: long-term follow-up in a single center. J Thorac Cardiovasc Surg 2010;139:1306–15.

32. De Vleeschauwer S, Van Raemdonck D, Vanaudenaerde B, et al. Early outcome after lung transplantation from non-heart-beating donors is comparable to heart-beating donors. J Heart Lung Transplant 2009;28:380–7.

33. Cypel M, Sato M, Yildirim E, et al. Initial experience with lung donation after cardiocirculatory death in Canada. J Heart Lung Transplant 2009;28:753–8.

34. Puri V, Scavuzzo M, Guthrie T, et al. Lung transplantation and donation after cardiac death: a single center experience. Ann Thorac Surg 2009;88: 1609–14 [discussion: 1614–5].

35. Mason DP, Murthy SC, Gonzalez-Stawinski GV, et al. Early experience with lung transplantation using donors after cardiac death. J Heart Lung Transplant 2008;27:561–3.

36. Mason DP, Thuita L, Alster JM, et al. Should lung transplantation be performed using donation after cardiac death? The United States experience. J Thorac Cardiovasc Surg 2008;136:1061–6.

37. Snell GI, Levvey BJ, Oto T, et al. Early lung transplantation success utilizing controlled donation after cardiac death donors. Am J Transplant 2008;8: 1282–9.

38. Erasmus ME, Verschuuren EA, Nijkamp DM, et al. Lung transplantation from nonheparinized category III non-heart-beating donors. A single-centre report. Transplantation 2010;89:452–7.

39. Fischer S, Matte-Martyn A, De Perrot M, et al. Low-potassium dextran preservation solution improves lung function after human lung transplantation. J Thorac Cardiovasc Surg 2001;121:594–6.

40. Shemie SD, Baker AJ, Knoll G, et al. National recommendations for donation after cardiocirculatory death in Canada: Donation after cardiocirculatory death in Canada. CMAJ 2006;175:S1.

41. Hopkinson DN, Bhabra MS, Hooper TL. Pulmonary graft preservation: a worldwide survey of current clinical practi. J Heart Lung Transplant 1998;17:525–31.

42. Southard JH, Belzer FO. Organ preservation. Annu Rev Med 1995;46:235.

43. Muller C, Hoffmann H, Bittmann I, et al. Hypothermic storage alone in lung preservation for transplantation: a metabolic, light microscopic, and functional analysis after 18 hours of preservation. Transplantation 1997;63:625–30.

44. Pegg DE. Organ preservation. Surg Clin North Am 1986;66:617.

45. Brasile L, Stubenitsky BM, Kootstra G. Solving the organ shortage: potential strategies and the likelihood of success. ASAIO J 2002;48:211–5.

46. Brasile L, Stubenitsky BM, Booster MH, et al. Overcoming severe renal ischemia: the role of ex vivo warm perfusion. Transplantation 2002;73:897–901.

47. Brasile L, Buelow R, Stubenitsky BM, et al. Induction of heme oxygenase-1 in kidneys during ex vivo warm perfusion. Transplantation 2003;76:1145–9.

48. Brasile L, Stubenitsky BM, Booster MH, et al. The underlying mechanism preserving vascular integrity and during ex vivo warm kidney perfusion. Am J Transplant 2003;3:647–9.

49. Brasile L, Stubenitsky BM, Haisch CE, et al. Repair of damaged organs in vitro. Am J Transplant 2005; 5:300–6.

50. Imber CJ, St Peter SD, Lopez de Cenarruzabeitia I, et al. Advantages of normothermic perfusion over cold storage in liver preservation. Transplantation 2002;73:701–9.

51. Carrel A, Lindbergh CA. The culture of whole organs. Science 1935;81:621–3.

52. Wang LS, Yoshikawa K, Miyoshi S, et al. The effect of ischemic time and temperature on lung preservation in a simple ex vivo rabbit model used for functional assessment. J Thorac Cardiovasc Surg 1989;98: 333–42.

53. Wisser W, Oturanlar D, Minich R, et al. Closed circuit perfusion of an isolated rabbit lung. A new model for the evaluation of preservation quality of stored lungs. Eur J Cardiothorac Surg 1993;7:71–4.

54. Trejo H, Urich D, Pezzulo A, et al. Effect of using several levels of positive end-expiratory pressure over barotrauma's induced lung injury in a model of isolated and perfused rabbit lungs. Invest Clin 2006;47:49–64.

55. Broccard AF, Vannay C, Feihl F, et al. Impact of low pulmonary vascular pressure on ventilator-induced lung injury. Crit Care Med 2002;30:2183–90.

56. Petak F, Habre W, Hantos Z, et al. Effects of pulmonary vascular pressures and flow on airway and parenchymal mechanics in isolated rat lungs. J Appl Physiol 2002;92:169–78.

57. Hardesty RL, Griffith BP. Autoperfusion of the heart and lungs for preservation during distant procurement. J Thorac Cardiovasc Surg 1987;93:11–8.

58. Brandes H, Albes JM, Conzelmann A, et al. Comparison of pulsatile and nonpulsatile perfusion of the lung in an extracorporeal large animal model. Eur Surg Res 2002;34:321–9.

59. Steen S, Liao Q, Wierup PN, et al. Transplantation of lungs from non-heart-beating donors after functional assessment ex vivo. Ann Thorac Surg 2003; 76:244–52.

60. Aitchinson JD, Orr HE, Flecknell PA, et al. Functional assessment of non-heart-beating donor lungs: prediction of post-transplant function. Eur J Cardiothorac Surg 2001;20:187–94.

61. Rega FR, Vanaudenaerde BM, Wuyts WA, et al. IL-1beta in bronchial lavage fluid is a non-invasive marker that predicts the viability of the pulmonary graft from the non-heart-beating donor. J Heart Lung Transplant 2003;24:20–8.

62. Rega FR, Jannis NC, Verleden GM, et al. Long-term preservation with interim evaluation of lungs from a non-heart-beating donor after a warm ischemic interval of 90 minutes. Ann Surg 2003; 238:782–92.

63. Egan TM, Haitchcock JA, Nicotra WA, et al. Ex vivo evaluation of human lungs for transplant suitability. Ann Thorac Surg 2006;81:1205–13.

64. Snell GI, Oto T, Levvey B, et al. Evaluation of techniques for lung transplantation following donation after cardiac death. Ann Thorac Surg 2006;81: 2014–9.

65. Wierup P, Haraldsson A, Nilsson F, et al. Ex vivo evaluation of nonacceptable donor lungs. Ann Thorac Surg 2006;81:460–6.

66. Erasmus ME, Fernhout MH, Elstrodt JM, et al. Normothermic ex vivo lung perfusion of non-heart-beating donor lungs in pigs: from pretransplant function analysis towards a 6-h machine preservation. Transpl Int 2006;19:589–93.

67. Cypel M, Yeung JC, Hirayama S, et al. Technique for prolonged normothermic ex vivo lung perfusion. J Heart Lung Transplant 2008;27:1319–25.

68. Cypel M, Rubacha M, Yeung J, et al. Normothermic ex vivo perfusion prevents lung injury compared to extended cold preservation for transplantation. Am J Transplant 2009;9:2262–9.

69. Sakuma T, Gu X, Wang Z, et al. Stimulation of alveolar epithelial fluid clearance in human lungs by exogenous epinephrine. Crit Care Med 2006;34: 676–81.

70. Frank JA, Briot R, Lee JW, et al. Physiological and biochemical markers of alveolar epithelial barrier dysfunction in perfused human lungs. Am J Physiol Lung Cell Mol Physiol 2007;293:L52–9.

71. Ware LB, Wang Y, Fang X, et al. Assessment of lungs rejected for transplantation and implications for donor selection. Lancet 2002;360:619–20.

72. Inci I, Zhai W, Arni S, et al. Fibrinolytic treatment improves the quality of lungs retrieved from non-heart-beating donors. J Heart Lung Transplant 2007;26:1054–60.

73. Inci I, Ampollini L, Arni S, et al. Ex vivo reconditioning of marginal donor lungs injured by acid aspiration. J Heart Lung Transplant 2008;27:1229–36.

74. Karamanou DM, Perry J, Walden HR, et al. The effect of ex-vivo perfusion on the microbiological profile of the donor lung. J Heart Lung Transplant 2010;29(Suppl 2):S88.

75. Ritter T, Kupiec-Weglinski JW. Gene therapy for the prevention of ischemia/reperfusion injury in organ transplantation. Curr Gene Ther 2005;5(1):101–9.

76. Cassivi SD, Cardella JA, Fischer S, et al. Transtracheal gene transfection of donor lungs prior to organ procurement increases transgene levels at reperfusion and following transplantation. J Heart Lung Transplant 1999;18:1181–8.

77. Chapelier A, Danel C, Mazmanian M, et al. Gene therapy in lung transplantation: feasibility of ex vivo adenovirus-mediated gene transfer to the graft. Hum Gene Ther 1996;7:1837–45.

78. Pellegrini C, O'Brien T, Jeppsson A, et al. Influence of temperature on adenovirus-mediated gene transfer. Eur J Cardiothorac Surg 1998;13: 599–603.

79. Ingemansson R, Eyjolfsson A, Mared L, et al. Clinical transplantation of initially rejected donor lungs after reconditioning ex vivo. Ann Thorac Surg 2009;87: 255–60.

80. Lindstedt S, Hlebowicz J, Koul B, et al. Comparative outcome of double lung transplantation using conventional donor lungs and non-acceptable donor lungs reconditioned ex vivo. Interact Cardiovasc Thorac Surg 2011;12(2):162–5.

81. Cypel M, Yeung JC, de Perrot M, et al. Ex vivo lung perfusion in clinical lung transplantation—the "Help" trial. J Heart Lung Transplant 2010;29:s88.

Extracorporeal Life Support as a Bridge to Lung Transplantation

Marcelo Cypel, MD, MSc[a],
Shaf Keshavjee, MD, MSc, FRCSC[b],*

KEYWORDS

- Bridge to lung transplantation • Extracorporeal life support
- Extracorporeal membrane oxygenation

HISTORICAL PERSPECTIVES

Lung transplantation (LTx) is effective life-saving therapy for patients with end-stage lung disease.[1] However, patients who are otherwise excellent candidates for LTx often die on the waiting list because they are too sick to survive until an organ becomes available. Currently, these patients are supported by maximal mechanical ventilation in the intensive care unit, but this can further aggravate the lung injury[2] and often leads to remote organ dysfunction with subsequent high mortality before or after LTx.[3] For many of these patients, refractory hypercapnia or hypoxemia will develop despite maximal ventilatory support and therefore extracorporeal life support (ECLS) is their only chance to survive until a compatible donor lung becomes available. Initial attempts at using ECLS as a bridge to LTx were hindered by a high rate of complications and poor outcomes.[4] In fact, the initial attempts of lung transplantation were frequently performed in patients on ECLS. In 1975, the first case of extracorporeal membrane oxygenation (ECMO) as a bridge to lung transplantation was performed for posttraumatic respiratory failure. The patient was successfully weaned from ECMO after the transplant; however, he died 10 days after the transplant from a combination of sepsis, bronchial anastomotic leak, and size mismatch. Subsequently, in 1982 in Toronto, a further

case of ECMO as a bridge to lung transplant was attempted in a patient with severe paraquat poisoning, but the patient died 92 days after the procedure with a tracheal-innominate artery fistula.[5] Many centers came to view ECMO, and mechanical ventilation, as contraindications to lung transplantation as it was thought that both compromised bronchial healing, the Achilles heel of transplantation in the early days.[4] In addition, the use of adult ECMO for acute respiratory failure (ARF) significantly declined after a negative National Institutes of Health randomized trial in which survival after veno-arterial ECMO was only 10% in patients with severe ARF.[6] This combination of factors resulted in the concept of using ECMO as a bridge to lung transplant being largely discouraged. However, in the last decade, improvements in lung transplant outcomes and patient selection, a better understanding of ventilator-associated lung injury, and improvements in artificial lung device technologies have made it possible to bridge these sick patients to successful LTx.[7–11] In addition, recent studies have shown more promising results using ECLS for adults with ARF with survival rates ranging from 50% to 80%. This finding includes the experience from Michigan in 100 subjects,[12] the conventional ventilation or ECMO for severe adult respiratory failure trial,[13] and H1N1/Acute Respiratory Distress Syndrome (ARDS) reports.[14,15] The

[a] Division Thoracic Surgery, Toronto Lung Transplant Program, Toronto General Hospital, University of Toronto, 200 Elizabeth Street, 9n969, M5G2C4, Canada
[b] Toronto Lung Transplant Program, Latner Thoracic Research Laboratories, Division of Thoracic Surgery, Institute of Biomaterials and Biomedical Engineering, University of Toronto, 190 Elizabeth Street, RFE 1-408, Toronto, M5G 2C4, Canada
* Corresponding author.
E-mail address: shaf.keshavjee@uhn.on.ca

Clin Chest Med 32 (2011) 245–251
doi:10.1016/j.ccm.2011.02.005
0272-5231/11/$ – see front matter © 2011 Elsevier Inc. All rights reserved.

primary scope of this article is to review the indications, modes of application, and outcomes of ECLS when used as a bridge to LTx.

INDICATIONS

The main indications for ECLS as a bridge to LTx include patients with irreversible end-stage lung diseases presenting with rapid deterioration of respiratory status as reflected by refractory hypercapnic or hypoxemic respiratory failure (usually PCO_2 >80 mm Hg and PaO2/FIO2 <80 mm Hg). Another indication for ECLS in the pretransplant setting is in patients with severe pulmonary hypertension and hemodynamic collapse caused by severe dysfunction of the right ventricle.[10,16] Given the level of resource use and the scarcity of donor organs, careful patient selection is clearly needed. No specific criteria for this group of patients can yet be suggested because of the small number of reported cases, but in general, young age, absence of multiple-organ dysfunction, and good prospects for rehabilitation should be considered. Usually, these patients have already been assessed by the LTx team and listed for LTx; however, in exceptional instances, urgent assessments and listing can be performed. With increased experience, there is also a trend toward implementing ECLS earlier in the course of the respiratory failure to avoid the need for prolonged high-pressure mechanical ventilation leading to secondary organ dysfunction.[2,3] Furthermore, recent reports have shown the feasibility of ECLS as bridge to LTx in awake and nonintubated patients allowing them to ambulate and potentially be in better physical condition by the time of the transplant.[8,17]

CONTRAINDICATIONS

Contraindications for the use of ECLS in general include septic shock, multi-organ dysfunction, severe arterial occlusive disease, and heparin-induced thrombocytopenia type II. Unfavorable prognostic factors include acute renal failure, high vasopressor requirements, a long preceding duration of mechanical ventilation, advanced age, and obesity.[18]

COMPONENTS OF ECLS SYSTEMS AND TECHNOLOGICAL ADVANCES

The main components of the ECLS system include a membrane oxygenator, a pump, and tubing circuits (**Fig. 1**). In the last decade, several important advancements in technology have contributed to improved management and overall outcomes of these patients, as detailed later.

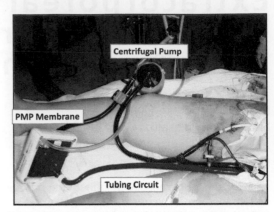

Fig. 1. Main components of a modern ECLS circuit.

Development of Polymethylpentene Membranes

In the past, most adult ECMO circuits used silicone membrane oxygenators and the remainder used polypropylene microporous oxygenators. Both these oxygenators had drawbacks. The introduction of polymethylpentene (PMP) membranes provided several technical advantages. Compared with silicone membrane oxygenators, the PMP oxygenator has reduced red blood cell and platelet transfusion requirements, significantly less plasma leakage, better gas exchange, lower resistance, and lower priming volume.[19,20] Compared with polypropylene microporous oxygenators, the PMP oxygenator has a reduced rate of oxygenator failure and can be functional for several weeks.[7] The PMP fibers are woven into a complex configuration of hollow fibers through which the oxygenated gas passes. The hollow fibers themselves are then arranged into mats and stacked into a configuration that allows blood to pass between the fibers with low resistance, which provides maximum blood/gas mixing and gas transfer can take place without direct contact with blood.

Introduction of Heparin-coated Circuits

Heparin-coated circuits led to reduced rates of platelet, complement, and granulocyte activation[8] and also significantly reduced heparin requirements.[21,22] Importantly, PMP oxygenators can also be readily heparin coated; whereas, the silicone membrane oxygenators cannot. Thus, the modern ECMO circuit can be entirely heparin coated and requires less systemic heparinization. In contrast, early ECMO circuits required full heparinization and consequently bleeding complications and daily blood product requirement were high.

Development of a New Generation of Centrifugal Pumps

Compared with traditional roller pumps, the centrifugal pumps have an improved performance and safety profile. They have virtually no risk of tubing rupture, require a smaller priming volume, do not require the use of a reservoir, and in general have a decreased incidence of hemolysis.[23,24]

MODES OF ECLS: CONFIGURATION OF DEVICE

In addition to the technical advances, device configuration can be individualized and tailored for specific patient ventilatory and hemodynamic requirements. The configuration and mode of ECLS will depend on the specific clinical scenario.

Hypercapnic Respiratory Failure

Refractory hypercapnic respiratory failure and acidosis is a common scenario in patients with cystic fibrosis (CF) waiting for lung transplantation. Noninvasive ventilation has become an important option as a treatment modality in ARF in CF, avoiding endotracheal intubation with its attendant complications.[25] If a suitable organ does not become available in time, respiratory failure progresses and mechanical ventilation becomes necessary. At that stage, management becomes increasingly difficult as high-pressure ventilation is required and alveolar hypoventilation and hypercapnia often persists despite it. Traditionally, patients with hypercapnia and respiratory acidosis required ECMO with the use of a pump. However, with the advent of an interventional lung assist device (iLA; Novalung, Heilbronn, Germany), the Hannover group demonstrated the feasibility of bridging these patients with the iLA in a *pumpless* arterio-venous (A-V) mode (**Fig. 2**).[7] This low-resistance (11mm Hg) PMP device is attached to the systemic circulation (usually femoral artery) and receives only part of the cardiac output (15% to 20% of cardiac output) for extracorporeal gas exchange, which allows prompt CO_2 removal and correction of respiratory acidosis. Varying the sweep of gas flow up to 15 L/min can control CO2 removal rates. The usual recommended rate of CO_2 clearance is 20 mm Hg/h. In order to use the pumpless device, patients must have an adequate mean arterial blood pressure to be able to sustain good flows through the device. Because only one-fifth of cardiac output is oxygenated in the membrane, PaO_2 is only augmented minimally with this mode of ECLS[7]; therefore, A-V iLA is not recommended in patients with severe hypoxia (PaO_2/FiO_2 <80 mm Hg). Cannulation is usually

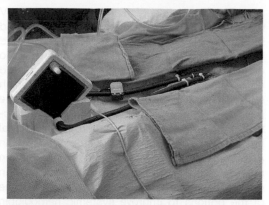

Fig. 2. Pumpless arterio-venous ECLS support. A low-resistance PMP device is attached to the systemic circulation (usually femoral artery) and receives part of the cardiac output (15%–20% of CO) for extracorporeal gas exchange. This procedure allows prompt CO_2 removal and correction of respiratory acidosis.

achieved percutaneously using a Seldinger technique in the femoral artery (13–15 Fr) and femoral vein (17 Fr). Because a centrifugal pump is not required, anticoagulation times (ACT) in the range of 150 to 180 seconds are acceptable.

Hypoxemic Respiratory Failure

Although CO_2 removal can be achieved with low membrane flows (0.5–1.0 L/min),[26] substantial oxygenation requires more physiologic flows through the membrane (3–5 L/min). In order to achieve that, veno-venous (V-V) or veno-arterial (V-A) pump-driven ECLS support is required. V-V mode is the preferred choice if patients are hypoxemic but hemodynamically stable. The advantages of the V-V mode in comparison to V-A mode are the decreased rate of complications, such as bleeding, arterial thrombosis, and neurologic complications. Generally, a 22-Fr cannula is inserted into a femoral vein for drainage and a 17-F single-stage cannula is inserted into an internal jugular vein percutaneously for patient inflow. More recently, a dual-lumen, single-cannula system has been developed for V-V ECLS that has the advantage of simplicity, and importantly, allows for patient mobilization.[17] Using this cannula, the inflow to the ECLS circuit occurs from the tip of the cannula, which is located in the inferior vena cava, and from fenestrations in the proximal part of the cannula located at the superior vena cava-right atrial junction. The outflow from ECLS (oxygenated blood) is located at the midpoint between these 2 intake points and is directed medially toward the tricuspid valve. Visualization with fluoroscopy or transesophageal echocardiography is recommended to facilitate accurate cannula insertion and positioning. In V-V mode, infused ECLS membrane oxygenated blood mixes with systemic venous return blood in the right atrium. At typical blood flow, the ratio of infused oxygenated blood to deoxygenated right atrial blood is usually around 3:1, which results in a hemoglobin saturation of 80% in the pulmonary artery. If there is no native lung function, this will be the oxygenation in the arterial blood. Although this can often be the case in ARDS, lungs from end-stage lung failure are often able to provide some degree of oxygenation contributing with better systemic saturation. One of the options to improve systemic hemoglobin saturation is to increase the pump flows, so that more blood flow bypasses the native lung. In all instances, hematocrit should be kept greater than 40% and cardiac function optimized to provide adequate systemic oxygen delivery. Usual ACTs should range from 160 to 200 seconds.

Hypoxemic Respiratory Failure and Hemodynamic Compromise

For patients with respiratory failure and hemodynamic compromise, V-A ECLS is the recommended option because it provides both cardiac and lung support. In fact, the initial experience with ECLS in LTx employed this mode.[5] Usually a femoral vein is cannulated for drainage and a femoral artery cannulated for blood return. Some investigators also propose the use of the axillary artery with an interposition graft.[27,28] Advantages of the axillary artery in this setting are the possibility of better patient mobilization and the low incidence of atherosclerosis in this vessel. Improved upper-body oxygenated perfusion is also an important advantage. During V-A femoral ECLS, fully saturated blood infused into the circulation from the ECLS circuit will preferentially perfuse the lower extremities and the abdominal viscera. Blood ejected from the heart will selectively perfuse the heart, brain, and upper extremities. As a result, the oxygen saturation of the blood perfusing the lower extremities and abdominal viscera may be substantially higher than that perfusing the upper body. Cardiac and cerebral hypoxia could exist and be unrecognized if oxygenation is monitored using blood from the lower extremity. Poor arterial saturations measured from the upper extremity should prompt adjustments to the mechanical ventilator to optimize pulmonary oxygenation or augmentation of blood flow through the ECLS circuit. Another option to improve central oxygenation is to insert another cannula into internal jugular vein and convert the circuit to a hybrid V (femoral vein)-VA

(jugular vein and femoral artery) ECLS. Conversely, V-VA ECMO can also be used to provide partial cardiac support when cardiac function is depressed and does not improve with improved oxygenation on V-V support alone.[29,30]

A recent report demonstrated the application of V-A ECLS in awake and spontaneously breathing subjects, avoiding the drawbacks and complications associated with intubation and prolonged mechanical ventilation. 4 out of 5 subjects were successfully bridged to LTx.[8]

Pulmonary Hypertension and Right Ventricular Failure

A novel mode of ECLS is the recently described pulmonary artery to left atrium (PA–LA) ECLS.[10,31] Although progress has been made for isolated lung failure, no truly effective solution existed for patients with severe pulmonary arterial hypertension (PAH). Compared with patients with lung failure caused by isolated lung parenchymal disorders, patients with end-stage PAH develop severe right heart failure. V-A or V-V ECLS does not effectively unload the right ventricle. An atrial septostomy is sometimes performed in the setting of severe right ventricular dysfunction; however, this leads to desaturated blood being systemically ejected as a result of the iatrogenic right to left shunt. Alternatively, the authors have demonstrated that the connection of a low-resistance gas exchange device (Novalung; Novalung, Heilbronn, Germany) between the main trunk of the pulmonary artery and the left atrium in a pumpless mode creates an effective *oxygenating* shunt that unloads the right ventricle much like an atrial septostomy (**Fig. 3**). The advantage, in this case, is that the membrane oxygenates the blood and thus the central hypoxemia seen with a simple septostomy is avoided. In the authors' experience, patients improve dramatically as soon as flow across the Novalung is instituted.[10] The elevated pressure in the pulmonary arteries serves as the driving force for the device and obviates the need for a pump. From a technical standpoint, patients are usually so severely unstable such that they usually require femoral-femoral V-A ECLS support just before anesthetic induction. This procedure is followed by median sternotomy and cannulation of the PA (Medtronic arterial cannula 21-24 Fr; Medtronic, Minneapolis, MN, USA). The LA is cannulated by inserting a 17-23 Fr Pacifico cannula (Bard Inc, Salt Lake City, UT, USA) into the right superior pulmonary vein. Extubation, physiotherapy, and ambulation are achievable while patients are on pumpless PA-LA ECLS awaiting a compatible donor lung. Eight

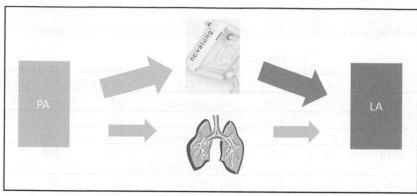

Fig. 3. Pumpless pulmonary artery to left atrium ECLS support for patients with pulmonary hypertension. An oxygenating shunt is created providing both right-ventricle decompression and oxygenation.

successful cases have been reported using this technique to bridge patients with PAH to LTx.[10,11,31] Of note, in most cases, heart-lung transplantation is not required because the unloaded right ventricle recovers on the Novalung and bilateral LTx provides ongoing remodeling and recovery of the right heart.[10]

PATIENT MANAGEMENT

Once ECLS is initiated, the ventilator should ideally be adjusted to resting lung settings with FiO_2 less than 0.6, end inspiratory pressure less than 35, PEEP 10 to 15, rate of 6/min. The ECLS flow should be maintained to sustain a venous blood saturation of 80% to 85% and an arterial saturation of 80% to 95%. Diuretics are given if required to maintain adequate urine output and remove excess fluid to maintain patients at dry weight (pre-illness weight). If negative fluid balance cannot be achieved with diuretics, hemofiltration should be initiated early. Neurologic status is frequently checked and any deterioration should prompt a head computed tomography scan. Cannulation sites and limb perfusion status are also frequently checked for bleeding and distal perfusion, respectively. Routine antibiotics and antifungal coverage should be given.

The general target guidelines used by the Toronto General Hospital ECLS/Lung Transplant Program are shown in **Table 1**.

OUTCOMES

The outcomes of patients bridged to LTx using mechanical support has been improving and is satisfactory considering the severity of their diseases and the overall survival of LTx recipients. A recent review from the UNOS experience totaling 51 subjects bridged to LTx from 1987 to 2008 using ECLS showed a 1-, 6-, 12-, and 24-month survival of 72%, 53%, 50%, and 45%, respectively compared with 93%, 85%, 79%, and 70% for unsupported patients, respectively.[32] Most recent reports from centers experienced in both LTx and ECLS have shown that 80% or more of patients can be successfully bridged to LTx and outcomes after LTx in these selected patients can approach that of conventional lung transplants.[7,8,10,11,33–36] These results demonstrate that outcomes in this patient population are better than the results of ECLS use to bridge patients to recovery from severe primary graft dysfunction after LTx,[18] although improved results have also been recently obtained in this latter group.[37,38] **Table 2** demonstrates reported case series of use of ECLS as a bridge to transplantation in which more than 4 subjects were included.[7,8,10,11,33–36]

Table 1	
Target guidelines for patients on ECLS	
Temperature	35.5°C–37.0°C
pH	7.35–7.45
pCO$_2$	35–45 mm Hg
pO$_2$	>100 mm Hg
Hemoglobin saturation	>85%
Hemoglobin	80–100 g/L
INR	<1.8 <1.5 if bleeding
Platelets	>80,000/mm^3 >100,000/mm^3 if bleeding
Fibrinogen	>1.5–4.0 g/L
Factor X concentration	0.4–0.6 u/mL
Anticoagulation time	160–200 sec
Pump flow	Aim 60 mL/kg/min

Abbreviation: INR, international normalized ratio.

Table 2
Experience with ECLS as a bridge to lung transplant (series with more than 4 cases)

Author	Number of Cases	Days on Device (Mean)	Mode ECLS	Bridged to LTx (%)	30-d Survival After LTx (%)	1-y Survival (%)
Fischer et al,[7] 2006	12	15.0	A-V pumpless	83	80	80
Olsson et al,[8] 2010	5	21.0	V-A	80	100	NA
Strueber et al,[10] 2009	4	17.0	PA-LA pumpless	100	100	75
Cypel et al,[11] 2010	12	7.0	V-A (3), V-V (1), A-V (4), PA-LA (4)	100	100	83
Yun et al,[33] 2010	7	7.0	V-V (5) V-A (2)	86	83	NA
Ricci et al,[34] 2010	12	13.5	A-V pumpless	25	NA	NA
Nosotti et al,[35] 2010	4	9.0	V-V	100	75	NA
Hämmäinen et al,[36] 2010	16	17.0	V-V (7) V-A (6)	81	100	92

Abbreviation: NA, not available.

COMPLICATIONS

The most common complications during ECLS include hemorrhage, complications at the cannulation site, renal failure, neurologic complications, and sepsis.[18] In an experience with 100 ECLS for ARF, cannula site and surgical site bleeding were the most common complications followed by arrhythmias and renal failure. In this series, 6 subjects died of gastrointestinal bleeding and 10 subjects developed irreversible brain damage caused by infarct or hemorrhage.[12] Patients on V-A ECLS have significantly higher rates of complications (especially neurologic complications and sepsis) when compared with V-V.[37]

SUMMARY

Although experience is still limited, ECLS clearly can be an effective tool to bridge patients to a life-saving lung transplant. Technological advances have permitted safer, less complicated application of ECLS for longer periods of time. Support can be tailored to minimize morbidity and provide the appropriate mode and level of cardiopulmonary support for each specific patient's physiologic requirements. Novel device refinements and further development of ECLS in an ambulatory and simplified manner will help to maintain these patients in better condition until transplantation. Further experience is required to ultimately define the optimal timing and criteria for initiation of ECLS in patients requiring bridging to lung transplantation.

REFERENCES

1. Christie JD, Edwards LB, Aurora P, et al. The Registry of the International Society for Heart and Lung Transplantation: Twenty-sixth Official Adult Lung and Heart-Lung Transplantation Report-2009. J Heart Lung Transplant 2009;28:1031–49.
2. Slutsky AS, Imai Y. Ventilator-induced lung injury, cytokines, PEEP, and mortality: implications for practice and for clinical trials. Intensive Care Med 2003; 29:1218–21.
3. Imai Y, Parodo J, Kajikawa O, et al. Injurious mechanical ventilation and end-organ epithelial cell apoptosis and organ dysfunction in an experimental model of acute respiratory distress syndrome. JAMA 2003;289:2104–12.
4. Jurmann MJ, Haverich A, Demertzis S, et al. Extracorporeal membrane oxygenation as a bridge to lung transplantation. Eur J Cardiothorac Surg 1991; 5:94–7 [discussion: 8].
5. Sequential bilateral lung transplantation for paraquat poisoning. A case report. The Toronto Lung Transplant group. J Thorac Cardiovasc Surg 1985;89:734–42.
6. Zapol WM, Snider MT, Hill JD, et al. Extracorporeal membrane oxygenation in severe acute respiratory failure. A randomized prospective study. JAMA 1979; 242:2193–6.
7. Fischer S, Simon AR, Welte T, et al. Bridge to lung transplantation with the novel pumpless interventional lung assist device NovaLung. J Thorac Cardiovasc Surg 2006;131:719–23.
8. Olsson KM, Simon A, Strueber M, et al. Extracorporeal membrane oxygenation in nonintubated patients as bridge to lung transplantation. Am J Transplant 2010;10:2173–8.
9. Aigner C, Wisser W, Taghavi S, et al. Institutional experience with extracorporeal membrane oxygenation in lung transplantation. Eur J Cardiothorac Surg 2007;31:468–73 [discussion: 73–4].
10. Strueber M, Hoeper MM, Fischer S, et al. Bridge to thoracic organ transplantation in patients with pulmonary arterial hypertension using a pumpless

lung assist device. Am J Transplant 2009;9:853–7.

11. Cypel M, Waddell TK, de Perrot M, et al. Safety and efficacy of the Novalung Interventional Lung Assist (iLA) Device as a bridge to lung transplantation. J Heart Lung Transplant 2010;29(Suppl 2):S88.

12. Kolla S, Awad SS, Rich PB, et al. Extracorporeal life support for 100 adult patients with severe respiratory failure. Ann Surg 1997;226:544–64 [discussion: 65–6].

13. Peek GJ, Mugford M, Tiruvoipati R, et al. Efficacy and economic assessment of conventional ventilatory support versus extracorporeal membrane oxygenation for severe adult respiratory failure (CESAR): a multicentre randomised controlled trial. Lancet 2009;374:1351–63.

14. Freed DH, Henzler D, White CW, et al. Extracorporeal lung support for patients who had severe respiratory failure secondary to influenza A (H1N1) 2009 infection in Canada. Can J Anaesth 2010;57:240–7.

15. Davies A, Jones D, Bailey M, et al. Extracorporeal membrane oxygenation for 2009 Influenza A (H1N1) Acute Respiratory Distress Syndrome. JAMA 2009;302:1888–95.

16. Puehler T, Philipp A, Schmid C. Paracorporeal artificial lung circuit as a possibility for bridge to lung transplantation. Ann Thorac Surg 2009;88:352 [author reply: 3].

17. Garcia JP, Iacono A, Kon ZN, et al. Ambulatory extracorporeal membrane oxygenation: a new approach for bridge-to-lung transplantation. J Thorac Cardiovasc Surg 2010;139:e137–9.

18. Fischer S, Bohn D, Rycus P, et al. Extracorporeal membrane oxygenation for primary graft dysfunction after lung transplantation: analysis of the Extracorporeal Life Support Organization (ELSO) registry. J Heart Lung Transplant 2007;26:472–7.

19. Peek GJ, Killer HM, Reeves R, et al. Early experience with a polymethyl pentene oxygenator for adult extracorporeal life support. ASAIO J 2002;48:480–2.

20. Khoshbin E, Roberts N, Harvey C, et al. Poly-methyl pentene oxygenators have improved gas exchange capability and reduced transfusion requirements in adult extracorporeal membrane oxygenation. ASAIO J 2005;51:281–7.

21. Tamim M, Demircin M, Guvener M, et al. Heparin-coated circuits reduce complement activation and inflammatory response to cardiopulmonary bypass. Panminerva Med 1999;41:193–8.

22. Moen O, Fosse E, Dregelid E, et al. Centrifugal pump and heparin coating improves cardiopulmonary bypass biocompatibility. Ann Thorac Surg 1996;62:1134–40.

23. Lawson DS, Ing R, Cheifetz IM, et al. Hemolytic characteristics of three commercially available centrifugal blood pumps. Pediatr Crit Care Med 2005;6:573–7.

24. Valeri CR, MacGregor H, Ragno G, et al. Effects of centrifugal and roller pumps on survival of autologous red cells in cardiopulmonary bypass surgery. Perfusion 2006;21:291–6.

25. Noone PG. Non-invasive ventilation for the treatment of hypercapnic respiratory failure in cystic fibrosis. Thorax 2008;63:5–7.

26. Zwischenberger BA, Clemson LA, Zwischenberger JB. Artificial lung: progress and prototypes. Expert Rev Med Devices 2006;3:485–97.

27. Iglesias M, Jungebluth P, Sibila O, et al. Experimental safety and efficacy evaluation of an extracorporeal pumpless artificial lung in providing respiratory support through the axillary vessels. J Thorac Cardiovasc Surg 2007;133:339–45.

28. Yokota K, Fujii T, Kimura K, et al. Life-threatening hypoxemic respiratory failure after repair of acute type a aortic dissection: successful treatment with venoarterial extracorporeal life support using a prosthetic graft attached to the right axillary artery. Anesth Analg 2001;92:872–6.

29. Chou NK, Chen YS, Ko WJ, et al. Application of extracorporeal membrane oxygenation in adult burn patients. Artif Organs 2001;25:622–6.

30. Madershahian N, Wittwer T, Strauch J, et al. Application of ECMO in multitrauma patients with ARDS as rescue therapy. J Card Surg 2007;22:180–4.

31. Camboni D, Philipp A, Arlt M, et al. First experience with a paracorporeal artificial lung in humans. ASAIO J 2009;55:304–6.

32. Mason DP, Thuita L, Nowicki ER, et al. Should lung transplantation be performed for patients on mechanical respiratory support? The US experience. J Thorac Cardiovasc Surg 2010;139:765–73, e1.

33. Yun JJ, Mangi AA, Benjamin LC, et al. ECMO as a bridge to lung transplantation: the Cleveland Clinic Experience. J Heart Lung Transplant 2010;29(Suppl 2):S31.

34. Ricci D, Boffini M, Del Sorbo L, et al. The use of CO2 removal devices in patients awaiting lung transplantation: an initial experience. Transplant Proc 2010;42:1255–8.

35. Nosotti M, Rosso L, Palleschi A, et al. Bridge to lung transplantation by venovenous extracorporeal membrane oxygenation: a lesson learned on the first four cases. Transplant Proc 2010;42:1259–61.

36. Hammainen P, Schersten H, Lemstrom K, et al. Usefulness of extracorporeal membrane oxygenation as a bridge to lung transplantation: a descriptive study. J Heart Lung Transplant 2011;30:103–7.

37. Hartwig MG, Appel JZ 3rd, Cantu E 3rd, et al. Improved results treating lung allograft failure with venovenous extracorporeal membrane oxygenation. Ann Thorac Surg 2005;80:1872–9 [discussion: 9–80].

38. Bermudez CA, Adusumilli PS, McCurry KR, et al. Extracorporeal membrane oxygenation for primary graft dysfunction after lung transplantation: long-term survival. Ann Thorac Surg 2009;87:854–60.

Survival and Quality of Life of Patients Undergoing Lung Transplant

Roger D. Yusen, MD, MPH

KEYWORDS

- Outcomes assessment (health care) • Lung transplant
- Survival analysis • Quality of life

Patients who have an advanced lung disease typically remain significantly symptomatic despite medical therapy, and they have a disturbingly high mortality rate. Such patients often desperately seek improved quality of life, and many would trade length of life for quality of life. Lung transplant offers hope for prolonged survival and improved quality of life. Unfortunately, the medical literature provides conflicting information regarding the effects of lung transplant on survival,[1,2] and it contains limited and often biased information regarding the effects of lung transplant on quality of life.[3,4]

Lung transplant registries primarily use descriptive analyses of survival on the waiting list[5,6] and after[5–7] transplant as the primary assessments of patient outcomes. Sophisticated statistical approaches have enabled analysts to assess the survival effects of lung transplant versus continued waiting.[5,6,8–11]

Although many patients live longer and better because of lung transplant, some die sooner than they would have without transplant, and a significant proportion of lung transplant recipients encounter adverse events and comorbidity.[7] Thus, survival assessment does not provide an adequate sole measure of the overall success or failure of lung transplant.[4] Unfortunately, the major lung transplant entities (eg, organizations that obtain data for registries) do not routinely collect extensive quality of life data.

This article addresses quality of life and survival outcomes associated with lung transplant. In addition to describing published data, the article focuses on pitfalls and challenges in studying patient outcomes in lung transplant.

LUNG TRANSPLANT: SURVIVAL
Descriptive Studies

A published large rigorous randomized controlled trial of lung transplant versus medical therapy does not exist. Registry reports and retrospective cohort studies provide the most evidence regarding the effects of lung transplant on survival.

Lung transplant registry reports typically describe the number and rates of deaths on the waiting list[5,6] and after lung transplant.[5–7] According to data from the Scientific Registry of Transplant Recipients (SRTR), in recent cohorts of recipients of deceased donor lungs in the US United Network for Organ Sharing (UNOS) system, recipients had 1-, 5-, and 10-year unadjusted survival rates of 83%, 54%, and 29%, respectively.[6] Survival rates at 1, 3, and 5 years posttransplant showed subtle improvement over the past 10 years.

According to the most recent publication from the Registry of the International Society for Heart

This work was supported, in part, by National Institutes of Health, National Heart, Lung, and Blood Institute (NIH/NHLBI), RO1 HL083067.

Divisions of Pulmonary and Critical Care Medicine and General Medical Sciences, Washington University School of Medicine, Campus Box 8052, 660 South Euclid Avenue, St Louis, MO 63110, USA

E-mail address: ryusen@dom.wustl.edu

& Lung Transplantation (ISHLT),[7] lung transplant recipients had an overall median survival or half-life of 5.3 years. Those who survived at least 1 year had an average (conditional) survival of 7.5 years after transplant. The Registry described unadjusted survival rates after lung transplant of 79% at 1 year, 63% at 3 years, 52% at 5 years, and 29% at 10 years (**Fig. 1**).

Survival outcomes for lung recipients remain inferior to those achieved after other solid-organ transplant procedures. Heart transplant recipients have survival rates of 88%, 75%, and 56% at 1, 5, and 10 years, respectively. Recipients of deceased donor livers have corresponding survival rates of 88%, 74%, and 60%.[5,6]

In a recent SRTR report of UNOS data, subgroups of patients had different unadjusted survival rates after lung transplant. However, adjustment for additional factors could have significantly affected the results, and UNOS does not collect data regarding all possible factors. For example, different primary lung diagnosis populations demonstrated modest differences in survival, and analyses of these subgroups showed a trend toward better long-term unadjusted survival among patients with cystic fibrosis (CF)-associated lung disease, idiopathic pulmonary arterial hypertension (IPAH), and chronic obstructive pulmonary disease (COPD) associated with alpha1-antitrypsin

deficiency (A1ATD) compared with patients with COPD not associated with A1ATD and idiopathic pulmonary fibrosis (IPF). Compared with most other primary lung diagnostic groups, patients with COPD not associated with A1ATD had relatively good short-term survival and relatively poor long-term survival. Alternatively, patients with IPAH had relatively poor short-term survival and relatively good long-term survival.[5,6]

Age did not have a major effect on 1- and 5-year unadjusted survival rates for adult recipients younger than 65 years, but recipients aged 65 years and older had lower survival rates than younger recipient groups at these time points. At 10 years posttransplant, cohorts of adult recipients younger than 50 years, aged 50 years to younger than 65 years, and aged 65 years and older at the time of transplant had survival rates of 38%, 23%, and 13%, respectively.[5,6]

Patients who underwent single or bilateral lung transplants had the same 1-year unadjusted survival of 83%. By 5 years, however, patients undergoing bilateral transplant had higher unadjusted survival than those undergoing single-lung transplant (57% vs 51%; $P<.001$); this trend became more pronounced at 10 years (37% vs 21%; $P<.001$).[5,6]

Patients in the intensive care unit (ICU) at the time of transplant had a lower unadjusted 1-year

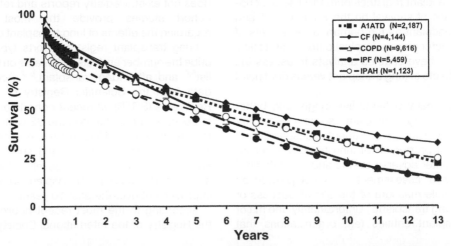

Fig. 1. ISHLT registry data for adult lung transplant survival, stratified by diagnosis, in patients who underwent transplant from January 1990 through June 2008. Although the registry incorporated data from transplant patients from whom they received follow-up information, loss to follow-up and lack of exact death dates affected the Kaplan-Meier survival estimates. A1ATD, alpha1-antitrypsin deficiency associated with chronic obstructive pulmonary disease (COPD); CF, cystic fibrosis (category includes non-CF bronchiectasis); COPD, chronic obstructive pulmonary disease (not associated with A1ATD); IPF, idiopathic pulmonary fibrosis (category includes other interstitial lung diseases); IPAH, idiopathic pulmonary arterial hypertension (category includes other pulmonary vascular diseases). (*Adapted from* Christie JD, Edwards LB, Kucheryavaya AY, et al. The registry of the International Society for Heart and Lung Transplantation: twenty-seventh official adult lung and heart-lung transplant report—2010. J Heart Lung Transplant 2010;29:1111; with permission.)

survival (57%) than hospitalized patients but not in ICU (84%) and nonhospitalized patients (86%). Using the metric of deaths per thousand patient-years at risk, these recipient groups demonstrated trends similar to those described above for the initial posttransplant year. For patients who underwent transplant in 2007, for example, patients in the ICU had a death rate of 699 deaths per thousand patient-years at risk; hospitalized patients but not in ICU, 237 deaths; and nonhospitalized patients, 172 deaths. The survival differential between the ICU and non-ICU groups became far less pronounced at 5 and 10 years after transplant.[5,6]

From the ISHLT report, which incorporates UNOS data and data from other non-US transplant systems, unadjusted analyses showed higher survival rates for bilateral versus single-lung transplant, most recent versus earlier eras, younger versus older recipients, transplant center high procedural (lung transplant) volume versus low volume, and recipients with cytomegalovirus (CMV) seronegative donors versus those with CMV seropositive donors. Patients with a pretransplant diagnosis of interstitial lung disease (ILD) or IPAH had lower early (ie, 3 months) unadjusted posttransplant survival rates compared with those with CF or COPD, whereas patients with ILD and COPD had lower late (ie, 5–10 years) posttransplant survival rates compared with those with other major disease categories.[7]

Similar to the ISHLT data, Thabut and colleagues[12] found an association between higher lung transplant volume and improved long-term survival among US lung transplant centers. However, variability in center performance remained significant after controlling for procedural volume, and this observation suggested that other factors had a significant effect on survival.

The major causes of death after lung transplant have remained constant over the decades. Graft failure and infection caused most early deaths (ie, first 30 days), whereas bronchiolitis obliterans syndrome (BOS) and infection caused most late deaths (ie, after the first year).[5,7]

The available registries typically do not report results from statistical models that assess the overall survival effects of lung transplant.[6,7] Some registries do not collect pretransplant outcomes data as rigorously as posttransplant data, thus preventing adequate estimation of the survival of a waiting-list control group.

Without having data from a randomized controlled trial of transplant versus no transplant, the best estimates of the survival effects of lung transplant come from studies that have used statistical models. However, such studies have limitations that include pretransplant primary diagnostic group misclassification, false model assumptions, and nongeneralizability to other types of organ allocation systems. The following paragraphs describe results of studies that used such models.

Hosenpud and colleagues[8] performed a retrospective cohort study of 1274 patients who were listed for lung transplant in 1992 to 1994 in the era of the previous UNOS time-dependent waiting-list donor lung allocation system. ABO blood type and body size compatibility and geographic distance between the donor and the recipient also affected donor lung allocation. The investigators calculated relative risks (RRs) over a 1-year period. The clearest survival benefit from lung transplant occurred in the group of patients with CF, and patients with IPF (ie, fibrotic lung diseases) experienced a smaller benefit. For patients with COPD, the risk of death after lung transplant always remained greater than that on the waiting list; therefore, the analysis did not support a survival benefit from lung transplant for patients with COPD under the previous UNOS donor lung allocation system.

A later retrospective cohort study by Liou and colleagues[1,13] used data from the US Cystic Fibrosis Foundation Patient Registry and the Organ Procurement and Transplantation Network (OPTN) to identify children with CF who underwent registration on the UNOS (time-dependent) waiting list for lung transplant during the period from 1992 through 2002. A total of 248 of the 514 children registered on the waiting list underwent lung transplant during the same period. Only a very small proportion of the children had an estimated improved survival associated with lung transplant. The controversial findings have undergone rigorous debate, and investigators representing the International Pediatric Lung Transplant Collaborative and other investigators have voiced concerns regarding the study methodology, results, and conclusions.[2]

On May 4, 2005, for adults and adolescents, the UNOS donor lung allocation system changed from one that prioritizes based on waiting time to one that prioritizes based on a lung allocation score (LAS).[14,15] Similar to the Eurotransplant and UK Transplant systems, the current UNOS donor lung allocation system prioritizes patients for lung transplant based on medical urgency. However, rather than using a clinician's perception of a patient's risk of dying on the waiting list, the current UNOS system objectively quantifies this assessment. In addition, the current UNOS system incorporates an objective measurement of expected survival after lung transplant. Thus, the

LAS system now makes some of the data from the pre-LAS UNOS donor lung allocation system obsolete.

To address survival outcomes under the LAS system, OPTN analysts calculated the predicted survival benefit of lung transplant for approximately 3500 adolescents and adults.[16] Using data reported to the OPTN as of March 10, 2008, the analysis included patients on the waiting list on February 22, 2008, and those individuals who had their first lung transplant between May 4, 2005, and November 3, 2007. The analysts used the same statistical models developed by the SRTR to predict waiting-list mortality and post-transplant survival for computation of the LAS. The analyses detected a survival benefit associated with lung transplant in all 4 major LAS diagnostic groups (group A, obstructive lung disease; group B, pulmonary vascular disease; group C, bronchiectasis; and group D, restrictive lung disease) when compared with no transplant (Edwards LB, PhD, Richmond, VA, USA, personal communication, September 2, 2008).

Using data from Eurotransplant, De Meester and colleagues[9] conducted a retrospective cohort study to assess the survival effect of lung transplant. The Eurotransplant system used medical urgency as the primary criterion for donor lung allocation in ABO blood type and size compatible potential recipients. The study evaluated data from adult patients registered for their first lung-only transplant from 1990 through 1996. The study assessed outcomes within the pretransplant diagnostic categories of COPD (n = 395), pulmonary fibrosis (n = 333), CF (n = 181), pulmonary hypertension (n = 130), and congenital heart disease (n = 46). All disease group cohorts, except for the cohort with congenital heart disease, had a lower risk of death with lung transplant than while remaining on the waiting list.

Using data only from Papworth Hospital in the UK Transplant system, Charman and colleagues[10] conducted another similar retrospective cohort study that included patients accepted for lung transplant between 1984 and 1999. Similar to the Eurotransplant system, and unlike the UNOS pre-LAS and LAS systems, the clinicians' subjective assessment of medical urgency helped to determine prioritization for lung transplant. The study categorized patients into pretransplant diagnostic categories of obstructive lung disease (n = 163), pulmonary fibrosis (n = 100), CF (n = 174), bronchiectasis (n = 51), and pulmonary hypertension (n = 68). Similar to the Eurotransplant study, the UK Transplant study showed a survival benefit for all disease groups except for Eisenmenger syndrome.

Recently, Titman and colleagues[11] reported their findings from a retrospective cohort statistical analysis of the UK lung transplant experience. The study used more up-to-date data than those in the single-center UK transplant study by Charman and colleagues[10] and extended the assessment to the entire UK transplant system. During the study period, the UK lung transplant system primarily allocated donor lungs according to local transplant center criteria. Using data from a UK cohort of 1997 first lung transplant candidates (listed from July 1995–July 2006, with follow-up till December 2007) aged 16 years and older, the investigators analyzed mortality relative to continued listing. They assessed survival within the primary lung disease diagnostic groups of COPD, diffuse parenchymal lung disease, CF-associated lung disease, non–CF associated bronchiectasis, pulmonary hypertension, and "other", although the UK lung transplant database may have had some diagnostic misclassification. **Table 1** shows data from the 3 largest primary lung disease diagnostic groups. Of the 1997 patients in the study, about 35% died before undergoing lung transplant, and the proportion of patients who died while listed varied significantly among diagnostic groups (range, 19% for COPD to 49% for diffuse parenchymal lung disease). Less than 10% of patients were still awaiting lung transplant at the end of follow-up. Approximately 57% of patients underwent lung transplant. All diagnostic groups had an initial increased risk of death at transplant which later fell below the waiting list risk of death (ie, the crossover point) within 4.3 months after transplant (**Fig. 2**). Thereafter, the hazard ratio for posttransplant risk of death relative to pretransplant risk of death ranged from 0.34 for CF to 0.64 for COPD ($P<.05$ for all groups except pulmonary hypertension). Transplant seemed to improve survival for all diagnostic groups (ie, all groups reached the equity point, the point at which the posttransplant initial increase in risk of death equaled the subsequent reduction in posttransplant risk).

Prospective and Retrospective Cohort Treatment Studies

Multiple prophylactic, empiric, and focused treatments exist for problems associated with lung transplant. For issues specific to lung transplant, few studies and fewer multicenter randomized controlled trials have been conducted. Retrospective studies have greatly outnumbered prospective studies. Some studies have assessed the effects of induction therapy, maintenance immunosuppression, and treatment of acute and chronic

Table 1
Waiting list and transplant activity in the United Kingdom from July 1995 to July 2006, by diagnostic group, with follow-up till December 2007

Diagnosis	CF	DPLD	COPD (includes A1ATD)
Number listed	430	564	647
Number who underwent transplant	234	257	483
Deaths pretransplant	157	274	125
Deaths posttransplant	78	146	239
Median survival posttransplant in days (95% CI)	2436 (1819, NA)	1474 (936, 1900)	1795 (1527, 2194)
Crossover point[a] in days (95% CI)	42 (27, 131)	59 (39, 110)	130 (94, 222)
Percentage surviving to crossover point[a]	91	82	83
Postcrossover[a] hazard ratio (95% CI)	0.34 (0.23, 0.51)	0.36 (0.26, 0.51)	0.64 (0.48, 0.86)
Equity point[b] in days (95% CI)	160 (87, 468)	170 (103, 330)	905 (551, 2251)

Abbreviations: CI, confidence interval; DPLD, diffuse parenchymal lung disease; NA, means upper limit could not be calculated from the current data set.
[a] Crossover point: the time point at which the risk of dying after lung transplant equals the risk of dying on the lung transplant waiting list.
[b] Equity point: the time at which the posttransplant initial increase in risk of death equals the subsequent posttransplant reduction in risk of death.
Data from Titman A, Rogers CA, Bonser RS, et al. Disease-specific survival benefit of lung transplantation in adults: a national cohort study. Am J Transplant 2009;9:1642, 1646.

rejection/BOS. Few studies have shown positive effects on survival.

A few studies of pharmacologic approaches to prevent or treat acute and chronic allograft rejection are noteworthy. Iacono and colleagues[17] conducted a single-center, randomized, double-blind, placebo-controlled trial of inhaled cyclosporine initiated within 6 weeks after transplant.

The study randomly assigned 58 patients to inhale either 300 mg of aerosolized cyclosporine (28 patients) or aerosolized placebo (30 patients) 3 days a week for the first 2 years after transplant. Patients otherwise received standard immunosuppression. The study used the rate of histologic acute rejection as the primary end point. The study showed similar rates of acute rejection of

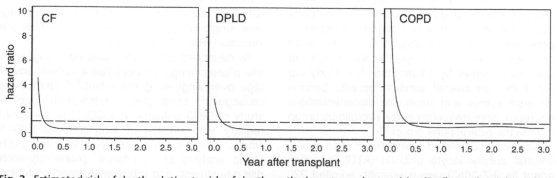

Fig. 2. Estimated risk of death relative to risk of death on the lung transplant waiting list (hazard ratio) in 3 lung transplant primary diagnostic groups. When the curve crosses the hazard ratio of 1, it graphically shows the crossover point, which represents the time point at which the risk of dying after lung transplant equals the risk of dying on the lung transplant waiting list. DPLD, diffuse parenchymal lung disease. (*Adapted from* Titman A, Rogers CA, Bonser RS, et al. Disease-specific survival benefit of lung transplantation in adults: a national cohort study. Am J Transplant 2009;9:1644; with permission.)

grade 2 or higher in the cyclosporine and placebo groups: 0.44 episodes (95% confidence interval [CI], 0.31–0.62) versus 0.46 episodes (95% CI, 0.33–0.64) per patient per year ($P = .87$ by Poisson regression). However, the study showed a higher survival rate for patients treated with aerosolized cyclosporine (3 deaths) than in those treated with placebo (14 deaths) (RR of death, 0.20; 95% CI, 0.06–0.70; $P = .01$). The aerosolized cyclosporine group also had higher chronic rejection-free survival than the placebo group as determined by spirometry (10 vs 20 events; RR of chronic rejection, 0.38; 95% CI, 0.18–0.82; $P = .01$) and histologic analysis (6 vs 19 events; RR, 0.27; 95% CI, 0.11–0.67; $P = .005$). Both treatment groups had similar risks of nephrotoxic effects and opportunistic infections. Although the study did not show a significant difference between treatment arms regarding the primary end point, the study did show improved survival and extended periods of chronic rejection-free survival in those treated with aerosolized cyclosporine in comparison to those treated with placebo. A larger randomized North American multicenter trial[18] further aims to assess the efficacy (BOS-free survival) and safety of inhaled cyclosporine. The study recently achieved its enrollment target of 300 patients, but the results remain unpublished.

One of the largest (n = 213) randomized controlled trials of maintenance immunosuppression in lung transplant evaluated everolimus versus azathioprine. The multicenter, international, double-blind clinical trial also used cyclosporine and corticosteroids for immunosuppression. The study had a primary composite end point (ie, efficacy failure) that consisted of lung function worsening (forced expiratory volume in the first second of expiration [FEV_1] decreased by >15%), graft loss, death, or loss to follow-up. The study showed a significantly lower composite end point rate in the everolimus group than in the azathioprine group (21.8% vs 33.9%, $P = .046$) at 12 months; however, the statistically significant difference waned by 24 months. The study did not show an overall survival benefit. Serious adverse events and treatment discontinuations occurred more frequently in the everolimus group than in the azathioprine group.[19]

A recently completed clinical trial[20] of an experimental antithymocyte globulin (ATG) induction agent (ie, EZ-2053) versus placebo enrolled 220 patients over 6 years. The study used a composite primary outcome measure of first occurrence of graft loss, acute rejection, loss to follow-up, or death. The investigators have not yet published the results.

Compared to the few completed clinical trials in lung transplant, investigators have published many cohort studies that have suggested that various treatment approaches prolong survival after transplant. Many biases exist in retrospective cohort studies, and they may not accurately estimate the treatment effects of randomized controlled trials. Large, multicenter, well-conducted, randomized controlled trials have not been conducted to confirm the findings of most of these retrospective studies. The following studies provide some compelling examples of interventions that might warrant further study.

To examine the effect of induction immunosuppression on survival after lung transplant, Hachem and colleagues[21] conducted a retrospective cohort study of patients in the ISHLT registry. The study divided a cohort of 3970 adult lung transplant recipients into 3 groups based on the use of induction: none, interleukin-2 receptor antagonist (IL-2 RA), and polyclonal ATG. The study estimated graft survival using the Kaplan-Meier method and constructed a multivariable Cox proportional hazards model to examine the independent effect of induction on graft survival. During the study period, 2249 patients received no induction, 1124 received an IL-2 RA, and 597 received an ATG. Four years after transplant, recipients treated with IL-2 RA had better Kaplan-Meier estimated graft survival (64%) than those treated with ATG (60%) and those who did not receive induction (57%; log rank $P = .0067$). The graft survival advantage persisted in the multivariable model for single and bilateral recipients treated with IL-2 RA when compared with those who did not receive induction (RR, 0.82; $P = .007$). Similarly, bilateral recipients treated with ATG had a graft survival advantage over bilateral recipients who did not receive induction (RR, 0.78; $P = .043$), but single-lung recipients treated with ATG did not have a graft survival advantage over single-lung recipients who did not receive induction (RR, 1.06; $P = .58$).

As described earlier, registries have suggested that bilateral lung transplant has a survival advantage over single-lung transplant.[5–7] Thabut and colleagues[22] conducted a retrospective cohort study of 9883 patients with COPD in the ISHLT registry who underwent lung transplant (64% single, 36% bilateral) between 1987 and 2006. Using analysis of covariance, propensity-score risk adjustment, and propensity-based matching, they found a survival benefit associated with bilateral lung transplant in those younger than 60 years compared with single-lung transplant.

Multiple cohort studies have suggested that azithromycin improves lung function in lung transplant recipients who develop BOS. To assess the effects of azithromycin on survival in this setting, Jain and colleagues[23] conducted a single-center retrospective cohort study of consecutive lung transplant recipients who developed BOS between 1999 and 2007. The study compared the time to death of 78 patients who received azithromycin (mainly since 2003) with that of the 95 patients who did not. The azithromycin-treated and untreated cohorts had similar baseline characteristics. Multivariate, time-dependent, Cox regression analysis showed a similar risk of death between the azithromycin-treated and untreated groups. However, for the 31 patients who were administered azithromycin after the development of BOS stage 1 and before the development of BOS stage 2, azithromycin treatment showed a reduced risk of death compared with no azithromycin treatment (adjusted hazard ratio, 0.30; 95% CI, 0.10–0.88; P = .03), after adjusting for FEV_1 at BOS stage 1 and bronchoscopic pseudomonas culture status. The study did not use a propensity score to adjust for the likelihood of receiving azithromycin, although the clinical practice switched from no azithromycin to azithromycin therapy for BOS in 2003 in most patients. The study did not adjust for all potentially significant covariates, and it had many potential biases associated with retrospective cohort analyses.

A retrospective cohort study by Johnson and colleagues[24] suggested that statin therapy in lung transplant recipients may improve survival. The retrospective design, the small cohort size, and other methodological issues limit the interpretation of the results.

LUNG TRANSPLANT: QUALITY OF LIFE

Multiple studies have provided a strong body of evidence that patients with lung disease severe enough to undergo listing for lung transplant have profoundly reduced quality of life and health-related quality of life (HRQOL).[25–60] Although a reasonable amount of published data exist, serious methodological limitations affect the ability to draw well-supported conclusions regarding the effects of lung transplant on quality of life. Missing data, usually because of noncompletion of questionnaires, and small sample sizes limit many of the studies. Because a significant proportion of patients die each year after lung transplant, the inability to account for deaths in the scoring of most non–utility based quality of life questionnaires significantly limits the interpretability of the quality of life data. Longitudinal cross-sectional designs have made it difficult to interpret

studies that have compared quality of life in post–lung transplant and pre–lung transplant unmatched cohorts. Many studies have typically not assessed results within subgroups of the primary lung disease indications for transplant or type of transplant, and small studies have lacked adequate power to detect significant findings and to perform meaningful subgroup analyses.

One type of subgroup analysis of lung transplant recipient quality of life has had relatively consistent results. After lung transplant, patients frequently develop BOS.[7] BOS has a high case-fatality rate, and it accounts for a large proportion of late deaths after lung transplant.[7] Studies have shown that patients with BOS have a significantly reduced quality of life compared with patients without BOS.[41,47,56,57,60]

Some studies have used utilities to assess the outcomes of lung transplant because they offer an important means for measuring the health benefit.[3,4,61] Utilities provide a means for quantitative measurement of patient preferences.[62] Utilities can capture degree of impairment, degree of bother, and willingness to undergo risk to reduce bother.[62,63] By convention, studies may score utilities on a continuous scale of 0.00 to 1.00, in which the most healthy state (top anchor) has a value of 1.00 and death (bottom anchor) has a value of 0.00. Studies determine utilities for other health states relative to the 2 anchors.

Direct utility assessment measures preferences about a patient's own health state or a theoretic health state. Studies typically use standard gamble, rating scale, time trade-off, and willingness to pay methods of preference assessment to directly estimate utilities. With *indirect* utility assessment, patients do not directly have their preferences elicited. Indirect utility assessment uses preferences for various health states from a sample of a population, and these preference values weigh the answers from completed questionnaires to produce estimates of utilities.[64,65]

Unlike non–preference based, disease-specific, and generic quality of life measures, preference measures typically allow deceased patients to receive a quality of life score and have their data used for analyses and interpretation. The inclusion of data from deceased patients removes a major bias associated with typical HRQOL studies of lung transplant. Preference data that estimate utilities take into consideration quantity as well as quality of life consequences of illnesses and their treatments and allow for the estimation of quality-adjusted survival and quality-adjusted life-years (QALYs). By determining QALYs, utilities may estimate the cost effectiveness or cost utility of a procedure.[26–30] Typical disease-specific or generic (nonutility) HRQL tools cannot similarly measure cost effectiveness.

Despite the advantages of utility assessment over other methods for estimating quality of life, only a few studies have directly assessed utilities in patients undergoing lung transplant.[26,30,31,34–36] Published studies have mainly used cross-sectional preoperative[26,30,31,34–36] and postoperative study designs,[26,35] and the literature has a miniscule amount of prospective longitudinal studies that directly assessed utilities in patients undergoing lung transplant.[25]

In 1995, Ramsey and colleagues[26] first reported results of direct utility assessment in lung transplant recipients. In their single-center (University of Washington) cross-sectional study of approximately 50 patients with various pretransplant diagnoses, trained interviewers assisted patients with standard gamble card-and-board prop-based interviews. The study assessed utility for current health on a scale of death (score equals zero) to perfect health (score equals 1). Patients on the waiting list who had various types of lung diseases (n = 16) had a mean ± SD utility score of 0.65 ± 0.26 and others (n = 22) who underwent lung transplant within 1 to 41 months prior had a utility score of 0.80 ± 0.24 ($P<.001$). The study excluded deceased patients from the scoring. When the interviewers asked posttransplant patients to perform their assessment imagining that they currently had their pretransplant health state, the recipients had an average imagined pretransplant utility score of 0.10 ± 0.31. The post–lung transplant patients had significantly lower imagined pre–lung transplant utility scores than the utility scores of patients who were actually on the lung transplant waiting list. Small sample size, cross-sectional design, and the likely utility score inflation due to the exclusion of deaths limited the interpretation of the study findings.

In 2002, Singer and colleagues[35] reported the cross-sectional results of a single-center (Stanford University) study of 6 pre–lung transplant candidates and 90 lung transplant recipients with COPD. The investigators obtained utility scores for use in a Markov decision analysis model. They used a computerized interactive interview[66,67] to assess utility for current health (scaled from death to ideal health) via the standard gamble technique. Ignoring deaths, the preoperative cohort had a median utility value of 0.48, whereas the postoperative cohort had a value of 0.73. The decision model assigned deceased patients a utility value of zero. Although the medical treatment strategy had a modeled survival better than that of the lung transplant treatment strategy (median survival, 55 months vs 48 months), lung transplant had a higher quality-adjusted survival than medical therapy (3.46 QALYs vs 2.63 QALYs, extrapolated over the remaining life span, assuming constant risks). This study suggested that quality of life (utility) gains outweigh the increased mortality associated with lung transplant, although it had methodological limitations similar to the study by Ramsey and colleagues.[26]

The medical literature lacks published results of longitudinal direct utility assessment before and after lung transplant. In 2005, the Washington University group reported results from a prospective (1997 through 2003) cohort study of a convenience sample of adult patients with COPD awaiting lung transplant. The study aimed to assess the effects of lung transplant on quality of life. Using a computerized, interviewer-assisted, standard gamble assessment (COPD titer),[34] they estimated utility scores for current health and current shortness of breath. They conservatively defined a minimally clinically important change in utility as 0.10, and they reported the change in utilities from before lung transplant to 6 months after lung transplant. Of 137 lung transplant candidates evaluated, 5 did not successfully complete the baseline interview, 22 remained alive on the waiting list, 9 died waiting for lung transplant, and 2 were removed from the lung transplant waiting list. The 99 patients who subsequently underwent lung transplant (88% bilateral, 12% unilateral) had a baseline mean ± SD utility for current health score of 0.51 ± 0.30 (median, 0.50) and a utility for current shortness of breath score of 0.51 ± 0.30 (median, 0.50). The investigators assigned the 5 patients who died after lung transplant a postoperative utility score of zero. For the 2 patients missing post–lung transplant utility scores, the investigators imputed the value of the lower limit of the 95% CI of the average post–lung transplant score of the survivors. At 6 months after lung transplant, the recipients had a utility for current health score of 0.78 ± 0.28 (median, 0.945) and a utility for current shortness of breath score of 0.79 ± 0.30 (median, 0.955). Regarding current health, 73% of recipients increased their utility score by the minimally important change of at least 0.10, 16% had no clinically significant change in utility, and 11% decreased their utility score by at least 0.10. Similar changes occurred with utility for current shortness of breath scores. The study demonstrated poor quality of life for patients with COPD on the lung transplant waiting list and statistically (Wilcoxon signed rank 2 tailed $P<.001$) and clinically significant improvements in disease-specific and general quality of life (utility scores) during the first 6 months after lung transplant.[25] The study did not address the important issue of response shift (change of internal standards, values, and the conceptualization of quality of life).

Similar to direct utility assessment, there are only a small number of published studies that used indirect utility assessment to assess patients undergoing lung transplant.[4,27–29,31,32,37] Based on study design, follow-up limitations, and missing data, significant biases may have affected the ability to adequately assess the effects of lung transplant on indirect utility scores. Importantly, exclusion of deceased patients from receiving a utility score biased the results of some of the studies upward, making utility scores seem higher than those obtained if the deceased patients were included in the analyses. All studies included a small number of patients, and this paucity significantly limited the ability to perform subgroup analyses. In addition, the studies did not frequently present results within pretransplant diagnostic groups. Because of these and other limitations, it becomes difficult to compare much of the data from the indirect utility assessments with data from direct utility assessments of patients.

INTEGRATING SURVIVAL AND QUALITY OF LIFE OUTCOMES

Patients with a far-advanced lung disease remain significantly symptomatic despite medical therapy, and they have a disturbingly high short-term mortality. Many such patients desperately seek symptomatic relief, and they would consider undergoing lung transplant to improve quality of life, whether or not it produces a survival benefit. Although many patients may live longer and better after lung transplant, a significant proportion experience adverse events and comorbidity, and some patients die sooner after transplant than they would have without transplant.

Lung transplant clearly has a significant early postoperative mortality rate, and the debate continues about whether it improves longevity.[1,2,8–11] Lung transplant has a great capacity to improve functioning, symptoms, satisfaction, bother, and other domains of quality of life. Unfortunately, lung transplant recipients may suffer from a great deal of morbidity associated with transplant and immunosuppression.[7]

After 2 decades of publications involving many large cohort studies and a few small randomized controlled trials, many questions remain unanswered; most importantly, do the benefits of lung transplant outweigh the harms? Exclusive use of survival to judge the success or failure of lung transplant remains inadequate because lung transplant provides significant palliation. Unfortunately, most studies that have assessed the quality of life and survival of patients undergoing lung transplant have not provided a formal mechanism for comparing the risks and the benefits. Most studies of quality of life have censored patients who died, as if they had neither good nor bad outcomes. This practice inflates the apparent benefits of lung transplant, and the bias worsens during long-term follow-up as the death rates increase. When studying the overall effects of lung transplant, it remains insufficient to measure survival *or* quality of life; studies should measure survival *and* quality of life and present the results as a package.[68] Some studies[69] in related fields have tried to address this issue by focusing on success rates and reporting proportions of patients improved, unchanged, and not improved (includes deceased and missing patients) within treatment groups. Such an approach in a study of quality of life of patients undergoing lung transplant would include all patients and would consider patients who underwent a retransplant, missing patients, and deceased patients as treatment failures.[3,4,68] However, one could question the appropriateness of equal weighting of such non-positive outcomes.

Only a few studies that assess outcomes in lung transplant have used instruments that incorporate quality of life and survival into one measure.[26–37,61] Formal mechanisms for combining quantity and quality of life information exist.[3,4] One approach adjusts the observed length of survival by a numeric factor that represents quality of life. For example, investigators may use certain types of quality of life (eg, preference or utility) data to generate quality scores for all patients. Investigators may then add up quality scores over time to estimate QALYs. When comparing groups of patients, the group with the most QALYs has the best quality-adjusted survival. For example, if 2 cohorts (eg, X and Y) undergoing comparison have equal survival rates, then the cohort with better quality of life will generate more QALYs. Alternatively, a relatively high mortality could be offset by excellent quality of life within cohort X, whereas a relatively low mortality and low quality of life in cohort Y might produce fewer QALYs than in cohort X. In this scenario, cohort X would live shorter and with better HRQOL, whereas cohort Y would live longer and with worse HRQOL.[3]

Lung transplant may require assessment of quality-adjusted survival to demonstrate its effectiveness. Cohort studies could miss this signal because of the lack of a control arm. For example, a cohort that has posttransplant quality-adjusted survival that is lower than its pretransplant quality-adjusted survival might suggest that transplant lacks benefit. However, a nontransplant control arm with a significantly worse trajectory would make transplant look beneficial. Thus, randomized controlled trials that compare lung transplant with non–lung transplant would provide the strongest evidence regarding the effects of lung transplant on quality-adjusted survival.

Assessment of outcomes using a single pretransplant baseline and one or multiple posttransplant follow-ups may also encounter bias. To assess the overall outcomes of lung transplant, the author proposes that patients should undergo assessment from the time of entry into the transplant system until death or their removal from the transplant system. Comprehensive assessment of lung transplant outcomes should not ignore outcomes on the waiting list. In addition, the intermittent assessment of outcomes may introduce bias because spaced out assessments may miss the highs and lows of quality of life.

The effects of lung transplant may depend on the system in which it occurs. For example, lung transplant in the current UNOS LAS system may function very differently than it did in the previous wait-time dependent donor lung allocation system. Also, lung transplant in UNOS may function differently than it does in the Eurotransplant or other systems. Patients, clinicians, researchers, and resource allocators face many challenges in making decisions about lung transplant. Clinicians should help patients understand the considerable risks and costs of lung transplant and balance these against the likely effects on longevity, symptoms, functioning, and other aspects of quality of life. Investigators need better tools for measuring patient outcomes. Policy makers need robust methods for evaluating the outcomes of lung transplant, so they can make informed judgments. Most lung transplant entities do not routinely collect robust quality of life data. However, the medical community and the public want to know how lung transplant affects quality of life. Given the huge stakes for the patients, the providers, and the health care systems, key stakeholders need to further support quality of life assessment in patients with advanced lung disease who enter into the lung transplant systems. Studies of lung transplant and its related technologies should assess patients with tools that integrate both survival and quality of life information. Higher-quality information leads to improved knowledge and more-informed decision making.[3]

REFERENCES

1. Liou TG, Adler FR, Cox DR, et al. Lung transplantation and survival in children with cystic fibrosis. N Engl J Med 2007;357:2143–52.
2. Sweet SC, Aurora P, Benden C, et al. International pediatric lung transplant collaborative. Lung transplantation and survival in children with cystic fibrosis: solid statistics–flawed interpretation. Pediatr Transplant 2008;12:129–36.
3. Yusen RD. Lung transplantation outcomes: the importance and inadequacies of assessing survival [editorial]. Am J Transplant 2009;9:1493–4.
4. Yusen RD. Technology and outcomes assessment in lung transplantation. Proc Am Thorac Soc 2009;6: 128–36.
5. Available at: http://www.ustransplant.org/annual_reports/current/113_surv-new_dh.htm. Accessed November 28, 2010.
6. Yusen RD, Shearon TH, Qian Y, et al. Lung transplantation in the United States, 1999–2008. Am J Transplant 2010;10(Part 2):1047–68.
7. Christie JD, Edwards LB, Kucheryavaya AY, et al. The Registry of the International Society for Heart and Lung Transplantation: twenty-seventh official adult lung and heart-lung transplant report–2010. J Heart Lung Transplant 2010;29:1104–18.
8. Hosenpud JD, Bennett LE, Keck BM, et al. Effect of diagnosis on survival benefit of lung transplantation for end-stage lung disease. Lancet 1998;351:24–7.
9. De Meester J, Smits JM, Persijn GG, et al. Listing for lung transplantation: life expectancy and transplant effect, stratified by type of end-stage lung disease, the Eurotransplant experience. J Heart Lung Transplant 2001;20:518–24.
10. Charman SC, Sharples LD, McNeil KD, et al. Assessment of survival benefit after lung transplantation by patient diagnosis. J Heart Lung Transplant 2002;21:226–32.
11. Titman A, Rogers CA, Bonser RS, et al. Disease-specific survival benefit of lung transplantation in adults: a national cohort study. Am J Transplant 2009;9:1640–9.
12. Thabut G, Christie JD, Kremers WK, et al. Survival differences following lung transplantation among US transplant centers. JAMA 2010;304:53–60.
13. Liou TG, Adler FR, Cahill BC, et al. Correction: lung transplantation and survival in children with cystic fibrosis. N Engl J Med 2008;359:536.
14. Egan TM, Murray S, Bustami RT, et al. Development of the new lung allocation system in the United States. Am J Transplant 2006;6:1212–27.
15. Available at: http://optn.transplant.hrsa.gov/resources/professionalResources.asp?index=88. Accessed November 28, 2010.
16. Available at: http://optn.transplant.hrsa.gov/Committee Reports/interim_main_ThoracicOrganTransplantation

Committee_5_1_2008_10_25.pdf. Accessed November 28, 2010.

17. Iacono AT, Johnson BA, Grgurich WF, et al. A randomized trial of inhaled cyclosporine in lung-transplant recipients. N Engl J Med 2006;354: 141–50.

18. Available at: http://clinicaltrials.gov/ct2/show/NCT00755781?term=nct00755781&rank=1 (Clinicaltrials.gov. Identifier NCT00755781). Accessed November 7, 2010.

19. Snell GI, Valentine VG, Vitulo P, et al. RAD B159 Study Group. Everolimus versus azathioprine in maintenance lung transplant recipients: an international, randomized, double-blind clinical trial. Am J Transplant 2006;6:169–77.

20. Available at: http://clinicaltrials.gov/ct2/show/NCT00105183?term=EZ-2053&rank=1. (Clinicaltrials.gov. Identifier NCT00105183). Accessed November 21, 2010.

21. Hachem RR, Edwards LB, Yusen RD, et al. The impact of induction on survival after lung transplantation: an analysis of the International Society for Heart and Lung Transplantation Registry. Clin Transplant 2008;22:603–8.

22. Thabut G, Christie JD, Ravaud P, et al. Survival after bilateral versus single lung transplantation for patients with chronic obstructive pulmonary disease: a retrospective analysis of registry data. Lancet 2008;371:744–51.

23. Jain R, Hachem RR, Morrell MR, et al. Azithromycin is associated with increased survival in lung transplant recipients with bronchiolitis obliterans syndrome. J Heart Lung Transplant 2010;29:531–7.

24. Johnson BA, Iacono AT, Zeevi A, et al. Statin use is associated with improved function and survival in lung allografts. Am J Respir Crit Care Med 2003; 167:1271–8.

25. Yusen RD, Brown KL, Habrock TE, et al. The impact of lung transplantation on quality of life in patients with COPD. J Heart Lung Transplant 2005;24: S156–7.

26. Ramsey S, Patrick D, Lewis S, et al. Improvement in quality of life after lung transplantation: a preliminary study. J Heart Lung Transplant 1995;14:870–7.

27. Gartner SH, Sevick MA, Keenan RJ, et al. Cost-utility of lung transplantation: a pilot study. J Heart Lung Transplant 1997;16:1129–34.

28. Al MJ, Koopmanschap MA, van Enckevort PJ, et al. Cost-effectiveness of lung transplantation in the Netherlands. A scenario analysis. Chest 1998;113: 124–30.

29. Anyanwu AC, McGuire A, Rogers CA, et al. Assessment of quality of life in lung transplantation using a simple generic tool. Thorax 2001;56:218–22.

30. Vasiliadis HM, Collet JP, Penrod JR, et al. A cost-effectiveness and cost-utility study of lung transplantation. J Heart Lung Transplant 2005;24:1275–8.

31. Busschbach JJ, Horikx PE, van den Bosch JM, et al. Measuring the quality of life before and after bilateral lung transplantation in patients with cystic fibrosis. Chest 1994;105:911–7.

32. Squier HC, Ries AL, Kaplan RM, et al. Quality of well-being predicts survival in lung transplantation candidates. Am J Respir Crit Care Med 1995;152: 2032–6.

33. van Enckevort PJ, TenVergert EM, Bonsel GJ, et al. Technology assessment of the Dutch Lung Transplantation Program. Int J Technol Assess Health Care 1998;14:344–56.

34. Yusen RD, Littenberg B, Brown K, et al. Validity of a computer-based patient preference instrument for assessing quality of life in COPD. Am J Respir Crit Care Med 1999;159:A815.

35. Singer LG, Gould MK, Glidden DV, et al. Effect of lung transplantation on quality-adjusted survival in emphysema. J Heart Lung Transplant 2002;21:154.

36. Singer LG, Theodore J. Validity of standard gamble utilities as measured by transplant readiness in lung transplant candidates. Med Decis Making 2003;23: 435–40.

37. Lobo FS, Gross CR, Matthees BJ. Estimation and comparison of derived preference scores from the SF-36 in lung transplant patients. Qual Life Res 2004;13:377–88.

38. Littlefield C, Abbey S, Fiducia D, et al. Quality of life following transplantation of the heart, liver, and lungs. Gen Hosp Psychiatry 1996;18:36S–47S.

39. Limbos MM, Chan CK, Kesten S. Quality of life in female lung transplant candidates and recipients. Chest 1997;112:1165–74.

40. TenVergert EM, Essink-Bot ML, Geertsma A, et al. The effect of lung transplantation on health-related quality of life. Chest 1998;113:358–64.

41. Cohen L, Littlefield C, Kelly P, et al. Predictors of quality of life and adjustment after lung transplantation. Chest 1998;113:633–44.

42. MacNaughton KL, Rodrigue JR, Cicale M, et al. Health-related quality of life and symptom frequency before and after lung transplantation. Clin Transplant 1998;12:320–3.

43. Lanuza DM, McCabe M, Norton-Rosko M, et al. Symptom experiences of lung transplant recipients: comparisons across gender, pretransplantation diagnosis, and type of transplantation. Heart Lung 1999;28:429–37.

44. Lanuza DM, Lefaiver C, Mc Cabe M, et al. Prospective study of functional status and quality of life before and after lung transplantation. Chest 2000; 118:115–22.

45. Stavem K, Bjørtuft O, Lund MB, et al. Health-related quality of life in lung transplant candidates and recipients. Respiration 2000;67:159–65.

46. van Den Berg JW, Geertsma A, van Der Bij W, et al. Bronchiolitis obliterans syndrome after lung

transplantation and health-related quality of life. Am J Respir Crit Care Med 2000;161:1937–41.

47. Matthees BJ, Anantachoti P, Kreitzer MJ, et al. Use of complementary therapies, adherence, and quality of life in lung transplant recipients. Heart Lung 2001; 30:258–68.

48. De Vito Dabbs A, Dew MA, Stilley CS, et al. Psychosocial vulnerability, physical symptoms and physical impairment after lung and heart-lung transplantation. J Heart Lung Transplant 2003;22:1268–75.

49. Vermeulen KM, Groen H, van der Bij W, et al. The effect of bronchiolitis obliterans syndrome on health related quality of life. Clin Transplant 2004;18: 377–83.

50. Gerbase MW, Spiliopoulos A, Rochat T, et al. Health-related quality of life following single or bilateral lung transplantation: a 7-year comparison to functional outcome. Chest 2005;128:1371–8.

51. Kugler C, Fischer S, Gottlieb J, et al. Health-related quality of life in two hundred-eighty lung transplant recipients. J Heart Lung Transplant 2005;24:2262–8.

52. Rodrigue JR, Baz MA, Kanasky WF Jr, et al. Does lung transplantation improve health-related quality of life? The University of Florida experience. J Heart Lung Transplant 2005;24:755–63.

53. Smeritschnig B, Jaksch P, Kocher A, et al. Quality of life after lung transplantation: a cross-sectional study. J Heart Lung Transplant 2005;24:474–80.

54. Rodrigue JR, Baz MA. Are there sex differences in health-related quality of life after lung transplantation for chronic obstructive pulmonary disease? J Heart Lung Transplant 2006;25:120–5.

55. Girard F, Chouinard P, Boudreault D, et al. Prevalence and impact of pain on the quality of life of lung transplant recipients: a prospective observational study. Chest 2006;130:1535–40.

56. Vermeulen KM, van der Bij W, Erasmus ME, et al. Long-term health-related quality of life after lung transplantation: different predictors for different dimensions. J Heart Lung Transplant 2007;26:188–93.

57. Gerbase MW, Soccal PM, Spiliopoulos A, et al. Long-term health-related quality of life and walking capacity of lung recipients with and without bronchiolitis obliterans syndrome. J Heart Lung Transplant 2008;27:898–904.

58. Vermeulen KM, TenVergert EM, Verschuuren EA, et al. Pre-transplant quality of life does not predict survival after lung transplantation. J Heart Lung Transplant 2008;27:623–7.

59. Limbos MM, Joyce DP, Chan CK, et al. Psychological functioning and quality of life in lung transplant candidates and recipients. Chest 2000;118:408–16.

60. Kugler C, Tegtbur U, Gottlieb J, et al. Health-related quality of life in long-term survivors after heart and lung transplantation: a prospective cohort study. Transplantation 2010;90(4):451–7.

61. Yusen RD. What outcomes should be measured in patients with COPD? Chest 2001;119:327–8.

62. von Neumann J, Morgenstern O. Theory of games and economic behavior. 3rd edition. New York: Wiley; 1953.

63. Nease RF Jr, Kneeland T, O'Connor GT, et al. Variation in patient utilities for outcomes of the management of chronic stable angina. Implications for clinical practice guidelines. JAMA 1995;273: 1185–90.

64. EuroQol Group. EuroQol—a new facility for the measurement of health-related quality of life. Health Policy 1990;16:199–208.

65. Kaplan R, Atkins C, Timms R. Validity of a quality of well-being scale as an outcome measure in chronic obstructive pulmonary disease. J Chronic Dis 1984; 37:85–95.

66. Sumner W, Nease R, Littenberg B. U-titer. A utility assessment tool. Med Decis Making 1991;11:327.

67. Sumner W, Nease R, Littenberg B. U-titer: a utility assessment tool. Fifteenth Annual Symposium on Computer Applications in Medical Care. Washington, DC; 1991. p. 710–5.

68. Yusen RD, Littenberg B. Integrating survival and quality of life data in clinical trials of lung disease. Chest 2005;127:1094–6.

69. Fishman A, Martinez F, Naunheim K, et al. A randomized trial comparing lung-volume-reduction surgery with medical therapy for severe emphysema. N Engl J Med 2003;348:2059–73.

Conventional and Novel Approaches to Immunosuppression

Timothy Floreth, MD[a], Sangeeta M. Bhorade, MD[a],
Vivek N. Ahya, MD[b],*

KEYWORDS

- Immunosuppression • Induction therapy
- Therapeutic drug monitoring • Lung transplantation

The introduction of potent immunosuppressive agents over the past thirty years is one of the factors that has led to significant improvements in posttransplant survival in the current era of solid organ transplantation. By targeting multiple pathways involved in the alloimmune response to the graft, rates of both acute and chronic rejection have declined. Unfortunately, these agents have not been as effective in lung transplantation where graft rejection remains a major obstacle to long-term survival. In this article, both conventional and novel approaches to preventing graft rejection are reviewed. Immunosuppressive therapy to treat established acute or chronic rejection is discussed elsewhere in this issue.

CONVENTIONAL APPROACHES

Although there is some variability in the medications used at different lung transplant centers, the approach to immunosuppression is generally similar. Maintenance regimens typically involve administration of three distinct classes of immunosuppressive agents: calcineurin inhibitors (CNIs; eg, cyclosporine, tacrolimus), antiproliferative agents (eg, azathioprine, mycophenolate mofetil [MMF], sirolimus), and corticosteroids. In addition, approximately 60% of lung recipients receive induction therapy to augment immunosuppression in the early posttransplant period. Institutional immunosuppression protocols are largely based

on evidence from methodologically flawed studies: retrospective single-center experiences and prospective studies that were not randomized, involved small numbers of patients, or compared outcomes to historical data. For many years, the strongest evidence has come from more robust studies in other solid organ transplant populations. In the past decade, however, several large, multicenter clinical trials have been performed in lung transplantation and have informed practice patterns.

Induction Therapy

Induction therapy involves the administration of a potent immunosuppressive agent in the perioperative or early postoperative period to reduce risk of acute rejection and permit more gradual initiation of maintenance immunosuppression. Several types of induction agents are currently in use and specifically target T-lymphocytes, the primary effector cells of the cell-mediated immune system.

The most common induction agents used in clinical practice are humanized or chimeric monoclonal antibodies to CD25 (eg, daclizumab, basiliximab), the alpha subunit of the interleukin-2 receptor (IL-2R).[1] By blocking signaling through the IL-2R, these drugs inhibit T-cell proliferation and differentiation, without inducing depletion. Both daclizumab and basiliximab are generally

[a] Section of Pulmonary and Critical Care Medicine, Department of Medicine, University of Chicago Medical Center, 5841 South Maryland Avenue, Chicago, IL 60637, USA
[b] Pulmonary, Allergy & Critical Care Division, Department of Medicine, University of Pennsylvania School of Medicine, 832 West Gates Building, Philadelphia, PA 19104, USA
* Corresponding author.
E-mail address: ahyav@uphs.upenn.edu

Clin Chest Med 32 (2011) 265–277
doi:10.1016/j.ccm.2011.02.012
0272-5231/11/$ – see front matter © 2011 Elsevier Inc. All rights reserved

chestmed.theclinics.com

well tolerated. However, there is concern that inhibition of IL-2 mediated signaling, which is also necessary for generation of CD4$^+$CD25$^+$FoxP3$^+$ T regulatory cells, may disrupt the delicate balance between alloreactivity and tolerance.[2]

In the latest report from the International Society of Heart and Lung Transplantation (ISHLT), approximately 13% of lung recipients in 2008 received induction therapy with polyclonal antithymocyte globulins (ATG) such as Thymoglobulin or Atgam.[1] These drugs were developed by immunizing rabbits or horses with human thymocytes to induce development of antibodies against a broad range of human T-cell markers.[3] Although the mechanisms responsible for their antirejection properties are not completely understood, administration of these agents results in profound depletion of T-cells, including alloreactive T-cells. It is not clear, however, what effect these drugs have on immunologic mechanisms that promote tolerance to the allograft. For example, animal studies have suggested that repopulation of the T-cell repertoire after initial depletion may consist of lymphocytes with a more alloreactive phenotype.[4] In contrast, other reports indicate that T-cell depletion may spare CD4$^+$CD25$^+$FoxP3$^+$ T-regulatory cells and thus promote immunologic tolerance.[5] Better understanding of the pleiotropic effects of antilymphocyte agents on the immune system is required to assess overall impact on the alloimmune response. Numerous clinical side effects associated with polyclonal antilymphocyte agents have been reported and include anaphylaxis, cytokine storm, serum sickness, leukopenia, anemia, and thrombocytopenia as well as increased risk of infection and malignancy.[3]

Alemtuzumab (Campath-1H) is a humanized monoclonal antibody to CD52, a cell surface marker found on all mononuclear lymphocytes. It is used by only a few transplant centers for induction therapy.[1] Alemtuzumab administration results in profound and prolonged T-cell depletion with variable effects on B-lymphocyte, natural killer cells, and monocyte populations. Thus, it is not surprising that infectious complications are among the most common adverse events reported. Similar to the polyclonal agents, a number of side effects have been reported with alemtuzumab use and include infusion-related anaphylaxis and profound cytopenias.[6]

Induction therapy in lung transplantation remains controversial and only about 60% receive this type of immunosuppression.[1] Although reports suggest that increased immunosuppression in the early posttransplant period reduces the risk of acute rejection, this potential benefit may be offset by an increased risk of infection or other induction therapy-associated adverse events. Unfortunately, published information from large, multicenter, prospective, randomized studies comparing induction therapy to placebo is lacking. Similarly, high quality studies comparing one regimen to another are also absent. Thus, transplant center practices regarding induction therapy are based largely on retrospective studies, registry reports, and small prospective single-center investigations as well as institutional experiences and expert opinion.[7–11] A few of these studies are reviewed below.

In the 2010 annual report of the ISHLT registry, induction therapy was associated with a small but statistically significant survival benefit (unadjusted for confounding effects) and decrease in the rate of bronchiolitis obliterans syndrome (BOS) in patients who survived at least 14 days.[1] In a more rigorous retrospective study of almost 4000 lung transplant recipients in the ISHLT registry transplanted between January 2000 and March 2004, induction therapy with either an IL-2R antagonist or polyclonal ATG remained independently associated with improved survival at 4 years (IL2R antagonist, 64%; ATG, 60%; no induction, 57%) even after adjustment for multiple donor and recipient specific variables. Interestingly, no differences in BOS rates were seen in the IL-2R antagonist treatment group compared with the no induction group, whereas BOS rates were slightly higher in the ATG treatment group. There was also a significantly higher rate of infection in both induction therapy groups compared with patients who did not receive induction therapy.[12] In a randomized single-center study of 50 lung transplant patients comparing induction therapy with ATG versus daclizumab, both treatment groups had comparable rates of acute and chronic rejection as well as survival after 1 year. Although cytomegalovirus (CMV) infection rates were higher in the daclizumab group, this may be explained by the significantly greater numbers of CMV-mismatched patients in the daclizumab group.[13]

Alemtuzumab (Campath-1H) induction has recently been studied in lung transplantation after experience in kidney transplantation suggested that it may allow use of lower levels of maintenance immunosuppression without increasing cellular rejection rates or infectious complications.[6] The first report was published by investigators at the University of Pittsburgh. They retrospectively compared short-term outcomes of 48 lung transplant patients who received either ATG or alemtuzumab induction followed by maintenance immunosuppression with tacrolimus with or without low-dose corticosteroids to 28 historical controls who received daclizumab induction and standard maintenance immunosuppression. Acute rejection rates (grade A2 or greater) were lowest in the alemtuzumab group and survival was similar in all three groups at 6 months posttransplant. In another study, 20 lung recipients treated with alemtuzumab and lower maintenance immunosuppression had survival, acute rejection and infection rates comparable to 20 historical controls.[14] Clearly, stronger evidence is needed before alemtuzumab induction can be recommended.

Maintenance Immunosuppression

Until the introduction of cyclosporine in the late 1970s and subsequent approval by the US Food and Drug Administration (FDA) in 1983, short-term outcomes after lung transplantation were poor. Immunosuppressive therapy options were limited in this era and included postoperative thymic irradiation, azathioprine, and high doses of corticosteroids.[15] In the 2 decades following Dr James Hardy's first human lung transplant procedure, approximately 40 lung transplant procedures were attempted. Most patients died within weeks to several months from infectious complications, graft rejection, or bronchial anastomotic dehiscence.[16] After performing a series of experiments in animal models demonstrating the deleterious effects of high doses of corticosteroids on bronchial anastomotic healing, in 1983 Dr Joel Cooper performed a unilateral lung transplant in a patient with idiopathic pulmonary fibrosis using a modified surgical technique and a cyclosporine-based immunosuppression regimen that initially did not include corticosteroids.[16] This patient survived 6 years, a dramatic improvement from previously reported outcomes. Since then, the triple combination of a CNI, an antiproliferative agent and low-dose prednisone has been the cornerstone of post–lung transplant immunosuppression.[1] Several of these agents are discussed in greater detail below.

CNIs

Cyclosporine A (CSA), is the first CNI approved for clinical use in transplantation. It exerts its immunosuppressive effects by forming a complex with the cytoplasmic carrier protein cyclophilin and binding to calcineurin to inactivate it. Calcineurin is a protein phosphatase capable of dephosphorylating and thereby activating the cytoplasmic transcription factor, nuclear factor of activated T cell (NFAT), and permitting it to migrate to the cell nucleus and enhance transcription of several proinflammatory cytokines (eg, IL-2) critical for T-cell activation and proliferation.[17]

CSA may be administered enterally or parenterally. Enteral absorption of CSA is variable. The initial oil-based oral preparation of CSA (Sandimmune) was highly lipophilic and characterized by significant intrapatient and interpatient pharmacokinetic variability related to erratic drug absorption and metabolism. A newer cyclosporine microemulsion formulation (Neoral) has significantly improved bioavailability. Thus, different CSA formulations cannot be readily interchanged and drug levels must be followed closely when one preparation is substituted for another.[17]

Tacrolimus is a newer, more potent (10- to 100-fold increased potency in vitro) CNI available for clinical use.[18] It has replaced cyclosporine in maintenance immunosuppression regimens at the majority of lung transplant centers around the world.[1] Its therapeutic effect is achieved by binding to the cytoplasmic protein FKBP-12 and forming an inactivating complex with calcineurin.[18] Tacrolimus can be administered orally, intravenously, or sublingually. Intravenous administration, however, is limited by an increased risk of renal toxicity. Oral administration of tacrolimus is also characterized by significant intrapatient and interpatient pharmacokinetic variability related to erratic drug absorption. Thus, this medication should be consistently taken in a similar manner (ie, always with food or always on an empty stomach). For patients unable take oral medication in the early postoperative period, therapeutic drug levels have been achieved by emptying the contents of the capsule under the patient's tongue. However, it is unclear whether resulting drug absorption occurs primarily through the sublingual mucosa or via the enteral route after swallowing of residual medication.[19,20]

Both CNIs have a narrow therapeutic window and drug levels must be monitored closely to avoid toxicity. CSA trough (C0) levels are the most commonly used tool to monitor drug levels; however, correlation with overall systemic exposure is poor.[21] CSA levels obtained 2 hours after CSA ingestion (C2) have been shown to be more predictive of total drug exposure during the dosing interval.[22] In a recent study of 50 consecutive lung transplant recipients, monitoring CSA with C2 levels was associated with lower rates of acute and chronic rejection as well as reduced toxicity compared with historical controls monitored with C0 levels.[23] Tacrolimus dosing is typically adjusted based on trough levels, although studies have again shown poor correlation with exposure over time. The ideal tacrolimus monitoring strategy is unknown, although reports have suggested that two measurements in the first 4 hours after drug administration allow for a better estimate of drug exposure during the 12-hour dosing interval.[24] This approach, unfortunately, is not practical for routine monitoring because patients are required to get multiple blood draws, but could be considered if there is concern that drug dosing is outside the therapeutic window.

For both CSA and tacrolimus, target serum immunosuppression levels will vary depending on a clinical estimate of the patient's overall state of immunosuppression and a number of factors that may warrant higher or lower levels of drug, including time after transplantation, and presence, severity, and frequency of acute rejection episodes, identification of infections or malignancies and evidence of drug toxicity.

CNI use is associated with frequent adverse events. One of the most common side effects is renal insufficiency. Several types of nephrotoxicity have been reported, including an acute, potentially reversible form mediated by vasoconstriction of the afferent arteriole and consequent reduction in the glomerular filtration rate (GFR).[25] Chronic nephrotoxicity is associated with long-term use of CNIs. Patients have progressive decline in renal function over years and may develop end-stage renal disease. The mechanism of damage is not well understood, but thought to be due to direct toxicity to renal tubules, ischemic injury related to recurrent hemodynamic effects, and perhaps CNI-induced production of profibrotic growth factors (eg, transforming growth factor-beta).[25] CNIs have also been infrequently associated with the hemolytic uremic syndrome.[26] If this condition is suspected, the medication should be stopped immediately. Other common side effects include hypertension, neurotoxicity (tremors, headaches, seizures, reversible posterior leukoencephalopathy), electrolyte abnormalities (hyperkalemia, hypomagnesemia), and hyperlipidemia. Tacrolimus is more strongly associated with the development of posttransplant diabetes although hirsutism and gingival hyperplasia are exclusively seen with cyclosporine.[27] CNIs are metabolized via the hepatic cytochrome P-450 system. Thus, any alteration of this system either by medications or hepatic dysfunction could potentially lead to increased toxicity. Inhibition of CNI metabolism (eg, azoles, calcium channel blockers, and macrolides) may result in overimmunosuppression and increased toxicity, whereas increased metabolism (eg, rifampin, phenytoin, phenobarbital) may be associated with inadequate immunosuppression.

Comparative studies of the CNIs suggest that a tacrolimus-based immunosuppression regimen may have greater efficacy than a CSA-based regimen. In a single-center, randomized trial of 133 lung recipients treated with a CNI, azathioprine, and prednisone, patients who received tacrolimus were statistically less likely to develop BOS compared with those who received CSA within 2 years (21.7% vs 38%; $P = .025$).[28] A trend toward reduced acute rejection rates and increased survival was also noted in the tacrolimus group, although this was not statistically significant. Notably, greater numbers of patients in the CSA group developed recurrent acute rejection and required crossover to the tacrolimus treatment group, with two-thirds of these patients demonstrating clinical resolution of graft rejection after the switch. No patients initially in the tacrolimus arm required crossover to CSA for recurrent acute rejection.[28] A smaller study comparing the two CNIs in conjunction with MMF and prednisone showed fewer acute rejection episodes per 100 patient-days in the tacrolimus group versus CSA (0.225 vs 0.426; $P<.05$), although 1-year survival rates were not different.[29] Longer-term follow-up (up to 9 years) of these patients did not reveal differences in acute rejection rates, BOS or survival rates.[30] More recently, in a single-center investigation of 90 patients treated with azathioprine and prednisone and randomized to receive either tacrolimus or CSA, the tacrolimus group demonstrated a lower cumulative burden of acute rejection and lymphocytic bronchiolitis over a median follow up period of approximately 2 years.[31] Although the data indicate that a tacrolimus-based maintenance immunosuppression regimen is somewhat more effective at reducing rejection rates without an attendant increased risk of infections or malignancies, it is not clear if this beneficial effect is maintained with different combinations of antiproliferative agents (eg, MMF vs azathioprine).[29,32] Furthermore, a positive impact on long-term outcomes has not been established.

Antiproliferative Agents

Maintenance immunosuppression regimens typically include at least one antiproliferative agent. Azathioprine is the oldest drug in this category and is still used by one-third of all transplant centers.[1] Newer agents such as MMF and sirolimus have been incorporated into immunosuppression protocols at many programs.

Azathioprine is a prodrug metabolized by glutathione to the "antimetabolite" 6-mercaptopurine (6MP) and inactivated by the enzyme thiopurine S-methyltransferase (TPMT). 6MP interferes with purine synthesis, consequently inhibiting DNA and RNA production and ultimately lymphocyte proliferation. Azathioprine may be administered orally or intravenously with a starting dose of 2 mg/kg. However, the dose may need to be adjusted if toxicity is evident (eg, myelosuppression, pancreatitis, cholestatic hepatitis). A dangerous hypersensitivity reaction characterized by a sepsis-like syndrome (fever, nausea, shock) has also been rarely reported and if recognized promptly, may resolve with drug cessation.[33]

Polymorphisms of TPMT that dramatically reduce 6-MP metabolism have been reported in approximately 10% of the population.[34] These patients are at particularly high risk for developing bone marrow toxicity. Thus, many centers routinely screen patients for TPMT deficiency and consider use of an alternative agent if reduced levels are identified. In the future, additional screening tools to identify patients at greater risk for azathioprine associated adverse events may become available (eg, genetic polymorphisms in the gene regulating inosine triphosphate pyrophosphatase) have recently been identified and shown to be associated with drug toxicity.[34]

Fewer drug interactions are noted with azathioprine compared with the CNIs. However, one notable example is with allopurinol, which inhibits 6MP metabolism and may result in a 5-fold increase in 6MP levels.[34] Because of this, the concurrent use of allopurinol with azathioprine should be avoided.

MMF is the most commonly used antiproliferative agent in post–lung transplant immunosuppression regimens.[1] It is hydrolyzed to mycophenolic acid, a potent inhibitor of B- and T-lymphocyte proliferation that blocks inosine monophosphate dehydrogenase, a critical enzyme for the de novo synthesis of guanosine nucleotides. MMF is usually administered twice a day with a total daily dose ranging from 1000 to 3000 mg. Recommendations for monitoring drug levels have not been established in the lung transplant population.

Major side effects of MMF include neutropenia, anemia, diarrhea, nausea, and abdominal pain. A new enteric coated formulation of MMF has recently been introduced and may decrease the incidence of gastrointestinal side effects. It has also has been found to have comparable efficacy to the previous formulation of MMF in renal and cardiac transplantation.[35,36]

Although data from other types of solid organ transplantation have demonstrated superior outcomes (including survival) with MMF compared with azathioprine, two prospective, randomized studies have shown no difference in either short-term (6-month rates of acute rejection and survival) or long-term (rates of acute rejection, BOS, and survival) outcomes.[37–39]

Sirolimus (rapamycin) is an antiproliferative agent structurally similar to tacrolimus. However, it exerts its immunosuppressive effects through a different mechanism. After entering the cytoplasm, sirolimus binds to FKBP forming an immunosuppressive complex that inhibits the mammalian target of rapamycin (mTOR). mTOR is a critical cell cycle regulator involved in cell growth, proliferation and survival. In addition to suppressing T- and B-cell proliferation, sirolimus appears to have a similar effect on proliferation of fibroblasts, vascular smooth muscle cells, and endothelial cells.[40] Numerous side effects have been associated with sirolimus, including diarrhea, nausea, edema, hyperlipidemia, and cytopenia as well as more serious complications such as impaired wound healing, bronchial anastomotic dehiscence, venous thromboembolism, and pneumonitis.[40–43]

In a recent prospective, randomized, controlled, multicenter study of 181 lung recipients comparing sirolimus (initiated 3-months posttransplantation to reduce risk of bronchial anastomotic dehiscence) with azathioprine in a tacrolimus-based immunosuppressive regimen, no differences in acute rejection, BOS, or survival rates at 1 or 3 years were noted.[44] However, there was a high early discontinuation rate in the sirolimus arm due to poor tolerance of the medication. Interestingly, CMV infection rates were lower in the sirolimus arm. Thus, beneficial role for routine use of sirolimus in lung transplantation as part of triple immunosuppression regimen that includes a CNI has not been established. However, in patients with renal insufficiency associated with chronic administration of CNIs, substitution of the CNI with sirolimus may improve renal function.[45] Patients who develop posttransplant malignancies, especially recurrent skin cancers, may also benefit from treatment with sirolimus.[46] In single-center, prospective, assessor-blinded, randomized trial of renal transplant recipients, transition to sirolimus treatment inhibited the progression of premalignant lesions and new nonmelanoma skin cancers.[47]

A second mTOR inhibitor, everolimus, a derivative of sirolimus with a shorter half-life, was recently approved by the FDA for use in renal transplantation. Its side effect profile appears to be similar to sirolimus. In a recent large, randomized, multicenter, double-blind study in lung transplantation comparing everolimus to azathioprine, in addition to cyclosporine and corticosteroids, pulmonary function, rates of BOS, and survival were similar. Adverse events, however, were increased in the everolimus group.[48]

Antihumoral Therapies

Standard maintenance immunosuppression regimens primarily suppress cell-mediated immunity.

However, over the past decade there has been increasing recognition of the important role of humoral immunity. Antibody-mediated rejection (AMR) in lung transplantation is a distinct form of graft dysfunction with potentially devastating impact on both short-term and long-term graft function. Although the mechanisms by which antibodies—usually donor-specific antibodies (DSA)—trigger lung injury are not well understood, it is thought that antibody-binding to HLA antigens in the graft induces complement-mediated and complement-independent inflammation and damage.[49,50] Preventative approaches include performance of a "virtual crossmatch" to avoid transplantation of a donor organ into a recipient with pre-existing anti-HLA antigens specific for the donor HLA type. However, between 11% and 56% of lung recipients have been reported to develop de novo DSA following transplantation.[51,52] Some centers have adopted the practice of routinely treating asymptomatic patients with antihumoral therapies such as intravenous immunoglobulin or the B-cell–depleting agent rituximab.[51] Whether or not specific interventions to reduce or eliminate these antibodies are effective and diminish the risk of AMR is uncertain and will be the subject of an upcoming randomized, placebo-controlled clinical trial funded by the National Institutes of Health.

NOVEL APPROACHES

Although improvement in surgical techniques, organ preservation methods, intensive care unit management, and current immunosuppressive therapy regimens have resulted in better early outcomes after lung transplantation, long-term survival remains poor. This has led to increased interest in alternative approaches to maintenance immunosuppression, treatment of graft rejection, and monitoring of immunosuppression to optimize efficacy and minimize toxicity.

Aerosolized Immunosuppression

Unlike other types of solid organ transplantation, the lung offers the unique opportunity to directly deliver high levels of immunosuppressive medications to the allograft through inhalation of aerosolized medications while limiting systemic exposure. Aerosolization of cyclosporine has been the subject of several recent and ongoing clinical trials in lung transplantation. In a single-center, randomized, double-blind, placebo-controlled trial of inhaled cyclosporine initiated within 6 weeks after transplantation and given in conjunction with a standard systemic immunosuppression regimen, 58 patients were randomized to receive either 300 mg of aerosol cyclosporine or aerosol placebo 3 days a week for the first 2 years after transplantation.[53] No differences were noted in the primary endpoint, rates of acute rejection (A2 or greater), between the two treatment groups. Notably, however, overall survival and BOS-free survival were significantly better in the treatment arm. Furthermore, there was no difference in rates of respiratory infections or other adverse events between the two groups.[53] Aerosolized cyclosporine is currently under investigation in a much larger phase III multicenter clinical trial that recently achieved its target enrollment of approximately 300 patients (ClinicalTrials.gov identifier: NCT00633373). Small case series have suggested that this agent may also have a role in the treatment of established BOS or persistent acute rejection; however, larger, better designed studies are needed to establish efficacy.[54,55] Aerosols of other immunosuppressive agents (eg, tacrolimus) are also being developed and currently are under investigation in preclinical trials.[56]

Inhaled corticosteroids have been the subject of several reports. The largest study included 30 lung recipients who were 3 to 9 months out from transplantation.[57] They were randomized to receive either 750 µg of fluticasone or placebo twice daily for 3 months. Twenty of these patients continued in the study for an additional 15 to 21 months. Neither short-term nor long-term administration of inhaled fluticasone resulted in significant differences in survival, rates of acute rejection, or development of BOS. Thus, the limited available evidence does not support routine use of inhaled corticosteroids for the prevention of graft rejection. Several investigators have advocated use of these agents for treatment of lymphocytic bronchiolitis or established BOS-based on data showing that inhaled corticosteroids reduce markers of airway inflammation and perhaps stabilize pulmonary function; however, their impact on more meaningful clinical outcomes is uncertain.[58–60]

Macrolides

Studies from patients with diffuse panbronchiolitis and cystic fibrosis have shown that macrolide antibiotics exhibit several immunomodulatory properties that have beneficial effects on pulmonary function.[61] Macrolides downregulate production of a number of proinflammatory cytokines (eg, IL-8, IL-6) and increase levels of anti-inflammatory cytokines (eg, IL-10). These agents may also reduce neutrophil adhesion and chemotaxis, decrease production of reactive oxygen species, and promote apoptosis of activated neutrophils. Their effects on bacterial adherence to airways, composition of airway biofilm, and bacterial cell-cell communication through quorum signaling may further protect the airways from infection and subsequent inflammation. Macrolides also increase gastric motility and it is possible that reduced gastroesophageal reflux disease (GERD) with macrolide treatment may contribute to its beneficial effects on pulmonary function.[62] The reader is referred to several recent reviews for further information on the immunomodulatory properties of macrolides.[61,63-65]

Investigators from Johns Hopkins were the first to evaluate the role of macrolides in lung transplantation. In a small open-label pilot study, six lung transplant recipients with clinical BOS stage 1 or greater who were treated with 250 mg of azithromycin three times per week after an initial loading dose of 500 mg per day for 3 days. Five patients demonstrated significant improvement in pulmonary function with a mean improvement in forced expiratory volume in 1 second [FEV1] of 630 mL.[66] The results of a large single-center retrospective study and several small prospective studies further support the beneficial effect of macrolides, although it appears that only about one-third to half of lung recipients with BOS respond to azithromycin treatment.[64] In a retrospective single-center analysis of 179 consecutive lung transplant recipients who developed at least stage 1 BOS, treatment with azithromycin before the development of BOS stage 2 was independently associated with a reduced risk for death.[67] The largest prospective study of azithromycin therapy involved 14 patients with varying degrees of BOS (stage 0-p to 3).[68] These patients were treated for 12 weeks with azithromycin (250 mg 3 times per week after a loading dose of 250 mg/day for 5 days). Six of 14 patients were noted to have improvement in pulmonary function defined by a greater than 10% increase in FEV1. Interestingly, compared with nonresponders, those patients who responded to azithromycin were noted to have increased bronchoalveolar lavage fluid (BALF) neutrophilia (>15% neutrophils was predictive of response to azithromycin) as well as higher levels of IL-8 mRNA. In responders, treatment with azithromycin reduced BALF neutrophilia and IL-8 levels.[68] Further studies are needed to better identify subsets of patients most likely to benefit from macrolide therapy.

The excellent safety profile of azithromycin and other macrolides has led to widespread use for treatment of BOS despite the absence of strong clinical evidence from larger randomized control trials. In fact, some centers have adopted use of azithromycin early after transplantation for prophylaxis against BOS. This practice is supported by a recent single-center, randomized, double-blind control trial of 83 patients.[69] Forty patients received azithromycin initiated within 30 days of transplantation and continued for 2 years. The treatment group had a lower incidence of BOS and improved BOS-free survival compared with 43 patients receiving placebo. Overall survival was not different between the two groups at 2 years. Interestingly rates of acute rejection, lymphocytic bronchiolitis, GERD, colonization with *Pseudomonas*, and CMV-pneumonitis were similar in both arms.[69] One emerging concern about chronic long-term use of macrolide antibiotics in lung transplant patients is the development of antimicrobial resistance.[64] This would be particularly worrisome for patients who develop aggressive infections with atypical mycobacterial species such as *Mycobacterium abscessus* for which macrolides are essential components of treatment regimens.[70]

Statins

There is emerging evidence that statins, or more specifically the 3-hydroxy-3-methylglutaryl coenzyme A reductase inhibitors, possess a number of antiinflammatory-immunomodulatory properties that may downregulate the alloimmune response, in addition to their effects on cholesterol synthesis. For example, in vitro studies have shown that statins reduce γ-interferon-induced expression of major histocompatibility complex (MHC) class II molecules on human endothelial cells and macrophages.[71] Because an important component of the adaptive immune response to the allograft is initiated by presentation of donor antigen by MHC class II molecules on antigen-presenting cells to recipient T-cells, statins, in theory, could reduce rates of graft rejection.[72] Additional evidence from other studies indicate that statins modulate T-cell activation and differentiation, increase numbers of $CD4^+CD25^+$ regulatory T cells, reduce lymphocyte adhesion and pulmonary neutrophil influx, and inhibit expression of proinflammatory cytokines.[73-76]

Clinical evidence supporting a potential benefit of statins in transplantation was first reported in cardiac transplantation.[77] In addition to lowering cholesterol levels, pravastatin was shown to reduce the incidence of cardiac rejection, coronary vasculopathy, and improve 1-year survival. Since then, clinical studies have indicated benefit in other transplant populations. Evidence in the lung transplantation population, however, is limited to one single-center retrospective study of 39 lung transplant recipients who were prescribed statins for treatment of hyperlipidemia and compared with a control group of 161 contemporary lung recipients who were not prescribed statins.[78] Six-year survival was significantly better in the statin group (91%) compared with the control group (54%). In addition, the treatment group had lower rates of acute rejection and BOS.[78] Although prospective randomized trials are needed to confirm these findings, some lung transplant centers have begun to use statins routinely for the treatment or prevention of pulmonary graft dysfunction.[62]

Extracorporeal Photopheresis

Extracorporeal photopheresis (ECP), also called extracorporeal photochemotherapy, is an immunomodulatory technique initially developed for the treatment of cutaneous T-cell lymphoma that is slowly gaining acceptance as a therapeutic modality for the treatment of refractory rejection or graft-versus-host disease after solid organ and hematopoietic stem cell transplantation.[79] ECP involves three steps: leukapheresis, ex vivo incubation of collected peripheral blood mononuclear cells with 8-methoxypsoralen (8-MOP), and subsequent photoactivation of 8-MOP with ultraviolet A (UVA) radiation. These "activated" white cells are subsequently reinfused into the patient. The therapeutic mechanism of this modality is not well understood. 8-MOP is a biologically inert compound until activated by UVA. Upon activation, it covalently binds and crosslinks DNA, ultimately triggering leukocyte apoptosis.[80] Since only about 5% to 10% of total circulating leukocytes are exposed to activated 8-MOP during each treatment cycle, it has been hypothesized that there may be other treatment-related effects on cell-mediated immunity besides T-cell depletion.[80] For example, data from animal models and human studies have suggested that ECP may modulate the alloimmune response by increasing the frequency of T-regulatory cells.[81–84] These and other potential therapeutic mechanisms of ECP in transplantation (eg, increased production of anti-inflammatory cytokines) have recently been reviewed.[80,85]

Clinical application of ECP in solid organ transplantation was first reported more than 20 years ago in a small nonrandomized study of kidney donors. Recipients of kidneys from donors pretreated with ECP had lower rates of acute rejection.[86] Since then, there have been numerous reports suggesting benefit for treatment of acute or chronic rejection after various solid organ transplant procedures. The first report in lung transplantation was published in 1995 and described stabilization or mild improvement in the pulmonary function of three patients with refractory BOS treated with ECP.[87]

The largest series in lung transplantation was recently published.[88] In a retrospective single-center review of all patients (n = 60) that received ECP in addition to other immunosuppressive therapies for treatment of progressive BOS between 2000 and 2007, the investigators found a significant reduction in the rate of decline in FEV1 in the 6 months preceding ECP initiation compared with the 6 months after ECP. This benefit appeared to be sustained when pulmonary function data was analyzed at 12 months after ECP initiation. ECP treatment appeared to be relatively safe. However, complications were noted in 10 of 60 patients including eight patients who developed bacteremia related to Hickman catheter infections. There were no malignancies or other life-threatening complications reported.[88]

Although experimental data and clinical reports are encouraging, there are a number of concerns regarding ECP. First, there is an absence of prospective, randomized controlled studies to confirm benefit. ECP is very inconvenient and could impair the patient's quality of life. For example, placement of an indwelling venous catheter is required. Each treatment is lengthy and may take up to 4 hours. ECP is also very expensive with one institution reporting ECP to cost $6,663 per treatment.[88] In addition, many insurance companies do not cover ECP for lung transplant recipients because it is deemed "investigational" in this population. Depending on outpatient availability and insurance requirements, inpatient hospitalization may be required, a particularly difficult issue because standard treatment protocols involve twice weekly ECP for several weeks with tapering of treatment cycles depending on clinical response. A typical regimen involves 24 ECP treatments over a 6-month period.

Investigational Agents

Improved understanding of T-cell biology and alloimmunity has led to the development several new immunosuppressive drugs that are currently in various stages of development. Only a few have been investigated in studies of solid organ transplant recipients. In the future, lung transplant specific clinical trials will be needed to determine if these new drugs will fulfill the promise of better outcomes and improved safety. Below, a few of these novel investigational agents are reviewed in greater detail.

Belatacept, perhaps one of the best studied of the novel immunosuppressive agents, is a second generation humanized cytotoxic T lymphocyte–associated antigen 4 (CTLA-4) fusion protein that blocks the costimulatory signal necessary for T-cell activation by binding CD80 and CD86 on antigen-presenting cells.[89] Two phase 3 clinical trials investigating the role of this agent in kidney transplantation are currently underway.[90,91] One of these trials, titled Belatacept Evaluation of Nephroprotection and Efficacy as Firstline Immunosuppression Trial (BENEFIT), is a 3-year, randomized, controlled, multicenter study comparing high-dose intravenous belatacept, low-dose intravenous belatacept, and oral cyclosporine (in addition to MMF and prednisone) in 686 renal transplant recipients.[90] Analysis of data at 1-year showed similar rates of patient and graft survival in all three study groups, superior renal function in the two belatacept treatment arms, but lower rates of acute rejection in the cyclosporine group. One concerning finding was higher rates of posttransplant lymphoproliferative disorder in the belatacept treatment groups.[90] Longer-term follow-up is needed to clarify the role of belatacept in kidney transplantation. Based on review of available data, the FDA Advisory Committee has recommended approval of belatacept for the prophylaxis of acute rejection in de novo kidney transplant recipients. Evidence from other solid organ transplant populations is currently unavailable, although a study in liver allograft recipients is underway (Clinicaltrials.gov Identifier: NCT00555321).

Voclosporin (Isotechnika; ISA247) is a semisynthetic analog of cyclosporine reported to be a more potent inhibitor of calcineurin. In addition, its potentially nephrotoxic metabolites have been reported to be cleared more rapidly than what has been observed with currently available CNIS. Animal models of transplantation have indicated that Voclosporin prolongs graft survival and is associated with less renal toxicity when compared with cyclosporine.[92] Unfortunately, data from human trials have been less impressive. In a phase IIb dose-ranging, multicenter, open-label clinical trial of 336 kidney transplant recipients, no significant differences in acute rejection rates or GFR was noted.[93] Phase III studies are currently underway.

CP-690,550 (Tasocitinib) is a synthetic orally administered Janus Kinase 3 (JAK3) inhibitor. JAK3s are activated by signaling through cell surface cytokine receptors (eg, IL-2 receptor γ-chain) and play an important role in intracellular signal transduction. Signaling through JAK3 is largely restricted to lymphocytes and has been shown to be important for lymphocyte proliferation, differentiation, survival, and function.[94] In humans, genetic abnormalities resulting in defects of JAK3 protein have been associated with the development of severe combined immunodeficiency.[94] Thus, JAK3 inhibition may lead to profound immunosuppression and potentially have a therapeutic role in the posttransplant setting.

In a phase II clinical trial of two doses of CP-690,550 compared with cyclosporine in 61 renal transplant recipients who also received MMF and prednisone for maintenance immunosuppression, treatment with low-dose (15 mg twice a day) CP-690, 550 resulted in comparable rates of acute rejection and renal function after 6 months. The high-dose (30 mg twice a day) regimen was associated with increased rates of CMV infection and BK nephropathy.[95] Clinical trials evaluating the long-term safety and efficacy of this agent are currently underway.

Most of these newer immunosuppressive agents broadly suppress the immune system rather than selectively targeting the alloimmune response. Thus complications such as opportunistic infections and malignancies will likely continue to threaten quality of life and survival.

Therapeutic Drug Monitoring

Current laboratory approaches to monitor the effects of immunosuppression are inadequate and depend upon suboptimal surrogate markers such as serum drug levels to assess the impact of these agents on an individual's immune system. The development of new techniques to better assess the net effect of combination immunosuppression regimens is essential to reducing adverse events and graft rejection.

The Immune Cell Function Assay (ImmuKnow; Cylex, Columbia, MD, USA) is a novel tool used to monitor the level of immunosuppression in transplant patients. The assay attempts to measure T-cell inhibition by coculturing the transplant recipient's T-cells with phytohemagglutinin, a nonspecific mitogen that stimulates lymphocytes to produce ATP. In theory, high levels of ATP production would suggest inadequate immunosuppression and thus increased risk of graft rejection, whereas low levels of ATP production would indicate excessive immunosuppression and increased risk for infectious complications. Limited data from the lung transplantation population, however, has not confirmed the correlation of rejection rates with high levels of ATP production, although low levels may be associated with higher rates of infection.[96,97] Hopefully, newer pharmacodynamic or pharmacogenetic approaches will lead to development of better tools for therapeutic drug monitoring of immunosuppression.[98]

SUMMARY

Immunosuppressive therapy has contributed significantly to improved survival after solid organ transplantation. Nevertheless, treatment-related adverse events and persistently high risk of chronic graft rejection remain as major obstacles to long-term survival after lung transplantation. The development of new agents, refinements in techniques to monitor immunosuppression, and enhanced understanding of transplant immunobiology are essential for further improvements in outcome.

REFERENCES

1. Christie JD, Edwards LB, Kucheryavaya AY, et al. The Registry of the International Society for Heart and Lung Transplantation: twenty-seventh official adult lung and heart-lung transplant report—2010. J Heart Lung Transplant 2010;29(10):1104–18.

2. Rech AJ, Vonderheide RH. Clinical use of anti-CD25 antibody daclizumab to enhance immune responses to tumor antigen vaccination by targeting regulatory T cells. Ann N Y Acad Sci 2009;1174:99–106.

3. Deeks ED, Keating GM. Rabbit antithymocyte globulin (thymoglobulin): a review of its use in the prevention and treatment of acute renal allograft rejection. Drugs 2009;69(11):1483–512.

4. Neujahr DC, Chen C, Huang X, et al. Accelerated memory cell homeostasis during T cell depletion and approaches to overcome it. J Immunol 2006; 176(8):4632–9.

5. Yeung MY, Sayegh MH. Regulatory T cells in transplantation: what we know and what we do not know. Transplant Proc 2009;41(Suppl 6):S21–6.

6. Ciancio G, Burke GW 3rd. Alemtuzumab (Campath-1H) in kidney transplantation. Am J Transplant 2008; 8(1):15–20.

7. Palmer SM, Miralles AP, Lawrence CM, et al. Rabbit antithymocyte globulin decreases acute rejection after lung transplantation: results of a randomized, prospective study. Chest 1999;116(1):127–33.

8. Hartwig MG, Snyder LD, Appel JZ 3rd, et al. Rabbit anti-thymocyte globulin induction therapy does not prolong survival after lung transplantation. J Heart Lung Transplant 2008;27(5):547–53.

9. Burton CM, Andersen CB, Jensen AS, et al. The incidence of acute cellular rejection after lung transplantation: a comparative study of anti-thymocyte globulin and daclizumab. J Heart Lung Transplant 2006;25(6):638–47.

10. Garrity ER Jr, Villanueva J, Bhorade SM, et al. Low rate of acute lung allograft rejection after the use of daclizumab, an interleukin 2 receptor antibody. Transplantation 2001;71(6):773–7.

11. Moffatt SD, Demers P, Robbins RC, et al. Lung transplantation: a decade of experience. J Heart Lung Transplant 2005;24(2):145–51.

12. Hachem RR, Edwards LB, Yusen RD, et al. The impact of induction on survival after lung transplantation: an analysis of the International Society for Heart and Lung Transplantation Registry. Clin Transplant 2008;22(5):603–8.

13. Mullen JC, Oreopoulos A, Lien DC, et al. A randomized, controlled trial of daclizumab vs anti-thymocyte globulin induction for lung transplantation. J Heart Lung Transplant 2007;26(5):504–10.

14. van Loenhout KC, Groves SC, Galazka M, et al. Early outcomes using alemtuzumab induction in lung transplantation. Interact Cardiovasc Thorac Surg 2010;10(2):190–4.

15. Hardy JD, Webb WR, Dalton ML Jr, et al. Lung homotransplantation in man. JAMA 1963;186:1065–74.

16. Unilateral lung transplantation for pulmonary fibrosis. Toronto Lung Transplant Group. N Engl J Med 1986;314(18):1140–5.

17. Dunn CJ, Wagstaff AJ, Perry CM, et al. Cyclosporin: an updated review of the pharmacokinetic properties, clinical efficacy and tolerability of a microemulsion-based formulation (neoral)1 in organ transplantation. Drugs 2001;61(13):1957–2016.

18. Monchaud C, Marquet P. Pharmacokinetic optimization of immunosuppressive therapy in thoracic transplantation: part I. Clin Pharmacokinet 2009;48(7): 419–62.

19. Reams BD, Palmer SM. Sublingual tacrolimus for immunosuppression in lung transplantation: a potentially important therapeutic option in cystic fibrosis. Am J Respir Med 2002;1(2):91–8.

20. van de Plas A, Dackus J, Christiaans MH, et al. A pilot study on sublingual administration of tacrolimus. Transpl Int 2009;22(3):358–9.

21. Levy G, Thervet E, Lake J, et al. Patient management by Neoral C(2) monitoring: an international consensus statement. Transplantation 2002;73 (Suppl 9):S12–8.

22. Iversen M, Nilsson F, Sipponen J, et al. Cyclosporine C2 levels have impact on incidence of rejection in de novo lung but not heart transplant recipients: the NOCTURNE study. J Heart Lung Transplant 2009; 28(9):919–26.

23. Glanville AR, Aboyoun CL, Morton JM, et al. Cyclosporine C2 target levels and acute cellular rejection after lung transplantation. J Heart Lung Transplant 2006;25(8):928–34.

24. Ragette R, Kamler M, Weinreich G, et al. Tacrolimus pharmacokinetics in lung transplantation: new strategies for monitoring. J Heart Lung Transplant 2005; 24(9):1315–9.

25. Hesselink DA, Bouamar R, van Gelder T. The pharmacogenetics of calcineurin inhibitor-related nephrotoxicity. Ther Drug Monit 2010;32(4):387–93.

26. Schwimmer J, Nadasdy TA, Spitalnik PF, et al. De novo thrombotic microangiopathy in renal transplant recipients: a comparison of hemolytic uremic syndrome with localized renal thrombotic microangiopathy. Am J Kidney Dis 2003;41(2):471–9.

27. McShane P, Bhorade SM. Maintenance immunosuppression in lung transplantation. In: Vigneswaran WT, Garrity ER, editors. Lung transplantation. London: Informa Health Care; 2010. p. 272–84.

28. Keenan RJ, Konishi H, Kawai A, et al. Clinical trial of tacrolimus versus cyclosporine in lung transplantation. Ann Thorac Surg 1995;60(3):580–4 [discussion: 584–5].

29. Treede H, Klepetko W, Reichenspurner H, et al. Tacrolimus versus cyclosporine after lung transplantation: a prospective, open, randomized two-center trial comparing two different immunosuppressive protocols. J Heart Lung Transplant 2001;20(5):511–7.

30. McCurry K, Zaldonis D, Keenan R, et al. Long term follow-up of a prospective randomized trial of tacrolimus versus cyclosporine in human lung transplantation. Am J Transplant 2002;2(Suppl 3):159 [abstract: 87].

31. Hachem RR, Yusen RD, Chakinala MM, et al. A randomized controlled trial of tacrolimus versus cyclosporine after lung transplantation. J Heart Lung Transplant 2007;26(10):1012–8.

32. Zuckermann A, Reichenspurner H, Birsan T, et al. Cyclosporine A versus tacrolimus in combination with mycophenolate mofetil and steroids as primary immunosuppression after lung transplantation: one-year results of a 2-center prospective randomized trial. J Thorac Cardiovasc Surg 2003;125(4):891–900.

33. Fields CL, Robinson JW, Roy TM, et al. Hypersensitivity reaction to azathioprine. South Med J 1998; 91(5):471–4.

34. Sahasranaman S, Howard D, Roy S. Clinical pharmacology and pharmacogenetics of thiopurines. Eur J Clin Pharmacol 2008;64(8):753–67.

35. Kobashigawa JA, Renlund DG, Gerosa G, et al. Similar efficacy and safety of enteric-coated mycophenolate sodium (EC-MPS, myfortic) compared with mycophenolate mofetil (MMF) in de novo heart transplant recipients: results of a 12-month, single-blind, randomized, parallel-group, multicenter study. J Heart Lung Transplant 2006;25(8):935–41.

36. Budde K, Curtis J, Knoll G, et al. Enteric-coated mycophenolate sodium can be safely administered in maintenance renal transplant patients: results of a 1-year study. Am J Transplant 2004;4(2):237–43.

37. McNeil K, Glanville AR, Wahlers T, et al. Comparison of mycophenolate mofetil and azathioprine for prevention of bronchiolitis obliterans syndrome in de novo lung transplant recipients. Transplantation 2006;81(7):998–1003.

38. Eisen HJ, Kobashigawa J, Keogh A, et al. Three-year results of a randomized, double-blind, controlled trial of mycophenolate mofetil versus azathioprine in cardiac transplant recipients. J Heart Lung Transplant 2005;24(5):517–25.

39. Palmer SM, Baz MA, Sanders L, et al. Results of a randomized, prospective, multicenter trial of mycophenolate mofetil versus azathioprine in the prevention of acute lung allograft rejection. Transplantation 2001;71(12):1772–6.

40. Augustine JJ, Bodziak KA, Hricik DE. Use of sirolimus in solid organ transplantation. Drugs 2007; 67(3):369–91.

41. Ahya VN, McShane PJ, Baz MA, et al. Increased risk of venous thromboembolism with a sirolimus-based immunosuppression regimen in lung transplantation. J Heart Lung Transplant 2011;30(2):175–81.

42. Champion L, Stern M, Israel-Biet D, et al. Brief communication: sirolimus-associated pneumonitis: 24 cases in renal transplant recipients. Ann Intern Med 2006;144(7):505–9.

43. King-Biggs MB, Dunitz JM, Park SJ, et al. Airway anastomotic dehiscence associated with use of sirolimus immediately after lung transplantation. Transplantation 2003;75(9):1437–43.

44. Bhorade S, Ahya VN, Baz MA, et al. Comparison of Sirolimus to Azathioprine in a Tacrolimus based immunosuppressive Regimen in Lung Transplantation. Am J Respir Crit Care Med 2011;183(3):379–87.

45. Snell GI, Levvey BJ, Chin W, et al. Sirolimus allows renal recovery in lung and heart transplant recipients with chronic renal impairment. J Heart Lung Transplant 2002;21(5):540–6.

46. Ciuffreda L, Di Sanza C, Incani UC, et al. The mTOR pathway: a new target in cancer therapy. Curr Cancer Drug Targets 2010;10(5):484–95.

47. Salgo R, Gossmann J, Schofer H, et al. Switch to a sirolimus-based immunosuppression in long-term renal transplant recipients: reduced rate of (pre-) malignancies and nonmelanoma skin cancer in a prospective, randomized, assessor-blinded, controlled clinical trial. Am J Transplant 2010;10(6): 1385–93.

48. Snell GI, Valentine VG, Vitulo P, et al. Everolimus versus azathioprine in maintenance lung transplant recipients: an international, randomized, double-blind clinical trial. Am J Transplant 2006;6(1):169–77.

49. Colvin RB, Smith RN. Antibody-mediated organ-allograft rejection. Nat Rev Immunol 2005;5(10): 807–17.

50. Glanville AR. Antibody-mediated rejection in lung transplantation: myth or reality? J Heart Lung Transplant 2010;29(4):395–400.

51. Hachem RR, Yusen RD, Meyers BF, et al. Anti-human leukocyte antigen antibodies and preemptive antibody-directed therapy after lung transplantation. J Heart Lung Transplant 2010;29(9):973–80.

52. Palmer SM, Davis RD, Hadjiliadis D, et al. Development of an antibody specific to major histocompatibility antigens detectable by flow cytometry after lung transplant is associated with bronchiolitis obliterans syndrome. Transplantation 2002;74(6):799–804.

53. Iacono AT, Johnson BA, Grgurich WF, et al. A randomized trial of inhaled cyclosporine in

lung-transplant recipients. N Engl J Med 2006; 354(2):141–50.

54. Iacono AT, Smaldone GC, Keenan RJ, et al. Dose-related reversal of acute lung rejection by aerosolized cyclosporine. Am J Respir Crit Care Med 1997;155(5):1690–8.

55. Iacono AT, Keenan RJ, Duncan SR, et al. Aerosolized cyclosporine in lung recipients with refractory chronic rejection. Am J Respir Crit Care Med 1996; 153(4 Pt 1):1451–5.

56. Deuse T, Blankenberg F, Haddad M, et al. Mechanisms behind local immunosuppression using inhaled tacrolimus in preclinical models of lung transplantation. Am J Respir Cell Mol Biol 2010; 43(4):403–12.

57. Whitford H, Walters EH, Levvey B, et al. Addition of inhaled corticosteroids to systemic immunosuppression after lung transplantation: a double-blind, placebo-controlled trial. Transplantation 2002; 73(11):1793–9.

58. Speich R, Boehler A, Russi EW, et al. A case report of a double-blind, randomized trial of inhaled steroids in a patient with lung transplant bronchiolitis obliterans. Respiration 1997;64(5):375–80.

59. Takao M, Higenbottam TW, Audley T, et al. Effects of inhaled nebulized steroids (budesonide) on acute and chronic lung function in heart-lung transplant patients. Transplant Proc 1995;27(1):1284–5.

60. De Soyza A, Fisher AJ, Small T, et al. Inhaled corticosteroids and the treatment of lymphocytic bronchiolitis following lung transplantation. Am J Respir Crit Care Med 2001;164(7):1209–12.

61. Kanoh S, Rubin BK. Mechanisms of action and clinical application of macrolides as immunomodulatory medications. Clin Microbiol Rev 2010;23(3):590–615.

62. Robertson AG, Griffin SM, Murphy DM, et al. Targeting allograft injury and inflammation in the management of post-lung transplant bronchiolitis obliterans syndrome. Am J Transplant 2009;9(6):1272–8.

63. Altenburg J, de Graaff CS, van der Werf TS, et al. Immunomodulatory effects of macrolide antibiotics - Part 1: biological mechanisms. Respiration 2011; 81(1):67–74.

64. Crosbie PA, Woodhead MA. Long-term macrolide therapy in chronic inflammatory airway diseases. Eur Respir J 2009;33(1):171–81.

65. Friedlander AL, Albert RK. Chronic macrolide therapy in inflammatory airways diseases. Chest 2010;138(5):1202–12.

66. Gerhardt SG, McDyer JF, Girgis RE, et al. Maintenance azithromycin therapy for bronchiolitis obliterans syndrome: results of a pilot study. Am J Respir Crit Care Med 2003;168(1):121–5.

67. Jain R, Hachem RR, Morrell MR, et al. Azithromycin is associated with increased survival in lung transplant recipients with bronchiolitis obliterans syndrome. J Heart Lung Transplant 2010;29(5):531–7.

68. Verleden GM, Vanaudenaerde BM, Dupont LJ, et al. Azithromycin reduces airway neutrophilia and interleukin-8 in patients with bronchiolitis obliterans syndrome. Am J Respir Crit Care Med 2006; 174(5):566–70.

69. Vos R, Vanaudenaerde BM, Verleden SE, et al. A randomized placebo-controlled trial of azithromycin to prevent bronchiolitis obliterans syndrome after lung transplantation. Eur Respir J 2011;37(1):164–72.

70. Chernenko SM, Humar A, Hutcheon M, et al. Mycobacterium abscessus infections in lung transplant recipients: the international experience. J Heart Lung Transplant 2006;25(12):1447–55.

71. Kwak B, Mulhaupt F, Myit S, et al. Statins as a newly recognized type of immunomodulator. Nat Med 2000;6(12):1399–402.

72. Martinu T, Howell DN, Palmer SM. Acute cellular rejection and humoral sensitization in lung transplant recipients. Semin Respir Crit Care Med 2010;31(2): 179–88.

73. Steffens S, Mach F. Drug insight: immunomodulatory effects of statins—potential benefits for renal patients? Nat Clin Pract Nephrol 2006;2(7):378–87.

74. Young RP, Hopkins R, Eaton TE. Pharmacological actions of statins: potential utility in COPD. Eur Respir Rev 2009;18(114):222–32.

75. Mausner-Fainberg K, Luboshits G, Mor A, et al. The effect of HMG-CoA reductase inhibitors on naturally occurring CD4+CD25+ T cells. Atherosclerosis 2008;197(2):829–39.

76. Broady R, Levings MK. Graft-versus-host disease: suppression by statins. Nat Med 2008;14(11): 1155–6.

77. Kobashigawa JA, Katznelson S, Laks H, et al. Effect of pravastatin on outcomes after cardiac transplantation. N Engl J Med 1995;333(10):621–7.

78. Johnson BA, Iacono AT, Zeevi A, et al. Statin use is associated with improved function and survival of lung allografts. Am J Respir Crit Care Med 2003; 167(9):1271–8.

79. Edelson R, Berger C, Gasparro F, et al. Treatment of cutaneous T-cell lymphoma by extracorporeal photochemotherapy. Preliminary results. N Engl J Med 1987;316(6):297–303.

80. Knobler R, Barr ML, Couriel DR, et al. Extracorporeal photopheresis: past, present, and future. J Am Acad Dermatol 2009;61(4):652–65.

81. Maeda A, Schwarz A, Kernebeck K, et al. Intravenous infusion of syngeneic apoptotic cells by photopheresis induces antigen-specific regulatory T cells. J Immunol 2005;174(10):5968–76.

82. George JF, Gooden CW, Guo L, et al. Role for CD4 (+)CD25(+) T cells in inhibition of graft rejection by extracorporeal photopheresis. J Heart Lung Transplant 2008;27(6):616–22.

83. Gatza E, Rogers CE, Clouthier SG, et al. Extracorporeal photopheresis reverses experimental

graft-versus-host disease through regulatory T cells. Blood 2008;112(4):1515–21.

84. Biagi E, Di Biaso I, Leoni V, et al. Extracorporeal photochemotherapy is accompanied by increasing levels of circulating CD4+CD25+GITR+Foxp3+ CD62L+ functional regulatory T-cells in patients with graft-versus-host disease. Transplantation 2007; 84(1):31–9.

85. Hivelin M, Siemionow M, Grimbert P, et al. Extracorporeal photopheresis: from solid organs to face transplantation. Transpl Immunol 2009;21(3):117–28.

86. Oesterwitz H, Scholz D, Kaden J, et al. Photochemical donor pretreatment in clinical kidney transplantation—preliminary report. Urol Res 1987;15(4): 211–3.

87. Slovis BS, Loyd JE, King LE Jr. Photopheresis for chronic rejection of lung allografts. N Engl J Med 1995;332(14):962.

88. Morrell MR, Despotis GJ, Lublin DM, et al. The efficacy of photopheresis for bronchiolitis obliterans syndrome after lung transplantation. J Heart Lung Transplant 2010;29(4):424–31.

89. Larsen CP, Pearson TC, Adams AB, et al. Rational development of LEA29Y (belatacept), a high-affinity variant of CTLA4-Ig with potent immunosuppressive properties. Am J Transplant 2005;5(3):443–53.

90. Vincenti F, Charpentier B, Vanrenterghem Y, et al. A phase III study of belatacept-based immunosuppression regimens versus cyclosporine in renal transplant recipients (BENEFIT study). Am J Transplant 2010;10(3):535–46.

91. Durrbach A, Pestana JM, Pearson T, et al. A phase III study of belatacept versus cyclosporine in kidney transplants from extended criteria donors (BENEFIT-EXT study). Am J Transplant 2010;10(3):547–57.

92. Aspeslet L, Freitag D, Trepanier D, et al. ISA(TX)247: a novel calcineurin inhibitor. Transplant Proc 2001; 33(1–2):1048–51.

93. Gaber AO, Busque S, Mulgaonkar S, et al. ISA247: a phase IIB multicenter, open label, concentration-controlled trial in de novo renal transplantation. Am J Transplant 2008;8(Suppl 2):336 [abstract: #LB306].

94. Changelian PS, Flanagan ME, Ball DJ, et al. Prevention of organ allograft rejection by a specific Janus kinase 3 inhibitor. Science 2003;302(5646):875–8.

95. Busque S, Leventhal J, Brennan DC, et al. Calcineurin-inhibitor-free immunosuppression based on the JAK inhibitor CP-690, 550: a pilot study in de novo kidney allograft recipients. Am J Transplant 2009; 9(8):1936–45.

96. Bhorade SM, Janata K, Vigneswaran WT, et al. Cylex ImmuKnow assay levels are lower in lung transplant recipients with infection. J Heart Lung Transplant 2008;27(9):990–4.

97. Husain S, Raza K, Pilewski JM, et al. Experience with immune monitoring in lung transplant recipients: correlation of low immune function with infection. Transplantation 2009;87(12):1852–7.

98. Wieland E, Olbricht CJ, Susal C, et al. Biomarkers as a tool for management of immunosuppression in transplant patients. Ther Drug Monit 2010;32(5): 560–72.

Primary Graft Dysfunction

James C. Lee, MD[a],*, Jason D. Christie, MD, MS[a,b]

KEYWORDS

- Lung transplantation • Primary graft dysfunction
- Bronchiolitis obliterans syndrome • Biomarkers

Primary graft dysfunction (PGD), a form of acute lung injury analogous to acute respiratory distress syndrome (ARDS), arises within the first 72 hours following lung transplantation, and is a leading cause of early morbidity and mortality. Previously known as "primary graft failure" or "reperfusion edema," PGD affects up to 25% of all lung transplant procedures and currently has no proven preventive therapy.[1–7] When compared with lung transplant recipients who do not develop PGD, 30-day mortality rates are up to eightfold higher in patients with the most severe form of PGD. Lung transplant recipients who recover from significant PGD may have impaired long-term function[5] and an increased risk of bronchiolitis obliterans syndrome (BOS).[8] Several reviews of PGD have recently been published[9,10]; this article aims to provide a state-of-the-art update on the current epidemiology, risk factors, biomarker studies, and intervention trials on PGD.

DEFINITION AND EPIDEMIOLOGY

In its severe forms, PGD results in impaired oxygenation and decreased lung compliance. Diffuse pulmonary infiltrates are seen radiographically (**Fig. 1**), and pathology reveals diffuse alveolar damage. This pattern of lung injury is clinically analogous to the spectrum of acute lung injury and ARDS, and similarly, treatment for PGD remains largely supportive. In 2005, to standardize clinical and research efforts related to PGD that had previously been inconsistent and variable, the International Society for Heart and Lung Transplantation (ISHLT) Working Group on PGD proposed a definition and grading system. Similar to that for acute lung injury and ARDS, the proposed definition of PGD was based on $Pa_{O_2}/F_{I_{O_2}}$ (P/F) ratio and radiographic infiltrates assessed at several time points up to 72 hours after transplant (**Table 1**).[7]

Studies published prior to the ISHLT guidelines report varying incidences of PGD.[6] Using a definition of PGD similar to the definition of ARDS (Grade 3 PGD), the reported incidence of PGD ranges from 10% to 25%, with 30-day mortality close to 50%.[1–3,11,12] If a less stringent definition of PGD is used, reported incidences of PGD increase to up to 57% of all lung transplants, with no significant mortality differences between patients who developed PGD and those who did not.[13]

Shortly after the ISHLT guidelines for PGD were published, Prekker and colleagues[14] validated the grading system in a retrospective review of 402 lung transplants performed at a single academic institution over 12 years. The investigators showed that short-term and long-term mortality and length of intensive care unit (ICU)/hospital stay were significantly associated with Grade 3 PGD based on the worst P/F measured within the first 48 hours after transplant. Prekker and colleagues also showed no significant differences in long-term survival between PGD Grades 1 and 2.[14] Survival at 90 days post transplant for the lower grade PGD groups was similar when compared with the program's overall survival rate (10% and 8%, respectively for PGD Grades 1 and 2 vs 12% overall 90-day mortality).[14]

[a] Division of Pulmonary, Allergy and Critical Care Medicine, University of Pennsylvania School of Medicine, 826 West Gates Building, 3400 Spruce Street, Philadelphia, PA 19104, USA
[b] Department of Biostatistics and Epidemiology, Center for Clinical Epidemiology and Biostatistics, University of Pennsylvania School of Medicine, 423 Guardian Drive, 719 Blockley Hall, Philadelphia, PA 19104, USA
* Corresponding author.
E-mail address: james.lee@uphs.upenn.edu

Clin Chest Med 32 (2011) 279–293
doi:10.1016/j.ccm.2011.02.007
0272-5231/11/$ – see front matter © 2011 Elsevier Inc. All rights reserved.

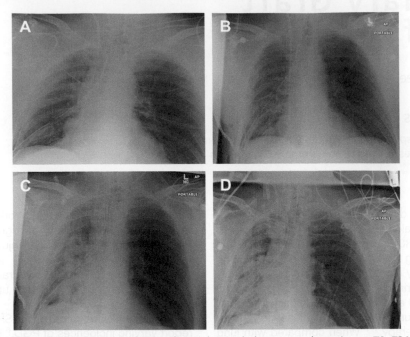

Fig. 1. (*A–D*) Radiographic progression of PGD after right single lung transplantation at T0, T24, T48, and T72.

More recently, the authors' group[15] published a study from the multicenter Lung Transplant Outcomes Group examining the discriminatory validity of the ISHLT PGD definition using previously described biomarker profiles and by conducting a survival analysis of a cohort of 450 patients. In this study, PGD Grade 3 was associated with greater differences in levels of biomarkers known to be altered in severe PGD, regardless of time point used for grading. Furthermore, PGD graded at 48 and 72 hours discriminated mortality better than PGD graded at 24 hours (**Fig. 2**).[15] These findings illustrate the discriminatory ability of the ISHLT PGD definition and its utility for use in clinical studies, suggesting that PGD Grade 3 at any point in time represents a useful threshold for the most severe form of lung injury. However, in this study the intermediate grades of injury (Grades 1 and 2) showed worse mortality compared with Grade 0. These findings, taken together with the links of intermediate grade PGD with BOS[16] (see later discussion), provide evidence for continuing classification of Grades 0, 1, 2, and 3.

The PGD definition and grading system are relatively new and could potentially be improved upon. Several proposed changes to the PGD grading system have been suggested, and are summarized in **Table 2**. These proposed refinements involve timing of P/F measurements, adding earlier time points for grading, examining trends of P/F, and evaluating PGD differently in single and bilateral lung transplant recipients.[17,18] There is sound physiologic basis behind these distinctions, and such refinements to the 2005 ISHLT PGD definition and guidelines represent fertile ground for future investigation.[19]

OUTCOMES

Several studies have investigated PGD patient outcomes since the ISHLT guidelines were published, adding evidence to the large impact of PGD on both short-term and long-term outcomes following lung transplantation. In a retrospective

Table 1
ISHLT PGD grading schema

Grade	Pao_2/Fio_2	Radiographic Infiltrates Consistent with Pulmonary Edema
0	>300	Absent
1	>300	Present
2	200–300	Present
3	<200	Present

Time points for assessment: T (0 to within 6 hours of reperfusion, 24, 48, and 72 hours).
Data from Christie JD, Carby M, Bag R, et al. Report of the ISHLT Working Group on Primary Lung Graft Dysfunction part II: definition. A consensus statement of the International Society for Heart and Lung Transplantation. J Heart Lung Transplant 2005;24:1458.

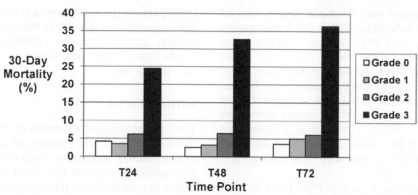

Fig. 2. Impact of primary graft dysfunction on 30-day mortality at different time points. (*Reproduced from Christie JD, Bellamy S, Ware LB, et al. Construct validity of the definition of primary graft dysfunction after lung transplantation. J Heart Lung Transplant 2010;29:1236; with permission.*)

review of 255 consecutive lung transplant procedures employing an outcome definition of Grade 3 PGD within 72 hours, Christie and colleagues[5] showed that all-cause 30-day mortality in patients with PGD versus those without was 63.3% versus 8.8%, hospital length of stay was 47 days versus 15 days, duration of mechanical ventilation was 15 days versus 1 day, and only 28.5% of survivors achieved normal 6-minute walk test distance at 12 months after transplant versus 71.4% of those without PGD. With the aim of examining the effect of PGD on long-term outcomes, Whitson and colleagues[20] reviewed 374 lung transplant procedures and graded PGD over the first 48 hours after transplant. Survival rates were 51% and 11% at 5 and 10 years in those patients who developed Grade 3 PGD at the time of transplant. In addition, BOS-free survival was lower in the severe PGD group, though the effect was limited to bilateral transplants.

Prior studies yielded conflicting results about the association between PGD and BOS,[21–25] but recent evidence has shown this link between PGD and BOS to be significant, even for intermediate grades of PGD. Examining a retrospective cohort of 337 lung transplant recipients, Daud and colleagues[8] showed that the risk of developing stage 1 BOS was directly related to PGD grade immediately after transplant (T0) and was independent of acute rejection, lymphocytic bronchiolitis, and community-acquired respiratory infection (3 widely accepted risk factors for BOS). More recent work by this group evaluated the association between PGD graded at 24, 48, and 72 hours (T24, T48, T72) after transplant and the risk of BOS 1, and progression to BOS 2 and 3. There was a direct relationship between the severity of PGD and the risk of BOS at all time points,[16] again independent of other recognized BOS risk factors. Grade 3 PGD was associated with the highest risk for BOS development at all time points (relative risk of 3.31 at T24).[16]

While the differences in both short-term and long-term survival following lung transplant seem

Table 2
Proposed refinements to the ISHLT PGD Grading system

	ISHLT PGD Guidelines	Proposed Refinement
Definition of T0	<6 hours after final reperfusion (at the time of ICU admission)	At the time of ICU admission
Time points	T0, T24, T48, T72: use worse P/F (when multiple readings are available)	T0, T6, T12, T24, T48, T72: use P/F closest to these time points
CXR: unilateral infiltrates in BLT	No suggestions	Consider infiltrates only if bilateral
Type of transplant	Apply same criteria	Apply SLT and BLT separately

Abbreviations: BLT, bilateral lung transplant; CXR, chest radiograph; SLT, single lung transplant.
Data from Oto T, Levvey BJ, Snell GI. Potential refinements of the International Society for Heart and Lung Transplantation primary graft dysfunction grading system. J Heart Lung Transplant 2007;26:435.

most pronounced with the most severe form of lung injury as defined by PGD Grade 3, less severe forms of lung injury (PGD Grades 1 and 2) are also associated with higher risk of death and worse long-term outcomes. As already described, when graded at 72 hours post transplant, PGD Grades 1 and 2 were associated with a higher risk of 30-day and overall mortality when compared with Grade 0 PGD.[15] This result is consistent with findings by Daud and colleagues[8] that increasing PGD grade was associated with increasing BOS risk.

The mechanisms by which PGD leads to BOS are not fully understood and require further investigation. In addition to as yet unidentified genetic factors that predispose certain lung transplant recipients to develop both PGD and BOS, there are several plausible mechanisms for this relationship, as summarized in **Table 3**. These mechanisms highlight the multiple pathogenic factors that underlie PGD-induced lung injury in the immediate posttransplant period. However, the subsequent perpetuation of these pathogenic mechanisms—perhaps not to the degree that is seen immediately after transplant—may contribute

Table 3
Potential mechanisms linking PGD to BOS

Proposed Mechanism	Details
Injury response	ROS generation
	Epithelial, endothelial, and stromal injury
	Aberrant and propagated injury response
	Activation of innate immune system
Initiation of a proinflammatory cascade	Cytokine and stimulatory chemokine release
	Activation of complement system
	Persistent elevation of cytokines after initial PGD injury
Humoral immunity	Pretransplant HLA antibodies potentially drive both PGD and BOS
	Development of novel HLA I and HLA II alloantibodies
	Development of alloantibodies to sequestered antigens

Abbreviations: BOS, bronchiolitis obliterans syndrome; HLA, human leukocyte antigen; PGD, primary graft dysfunction; ROS, reactive oxygen species.

to BOS development. A thorough understanding of the pathogenesis of PGD is therefore relevant to guiding prophylactic or immediate treatment efforts that may then also have an impact on long-term outcomes.

PATHOGENESIS

The multifactorial pathogenesis of PGD is conceptualized in **Fig. 3** and involves all aspects of the lung transplant procedure, beginning with pathophysiologic changes in the donor following brain death, to cold ischemia during organ preservation, and ultimately reperfusion in the recipient. Central to this process is ischemia-reperfusion injury with subsequent generation of damaging reactive oxygen species (ROS).[26] These ROS cause direct injury to pulmonary endothelium and epithelium, resulting in capillary and alveolar leakiness that manifests clinically as hypoxia and radiographic infiltrates seen on chest radiograph. In addition, a complex proinflammatory cascade resulting from the influx of donor macrophages also causes upregulation of chemokines and cytokines. This process leads to the recruitment, localization, and activation of recipient T cells and neutrophils, perpetuating the injury pattern of PGD.[26] Downstream effects also include activation of the classic complement system[27] and the release of platelet-activating factors, further causing leukocytes to release cytokines and express cell adhesion molecules, and causing platelet aggregation and microvascular thrombi.[28–31]

Of importance, many of these pathogenic pathways can be used to identify circulating biomarkers and mediators for those patients who are actively experiencing significant PGD, ideally as early as possible after transplant (and perhaps even before transplant) so as to guide therapy. As discussed later, an understanding of these biomarkers in combination with well-defined clinical risk factors has the potential to affect PGD treatment strategies as well as approaches to organ allocation.

CLINICAL RISK FACTORS

Studies identifying the clinical risk factors for PGD development have been limited by small sample sizes. While larger, longitudinal series have been reported, they are often drawn from several different treatment eras, making firm conclusions difficult.[32,33] Despite these limitations, there are clinical risk factors that have been consistently identified in the literature and can be categorized as donor, recipient, and operative risk factors (**Table 4**). Adding to this literature, Kuntz and

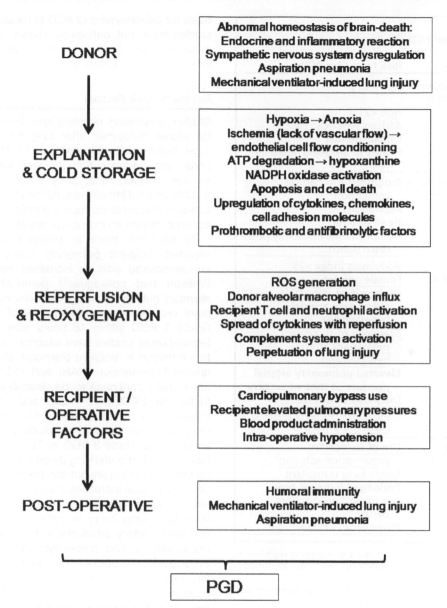

DONOR

> Abnormal homeostasis of brain-death:
> Endocrine and inflammatory reaction
> Sympathetic nervous system dysregulation
> Aspiration pneumonia
> Mechanical ventilator-induced lung injury

EXPLANTATION & COLD STORAGE

> Hypoxia → Anoxia
> Ischemia (lack of vascular flow) →
> endothelial cell flow conditioning
> ATP degradation → hypoxanthine
> NADPH oxidase activation
> Apoptosis and cell death
> Upregulation of cytokines, chemokines,
> cell adhesion molecules
> Prothrombotic and antifibrinolytic factors

REPERFUSION & REOXYGENATION

> ROS generation
> Donor alveolar macrophage influx
> Recipient T cell and neutrophil activation
> Spread of cytokines with reperfusion
> Complement system activation
> Perpetuation of lung injury

RECIPIENT / OPERATIVE FACTORS

> Cardiopulmonary bypass use
> Recipient elevated pulmonary pressures
> Blood product administration
> Intra-operative hypotension

POST-OPERATIVE

> Humoral immunity
> Mechanical ventilator-induced lung injury
> Aspiration pneumonia

PGD

Fig. 3. Conceptualization of pathophysiology of PGD. ATP, adenosine triphosphate; NADPH, nicotinamide adenine dinucleotide phosphate; ROS, reactive oxygen species. (*Reproduced from* Lee JC, Christie JD. Primary graft dysfunction. In: Vigneswaran W, Garrity E, editors. Lung transplantation. London (UK): Informa Healthcare; 2010. p. 242; with permission.)

colleagues recently published a large, retrospective registry study of 6984 transplants performed between 1994 and 2002, with similar findings to previous smaller studies of PGD risk factors (highlighted in **Table 4**). The findings from this study are limited by the coarseness of the PGD definition but are nonetheless consistent with prior studies. As more multicenter, single-era studies are published, these risk factors will likely be further refined. Several important findings related to clinical risk factors for PGD are now discussed.

Donor Risk Factors

Similar to experience in other solid organ transplant procedures, older donor age has been associated with an increased risk of PGD, particularly in donors older than 32 to 45 years.[3,34,35] The

Table 4
Suggested PGD risk factors

Category	Risk Factor for PGD
Donor variables (inherent):	**Age >45 y**
	Age <21 y
	African American race
	Female gender
	History of smoking >10 pack years
Donor variables (acquired):	Prolonged mechanical ventilation
	Aspiration
	<u>Head trauma</u>
	Hemodynamic instability post brain death
Recipient variables:	<u>Body mass index >25</u>
	<u>Female gender</u>
	Diagnosis of idiopathic pulmonary arterial hypertension
	<u>Diagnosis of secondary pulmonary arterial hypertension</u>
	Elevated pulmonary arterial pressure at time of surgery
	<u>Diagnosis of diffuse parenchymal lung disease: pulmonary fibrosis</u>
Operative variables:	<u>Use of Eurocollins preservation solution</u>
	<u>Single lung transplant</u>
	Prolonged ischemic time
	Use of cardiopulmonary bypass
	Blood product transfusion

Bold indicates risk factors most consistently reported in the literature. <u>Underlining</u> indicates risk factors identified in Kuntz et al.[85]

Data from Lee JC, Christie JD. Primary graft dysfunction. Proc Am Thorac Soc 2009;6:40.

youngest donor ages (<21 years), donor African American race, and donor female gender have also been identified as potential risk factors for PGD, though these findings have not been consistently reproduced. Mechanisms for such associations remain speculative.[3] A positive donor smoking history has not consistently been identified as a risk factor for PGD.[33,36] Noninnate donor-acquired risk factors that potentially contribute to the development of PGD include prolonged mechanical ventilation, aspiration pneumonitis/pneumonia or ventilator-associated pneumonia, trauma, and hemodynamic instability/systemic inflammatory response following brain death.[33] Despite a theoretical pathogenic

basis for development of PGD in these situations, studies have not definitively shown such donor acquired risk factors to be associated with increased PGD incidence.

Recipient Risk Factors

Studies examining recipient-specific risk factors for worse outcomes after lung transplantation have been previously reviewed.[32] There is no consistent evidence that recipient factors such as age, gender, race, body weight, underlying hepatic or renal impairment, left heart disease, diabetes, or steroid or inotrope use before surgery are associated with an increased risk of PGD.[32]

By contrast, there is strong evidence that elevated recipient pulmonary artery pressures are associated with an increased risk of PGD. Whitson and colleagues[35] demonstrated that elevated pulmonary artery pressure in the transplant recipient increased the risk of developing Grade 3 PGD within 48 hours after transplant. Several other studies have described an association between a recipient diagnosis of pulmonary arterial hypertension (PAH) and PGD, and this association continues to be described as a risk factor for PGD.[2,3,37–39] Lee and colleagues[40] described an association between elevated mean pulmonary arterial pressures at the time of surgery and Grade 3 PGD at 72 hours that was independent of underlying diagnosis. The reasons for this association are not completely understood, but may involve increased mechanical endothelial shear stress experienced during reperfusion leading to lung injury in patients with elevated pulmonary artery pressures at the time of transplantation, shared pathophysiology or genetic predisposition in both PAH and PGD, or confounding factors such as use of cardiopulmonary bypass or use of blood products.[28,39] Other recipient disease associations with PGD are less consistent across studies. Patients with chronic obstructive pulmonary disease may have the lowest risk of PGD[3,12,41] whereas patients with a diffuse parenchymal lung disease such as idiopathic pulmonary fibrosis (IPF) may have an increased risk of PGD.[32,40,42] The association between secondary elevated pulmonary arterial pressures due to parenchymal lung disease and PGD was recently investigated by Fang and colleagues.[43] In a cohort of 126 lung transplant procedures for IPF, these investigators showed an increased odds ratio of 1.64 for PGD Grade 3 at 72 hours for each 10 mm Hg increase in mean pulmonary arterial pressure measured by right heart catheterization performed at the time of lung transplantation. The use of cardiopulmonary bypass (CPB) partially attenuated this relationship, indicating that CPB use may contribute to PGD in this circumstance.[43]

Operative Risk Factors

The type of transplant procedure performed (single vs bilateral) has not consistently been shown to be an independent risk factor for PGD development. Of importance, potential confounding by more frequent use of CPB in bilateral transplant procedures and a higher percentage of PAH patients undergoing bilateral lung transplant procedures precludes drawing firm conclusions about an association between bilateral lung transplantation and PGD risk. The association between PGD and CPB is also unclear; a recipient diagnosis of PAH is more common in lung transplant procedures that require CPB and also then go on to develop PGD.[44] It has been shown that in lung transplant recipients without an underlying diagnosis of PAH, the need for CPB during surgery was associated with worse early outcomes and death.[41] In contrast to these findings, however, other groups have suggested that CPB use is not an independent risk factor for PGD and that similar early outcomes are attained when CPB use is not dictated by pulmonary hypertension or other factors.[3,45] Variability in the indication for CPB use may contribute to these inconsistencies, such as whether the CPB was employed in a planned fashion or as a result of unforeseen surgical events.

Another operative risk factor of interest in PGD is perioperative blood product transfusions, specifically the risk for transfusion-related lung injury (TRALI) as a potential contributor to PGD incidence. As has been well documented, in its severe forms TRALI can result in an ARDS-like picture identical to that seen in PGD. In the majority of cases, TRALI is thought to be mediated by alloantibodies contained in the transfused blood (ie, derived from the blood donor) that react against recipient-specific leukocyte antigens.[46] In a small proportion of cases (<10%), alloantibodies of recipient origin may be directed against leukocytes from the blood donor.[46] In addition, there are other proposed mechanisms for augmentation of lung injury by blood product transfusion that may not fit the strict TRALI definition.[47–49] Wang and colleagues[50] have shown that bilateral lung transplant procedures, use of CPB, and recipients with a diagnosis of Eisenmenger syndrome or cystic fibrosis had a need for significantly more blood products in the first 24 hours after surgery in comparison with other lung transplant procedures. This study did not directly assess PGD

incidence, but illustrates another potential confounder of blood product transfusion similar to CPB use and PAH diagnosis in the recipient. Recent multicenter studies have also demonstrated the independent association between blood product administration and an increased risk for PGD, but the exact relationship between the two is not yet clear, partially because of the collinear effects of pulmonary hypertension and CPB use.[28,42] A recent communication illustrates the feasibility of conducting human leukocyte antigen (HLA) screening of the sera of pooled blood product donors and transplant recipients in cases of suspected TRALI complicating PGD in order to detect the presence of antibodies transmitted through blood product transfusion that are directed against either the allograft tissue or the lung transplant recipient leukocyte pool.[51] Such a process would help determine the proportion of TRALI cases that are undiagnosed and otherwise labeled as PGD following lung transplantation.

BIOMARKERS OF PGD

A combination of well-defined clinical risk factors with feasible point-of-care testing for biochemical and genetic risk factors in both the donor and recipient could potentially allow for earlier detection of PGD, targeted therapy, or different management strategies. A better understanding of those transplant recipients at highest and lowest risk for developing PGD might allow for the safe extension of the donor pool in select cases, given the perennial short supply of donor organs. At present, there are no well-established nor widely accepted molecular or genetic markers to predict PGD, but with advances in molecular and genetic techniques, measurement of such biomarkers may eventually provide both greater understanding of the pathogenesis and natural history of PGD as well as allow for earlier identification and better prognostication of PGD patients.

Molecular fingerprinting techniques with microarray technology and functional genomics have been applied to acute lung injury.[52] Such techniques are being employed in ischemia-reperfusion injury, though the clinical application of such information is not yet clear.[53] Although there have been no definitive studies illustrating consistent donor clinical risk factors for PGD, several studies have evaluated genetic expression changes in donor lung tissue that are associated with PGD. Ray and colleagues[54] observed changes in gene expression in donor lungs that developed PGD, showing differences in genes involved in signaling, apoptosis, and stress-activated pathways as compared with those that did not. Similarly, Anraku and colleagues[55] identified 4 upregulated genes in donor lung samples in cases of severe PGD that were associated with either death within 30 days or requirement for extracorporeal membrane oxygenation (ECMO) for severe hypoxia. The investigators also measured expression of these genes in donor lung tissue from a group of lung transplant subjects felt to have a poor prognosis (death within 30 days but not definitively attributed to PGD). Compared with controls, the 4 genes were similarly upregulated in this group, illustrating the feasibility of assaying gene expression patterns in donor lungs before implantation to help predict posttransplant PGD.

An incomplete area of investigation in PGD risk involves preexisting humoral immunity in the lung transplant recipient. Elevations in pretransplant panel reactive antibody testing have been shown to be associated with worse posttransplant outcomes.[56] Recent work has focused on detecting specific autoimmunity to newly identified and normally sequestered lung antigens. One such antigen is collagen type V. Using a rodent model, Yoshida and colleagues[57] showed that ischemia-reperfusion injury unmasks antigenic collagen type V, a form of collagen normally intercalated with the more prevalent collagen type I. After exposure of this antigen during ischemia-reperfusion injury, a proliferation of collagen V–specific Th-1 cells follows, thereby mediating PGD.[57] This group also showed that pretransplant collagen V–specific cellular immunity affects PGD. Delayed-type hypersensitivity to collagen V was assessed in 55 patients awaiting lung transplant, and P/F ratios were significantly decreased up to 72 hours after transplant in collagen V–reactive versus nonreactive patients.[58]

Such studies postulate that the injured PGD lung is more immunogenic, the so-called injury response hypothesis[59]—an attractive and plausible concept given that a robust inflammatory response is an important component of the pathophysiology of ischemia-reperfusion injury. The long-term effects of this increased immunogenicity are relevant to the association between PGD and BOS, as already discussed. Burlingham and colleagues[60] have shown that long-term collagen V–specific immune responses have also been associated with the incidence and severity of BOS. Bharat and colleagues[61] showed that 5 years after transplant, patients with a history of PGD had increased de novo anti-HLA type II alloantibodies. The investigators hypothesize that through induction of a proinflammatory state after transplant and increasing donor HLA-II

expression, clinically severe PGD promotes the development of donor-specific alloimmunity, again mechanistically linking PGD and BOS. The same group[62] recently published a follow-up investigation to this work that specifically examines the increased risk of PGD development in patients with antibodies to self-antigens k-α1 tubulin, collagen type V, and collagen I prior to transplant. In 142 lung transplant recipients prospectively enrolled between 1995 and 2005, patients with pretransplant self-antigen antibodies had an increased risk of PGD (odds ratio 3.09, confidence interval 1.2–8.1, $P = .02$) compared with those patients without pretransplant antibodies.[62] At 5-year follow-up, patients without pretransplant self-antigen antibodies had greater freedom from the development of HLA antibodies, and patients with pretransplant self-antigen antibodies had a relative risk of 2.3 for developing BOS.[62] The stress and injury from PGD therefore appears to lead to both increased self-antigen exposure and donor major histocompatibility complex expression that contributes to BOS over time. This work opens new avenues not only for assessing recipient risk for PGD by measuring antibodies to self-antigens but also for exploring novel therapeutics (ie, induction of tolerance to collagen V prior to transplant).

Several posttransplant recipient biochemical markers for PGD have been identified and may ultimately prove to be attractive candidates for PGD monitoring. Candidate biomarkers include cytokines and chemokines, indicators of hypercoagulability and impaired fibrinolysis, and markers of vascular permeability, as summarized in **Table 5**. With improving technology, recent studies illustrate how multiple candidate biomarkers can be simultaneously assayed over several perioperative time points.[63] Several potential biomarkers that have plausible connections to the multifactorial nature of PGD pathogenesis have received recent attention and are highlighted here. However, any candidate biomarkers need to be assessed with large cohorts of transplant patients before widespread use can be advocated.[64]

In a multicenter nested case control study, Kawut and colleagues[39] found higher soluble P-selectin levels at 6 and 24 hours post transplant in patients who developed Grade 3 PGD at 72 hours. P-selectin, a marker of platelet activation, is integral in localizing and activating neutrophils that perpetuate the PGD injury response. These investigators again show a relationship between elevated pulmonary arterial pressures at the time of transplant and PGD independent of CPB use; in the context of their findings on P-selectin

Table 5
Candidate biomarkers for PGD

	Biomarker	Function(s)
Hoffman et al[63]	MCP-1/CCL2 IP-10/CXC10	Chemokines involved in monocyte and lymphocyte recruitment
	IFN-γ	Anti-inflammatory and pleiotropic cytokine
	IL-13 IL-2R TNF-α	Proinflammatory cytokines that activate lymphocytes and neutrophils
Fisher et al[86] De Perrot et al[87]	IL-8	Chemokine involved in neutrophil recruitment
Kaneda et al[88]	IL-6	Anti-inflammatory and pleiotropic cytokine
Christie et al[38] Pelaez et al[69]	sRAGE	Marker of alveolar type I cell injury
Salama et al[70]	Endothelin-1	Vasoconstrictive peptide Regulator of vascular permeability
Krenn et al[89]	VEGF	Regulator of vascular permeability
Christie et al[90]	Protein C Type I plasminogen activator inhibitor	Anticoagulant Inhibitor of fibrinolysis
Covarrubias et al[28]	Plasma intercellular adhesion molecule 1 vWF	Adhesion molecule expressed by type-I pneumocytes, alveolar capillary endothelium, and neutrophils Glycoprotein on endothelium that stabilizes Factor VIII and initiates platelet aggregation

Abbreviations: IP-10/CXC10, interferon (IFN)-inducible protein 10/chemokine CXC motif ligand 10; MCP-1/CCL2, monocyte chemotactic protein 1/chemokine CC motif ligand 2; sRAGE, soluble receptor for advanced glycation end products; TNF-α, tumor necrosis factor α; vWF, von Willebrand factor.

Data from Lee JC, Christie JD, Keshavjee S. Primary graft dysfunction: definition, risk factors, short- and long-term outcomes. Semin Respir Crit Care Med 2010;31:166.

(elevation of which was not associated with mean pulmonary arterial pressures), they hypothesize that preoperative pulmonary vascular disease may result in baseline platelet defects, leading to an increased susceptibility to the activated pulmonary vascular milieu after transplantation.[39]

Elevated levels of receptor for advanced glycation end products (RAGE), a marker of alveolar type I epithelial cell injury, has received considerable recent attention as a candidate biomarker for PGD monitoring. Calfee and colleagues[65] demonstrated that higher levels of RAGE measured 4 hours after reperfusion was associated with a longer duration of mechanical ventilation and longer ICU stay after lung transplantation. Christie and colleagues[38] demonstrated that patients who developed PGD had higher levels of soluble RAGE at both 6 hours and 24 hours after transplant, and also showed that elevated soluble RAGE levels were associated with blood product transfusion and the use of CPB. With evidence that blood products contain elevated levels of advanced glycation end products that are also increased with duration of storage,[66] some investigators postulate that

posttransfusion binding to RAGE on endothelial cells could mediate vascular inflammation and contribute to PGD.[67,68] A recent study by Pelaez and colleagues[69] examined RAGE levels in bronchoalveolar lavage (BAL) fluid from 25 donors and 34 lung transplant recipients. There was an increased risk for PGD development in patients receiving donor lungs with elevated RAGE levels in BAL, and there was a significant correlation between donor RAGE level and PGD grade. Based on immunohistochemical assessment of transbronchial biopsies from patients with and without PGD, RAGE levels were elevated for at least 14 days after transplant in patients with severe, sustained PGD (PGD Grades 2 or 3 over 2 consecutive time points) compared with patients who had not developed PGD.[69]

A recent study by Salama and colleagues[70] illustrates the potential for combining biomarker analysis of both lung transplant donors and recipients. While individual risk factors in donors and recipients may not be well characterized, based on these investigators' findings the possibility of synergism between donor and recipient risk factors for PGD development should be considered. Salama's group measured levels of endothelin-1 (ET-1) in lung tissue and serum from both lung donors and recipients prior to transplant and correlated these measurements with PGD Grade 3 development. ET-1 is a major vasoconstrictive peptide that is expressed highly by activated alveolar macrophages, lymphocytes, and airway epithelial cells. Patients with cystic fibrosis, IPF, and PAH also have been shown to have elevated circulating ET-1 levels.[70] The investigators showed that ET-1 mRNA expression was significantly increased in both donor and recipient tissue in the PGD group, and serum pretransplant ET-1 levels were elevated in recipients who developed PGD.[70] Concomitant elevated donor ET-1 expression and elevated pretransplant serum ET-1 levels in recipients might then be used to predict severe PGD. Targeted ET-1 blockade may also be a feasible avenue of intervention.

PREVENTION AND TREATMENT OF PGD
Prevention

The first efforts aimed at preventing PGD focused on improving lung preservation techniques. Such efforts involved manipulating the volume, temperature, pressure, and composition of preservation solutions; and altering inflation and ventilation parameters of the organs during transport.[33] Unfortunately, lung preservation protocols following harvest are not universally standardized at transplant centers, making comparisons of efficacy difficult.[33] Several therapeutic agents have been investigated in an effort to reduce the incidence of PGD during lung transplantation, but there have been only a few randomized controlled trials conducted, with mixed results (Table 6).

Inhaled nitric oxide (iNO) has been an agent of great interest given its effects on pulmonary vasodilation, maintenance of capillary integrity, and prevention of leukocyte adhesion and platelet aggregation.[71] In a prospective, randomized, blinded clinical trial, Meade and colleagues[72] administered iNO to 84 transplant patients in an effort to affect the incidence of PGD. The investigators found no difference in PGD incidence when iNO was started 10 minutes after reperfusion. A similar trial was conducted by Botha and colleagues,[73] also showing no benefit of iNO administered at the onset of reperfusion on PGD Grade 3 incidence, gas exchange, neutrophil sequestration, or BAL concentration of proinflammatory cytokines. However, a recent trial in 29 lung transplant recipients conducted by Moreno and colleagues[74] demonstrated a decreased incidence of PGD Grade 3 within 72 hours after reperfusion if iNO was given from the start of the transplant procedure until 48 hours after transplantation. These investigators also showed a decrease in inflammatory cytokines interleukin (IL)-6, IL-8, and IL-10 in blood and BAL as a result of this duration of iNO exposure.[74]

Other agents investigated in both observational and randomized, placebo-controlled trials for PGD prevention are summarized in Table 6. Unfortunately, although some studies may have shown modest improvements in early clinical parameters, these often small trials illustrate the difficulty in conducting studies that are sufficiently robust to definitively affect PGD incidence and/or mortality. Preclinical studies employing animal models have suggested other novel therapeutics such as N-acetylcysteine[75] or activated protein C,[76] which show promise and will require evaluation in patients.

Treatment

Treatment of PGD is supportive. Management strategies are similar to those applied in patients with ARDS, include lung-protective ventilation strategies and avoidance of excess fluid administration to minimize edema from increased capillary permeability.[71] Currey and colleagues[77] showed that implementing protocolized respiratory and hemodynamic management guidelines in the ICU setting is feasible, safe, and effective in reducing the severity of PGD. While there are no studies systematically evaluating the application of strategies that have been specifically used in ARDS patients to lung transplant recipients with severe PGD, it is likely that a similar evidence-based, systematic approach to the postoperative care of the lung transplant recipient could have some impact on PGD incidence. Until then, PGD management is largely individualized by center.

Although iNO does not yet have an established role in prevention of PGD development, it may be beneficial in the support of patients with established PGD. There are several reports and case series that show improved outcomes with iNO administration in the setting of severe PGD and refractory hypoxemia after lung transplant.[78–80] However, there are also conflicting studies showing lack of efficacy for iNO use in the setting of already established severe PGD.[81] Without randomized clinical trials showing survival benefit for the use of iNO in the treatment of severe PGD, widespread application cannot yet be recommended. However, its use may be justified in selected cases of severe hypoxemia and/or elevated pulmonary artery pressures. Extrapolating data from iNO use in ARDS patients, the

Table 6
Summary of studies aimed at PGD prevention

Author	Design	Intervention	Effect
Meade et al[72]	RCT: 84 total patients	Inhaled NO (iNO): 20 ppm iNO within 10 min of reperfusion	No difference in PGD incidence, time to extubation, ICU LOS, and hospital LOS
Botha et al[73]	RCT: 20 total patients	20 ppm iNO at the onset of ventilation	No difference in PGD incidence, gas exchange, neutrophil sequestration, or BAL inflammatory cytokines
Moreno et al[74]	RCT: 49 total patients	10 ppm iNO from the start of transplant until 48 h	Lower incidence of PGD in the iNO group (17.2% vs 45%, $P<.035$); decreased levels of IL-6, IL-8, IL-10 in iNO group
Herrington et al[91]	RCT: 48 total patients	Perfadex + aprotinin vs placebo during procurement; Aprotinin vs placebo administered perioperatively to recipients	No difference in PGD incidence within 48 h after procedure; no excess renal failure seen with aprotinin administration
Marasco et al[92]	Retrospective review of 213 lung transplants	Aprotinin use assessed	Increased risk of PGD in the first 48 h in cohort that received aprotinin
Zamora et al[93]	Multicenter RCT: 59 total patients	Soluble complement receptor 1 inhibitor (sCR1)	50% vs 19% extubated within 24 h in treatment group; duration of MV and length of ICU stay trended lower; no effect on P/F, operative deaths, incidence of infection or rejection, or hospital LOS
Wittwer et al[94]	RCT: 24 patients	Platelet activating factor antagonist BN52021	Improved oxygenation scores and CXR findings in first 12 h

Abbreviations: BAL, bronchoalveolar lavage; CXR, chest radiograph; ICU, intensive care unit; LOS, length of stay; MV, mechanical ventilation; ppm, parts per million; RCT, randomized controlled trial.

Data from Lee JC, Christie JD. Primary graft dysfunction. Proc Am Thorac Soc 2009;6:42.

beneficial effects of iNO on oxygenation may be largely transient.[71]

ECMO has been studied in the setting of refractory hypoxemia following lung transplantation, particularly during hemodynamically unstable PGD.[12,82,83] ECMO currently is regarded as a salvage treatment option if started early in the course (no later than 7 days post transplant) of severe PGD refractory to traditional supportive therapies.[71] Recently, Bermudez and colleagues[84] described the University of Pittsburgh experience with ECMO in 763 lung or heart-lung transplant recipients over 15 years. Fifty-eight of 763 patients (7.6%) required institution of either venovenous or venoarterial ECMO for severe PGD. Not surprisingly, when compared with overall survival rates of 82% and 54% at 1 and 5 years in the entire cohort of 763 lung transplant recipients, survival rates in ECMO recipients at 30 days, 1 year, and 5 years were significantly lower at 56%, 40%, and 25%, respectively. PGD survivors who required ECMO and were able to be subsequently weaned from ECMO had slightly higher survival rates at 1 and 5 years of 59% and 33%. Patients receiving venovenous or venoarterial ECMO had similar long-term survival, suggesting no difference based on the mode of ECMO access.[84]

SUMMARY

PGD remains the most important cause of early mortality following lung transplantation, as well as having significant short-term and long-term morbidity and an increased BOS risk among survivors. As efforts to expand the lung donor pool are employed, such as increased use of donation after cardiac death and ex vivo lung conditioning (see the article by Keshavjee and colleagues elsewhere in this issue), the impact on PGD will need to be assessed and its grading system potentially refined. As increasingly sophisticated methods are employed to better understand the complex pathophysiology of PGD, accurate clinical and biomarker phenotyping will become possible in order to help increase donor pools, better match organs, develop novel therapeutics, and reduce the impact of PGD on lung transplant outcomes.

REFERENCES

1. Christie JD, Bavaria JE, Palevsky HI, et al. Primary graft failure following lung transplantation. Chest 1998;114(1):51–60.
2. King RC, Binns OA, Rodriguez F, et al. Reperfusion injury significantly impacts clinical outcome after pulmonary transplantation. Ann Thorac Surg 2000; 69(6):1681–5.
3. Christie JD, Kotloff RM, Pochettino A, et al. Clinical risk factors for primary graft failure following lung transplantation. Chest 2003;124(4):1232–41.
4. Arcasoy SM, Kotloff RM. Lung transplantation. N Engl J Med 1999;340(14):1081–91.
5. Christie JD, Van Raemdonck D, de Perrot M, et al. Report of the ISHLT working group on primary lung graft dysfunction part I: introduction and methods. J Heart Lung Transplant 2005;24(10):1451–3.
6. Arcasoy SM, Fisher A, Hachem RR, et al. Report of the ISHLT Working Group on Primary Lung Graft Dysfunction part V: predictors and outcomes. J Heart Lung Transplant 2005;24(10):1483–8.
7. Christie JD, Carby M, Bag R, et al. Report of the ISHLT Working Group on Primary Lung Graft Dysfunction part II: definition. A consensus statement of the International Society for Heart and Lung Transplantation. J Heart Lung Transplant 2005;24(10):1454–9.
8. Daud SA, Yusen RD, Meyers BF, et al. Impact of immediate primary lung allograft dysfunction on bronchiolitis obliterans syndrome. Am J Respir Crit Care Med 2007;175(5):507–13.
9. Lee JC, Christie JD. Primary graft dysfunction. Proc Am Thorac Soc 2009;6(1):39–46.
10. Lee JC, Christie JD, Keshavjee S. Primary graft dysfunction: definition, risk factors, short- and long-term outcomes. Semin Respir Crit Care Med 2010;31(2):161–71.
11. Christie JD, Sager JS, Kimmel SE, et al. Impact of primary graft failure on outcomes following lung transplantation. Chest 2005;127(1):161–5.
12. Fiser SM, Kron IL, McLendon Long S, et al. Early intervention after severe oxygenation index elevation improves survival following lung transplantation. J Heart Lung Transplant 2001;20(6):631–6.
13. Khan SU, Salloum J, O'Donovan PB, et al. Acute pulmonary edema after lung transplantation: the pulmonary reimplantation response. Chest 1999; 116(1):187–94.
14. Prekker ME, Nath DS, Walker AR, et al. Validation of the proposed International Society for Heart and Lung Transplantation grading system for primary graft dysfunction after lung transplantation. J Heart Lung Transplant 2006;25(4):371–8.
15. Christie JD, Bellamy S, Ware LB, et al. Construct validity of the definition of primary graft dysfunction after lung transplantation. J Heart Lung Transplant 2010;29:1231–9.
16. Huang HJ, Yusen RD, Meyers BF, et al. Late primary graft dysfunction after lung transplantation and bronchiolitis obliterans syndrome. Am J Transplant 2008;8(11):2454–62.
17. Prekker ME, Herrington CS, Hertz MI, et al. Early trends in PaO2/fraction of inspired oxygen ratio predict outcome in lung transplant recipients with severe primary graft dysfunction. Chest 2007; 132(3):991–7.

18. Oto T, Levvey BJ, Snell GI. Potential refinements of the International Society for Heart and Lung Transplantation primary graft dysfunction grading system. J Heart Lung Transplant 2007;26(5):431–6.

19. Christie J, Keshavjee S, Orens J, et al. Potential refinements of the International Society for Heart and Lung Transplantation primary graft dysfunction grading system. J Heart Lung Transplant 2008; 27(1):138.

20. Whitson BA, Prekker ME, Herrington CS, et al. Primary graft dysfunction and long-term pulmonary function after lung transplantation. J Heart Lung Transplant 2007;26(10):1004–11.

21. Fiser SM, Tribble CG, Long SM, et al. Ischemia-reperfusion injury after lung transplantation increases risk of late bronchiolitis obliterans syndrome. Ann Thorac Surg 2002;73(4):1041–7 [discussion: 1047–8].

22. Fisher AJ, Wardle J, Dark JH, et al. Non-immune acute graft injury after lung transplantation and the risk of subsequent bronchiolitis obliterans syndrome (BOS). J Heart Lung Transplant 2002; 21(11).1206–12.

23. Girgis RE, Tu I, Berry GJ, et al. Risk factors for the development of obliterative bronchiolitis after lung transplantation. J Heart Lung Transplant 1996; 15(12):1200–8.

24. Hachem RR, Khalifah AP, Chakinala MM, et al. The significance of a single episode of minimal acute rejection after lung transplantation. Transplantation 2005;80(10):1406–13.

25. Khalifah AP, Hachem RR, Chakinala MM, et al. Minimal acute rejection after lung transplantation: a risk for bronchiolitis obliterans syndrome. Am J Transplant 2005;5(8):2022–30.

26. de Perrot M, Liu M, Waddell TK, et al. Ischemia-reperfusion-induced lung injury. Am J Respir Crit Care Med 2003;167(4):490–511.

27. Frank MM. Complement in the pathophysiology of human disease. N Engl J Med 1987;316(24): 1525–30.

28. Covarrubias M, Ware LB, Kawut SM, et al. Plasma intercellular adhesion molecule-1 and von Willebrand factor in primary graft dysfunction after lung transplantation. Am J Transplant 2007;7(11):2573–8.

29. Moreno I, Vicente R, Ramos F, et al. Determination of interleukin-6 in lung transplantation: association with primary graft dysfunction. Transplant Proc 2007; 39(7):2425–6.

30. Miotla JM, Jeffery PK, Hellewell PG. Platelet-activating factor plays a pivotal role in the induction of experimental lung injury. Am J Respir Cell Mol Biol 1998;18(2):197–204.

31. Serrick C, Adoumie R, Giaid A, et al. The early release of interleukin-2, tumor necrosis factor-alpha and interferon-gamma after ischemia reperfusion injury in the lung allograft. Transplantation 1994; 58(11):1158–62.

32. Barr ML, Kawut SM, Whelan TP, et al. Report of the ISHLT working group on primary lung graft dysfunction part IV: recipient-related risk factors and markers. J Heart Lung Transplant 2005;24(10):1468–82.

33. de Perrot M, Bonser RS, Dark J, et al. Report of the ISHLT working group on primary lung graft dysfunction part III: Donor-related risk factors and markers. J Heart Lung Transplant 2005;24(10):1460–7.

34. Meyer DM, Bennett LE, Novick RJ, et al. Effect of donor age and ischemic time on intermediate survival and morbidity after lung transplantation. Chest 2000;118(5):1255–62.

35. Whitson BA, Nath DS, Johnson AC, et al. Risk factors for primary graft dysfunction after lung transplantation. J Thorac Cardiovasc Surg 2006;131(1): 73–80.

36. Oto T, Griffiths AP, Levvey B, et al. A donor history of smoking affects early but not late outcome in lung transplantation. Transplantation 2004;78(4):599–606.

37. Thabut G, Vinatier I, Stern JB, et al. Primary graft failure following lung transplantation: predictive factors of mortality. Chest 2002;121(6):1876–82.

38. Christie JD, Shah CV, Kawut SM, et al. Plasma levels of receptor for advanced glycation end-products (SRAGE), blood transfusion, and risk of primary graft dysfunction. Am J Respir Crit Care Med 2009;180(10):1010–5.

39. Kawut SM, Okun J, Shimbo D, et al. Soluble P-selectin and the risk of primary graft dysfunction after lung transplantation. Chest 2009;136(1):237–44.

40. Lee JC, Kuntz C, Kawut SM, et al. Clinical risk factors for the development of primary graft dysfunction. J Heart Lung Transplant 2008;27(2 Suppl 1):S67–8.

41. Cassivi SD, Meyers BF, Battafarano RJ, et al. Thirteen-year experience in lung transplantation for emphysema. Ann Thorac Surg 2002;74(5):1663–9 [discussion: 1669–70].

42. Lee JC, Hadjiliadis D, Aahya VN, et al. Risk factors for early vs late primary graft dysfunction [abstract]. Am J Respir Crit Care Med 2008;177:A396.

43. Fang A, Studer S, Kawut SM, et al. Elevated pulmonary artery pressure is a risk factor for primary graft dysfunction following lung transplantation for idiopathic pulmonary fibrosis Chest 2010. [Epub ahead of print].

44. Sommers KE, Griffith BP, Hardesty RL, et al. Early lung allograft function in twin recipients from the same donor: risk factor analysis. Ann Thorac Surg 1996;62(3):784–90.

45. Szeto WY, Kreisel D, Karakousis GC, et al. Cardiopulmonary bypass for bilateral sequential lung transplantation in patients with chronic obstructive pulmonary disease without adverse effect on lung function or clinical outcome. J Thorac Cardiovasc Surg 2002;124(2):241–9.

46. Webert KE, Blajchman MA. Transfusion-related acute lung injury. Transfus Med Rev 2003;17(4):252–62.

47. Silliman CC, Fung YL, Ball JB, et al. Transfusion-related acute lung injury (TRALI): current concepts and misconceptions. Blood Rev 2009;23(6):245–55.

48. Silliman CC, Boshkov LK, Mehdizadehkashi Z, et al. Transfusion-related acute lung injury: epidemiology and a prospective analysis of etiologic factors. Blood 2003;101(2):454–62.

49. Mangalmurti NS, Xiong Z, Hulver M, et al. Loss of red cell chemokine scavenging promotes transfusion-related lung inflammation. Blood 2009;113(5):1158–66.

50. Wang Y, Kurichi JE, Blumenthal NP, et al. Multiple variables affecting blood usage in lung transplantation. J Heart Lung Transplant 2006;25(5):533–8.

51. Goodwin J, Tinckam K, denHollander N, et al. Transfusion-related acute lung injury (TRALI) in graft by blood donor antibodies against host leukocytes. J Heart Lung Transplant 2010;29(9):1067–70.

52. dos Santos CC, Okutani D, Hu P, et al. Differential gene profiling in acute lung injury identifies injury-specific gene expression. Crit Care Med 2008;36(3):855–65.

53. Li J, Nie J, Chen G, et al. Gene expression profile of pulmonary tissues in different phases of lung ischemia-reperfusion injury in rats. J Huazhong Univ Sci Technolog Med Sci 2007;27(5):564–70.

54. Ray M, Dharmarajan S, Freudenberg J, et al. Expression profiling of human donor lungs to understand primary graft dysfunction after lung transplantation. Am J Transplant 2007;7(10):2396–405.

55. Anraku M, Cameron MJ, Waddell TK, et al. Impact of human donor lung gene expression profiles on survival after lung transplantation: a case-control study. Am J Transplant 2008;8(10):2140–8.

56. Hadjiliadis D, Chaparro C, Reinsmoen NL, et al. Pre-transplant panel reactive antibody in lung transplant recipients is associated with significantly worse post-transplant survival in a multicenter study. J Heart Lung Transplant 2005;24(7 Suppl):S249–54.

57. Yoshida S, Haque A, Mizobuchi T, et al. Anti-type V collagen lymphocytes that express IL-17 and IL-23 induce rejection pathology in fresh and well-healed lung transplants. Am J Transplant 2006;6(4):724–35.

58. Bobadilla JL, Love RB, Jankowska-Gan E, et al. Th-17, monokines, collagen type V, and primary graft dysfunction in lung transplantation. Am J Respir Crit Care Med 2008;177(6):660–8.

59. Halloran PF, Homik J, Goes N, et al. The "injury response": a concept linking nonspecific injury, acute rejection, and long-term transplant outcomes. Transplant Proc 1997;29(1–2):79–81.

60. Burlingham WJ, Love RB, Jankowska-Gan E, et al. IL-17-dependent cellular immunity to collagen type V predisposes to obliterative bronchiolitis in human lung transplants. J Clin Invest 2007;117(11):3498–506.

61. Bharat A, Kuo E, Steward N, et al. Immunological link between primary graft dysfunction and chronic lung allograft rejection. Ann Thorac Surg 2008;86(1):189–95 [discussion: 196–7].

62. Bharat A, Saini D, Steward N, et al. Antibodies to self-antigens predispose to primary lung allograft dysfunction and chronic rejection. Ann Thorac Surg 2010;90(4):1094–101.

63. Hoffman SA, Wang L, Shah CV, et al. Plasma cytokines and chemokines in primary graft dysfunction post-lung transplantation. Am J Transplant 2009;9(2):389–96.

64. Justice AC, Covinsky KE, Berlin JA. Assessing the generalizability of prognostic information. Ann Intern Med 1999;130(6):515–24.

65. Calfee CS, Budev MM, Matthay MA, et al. Plasma receptor for advanced glycation end-products predicts duration of ICU stay and mechanical ventilation in patients after lung transplantation. J Heart Lung Transplant 2007;26(7):675–80.

66. Lysenko L, Mierzchala M, Gamian A, et al. The effect of packed red blood cell storage on arachidonic acid and advanced glycation end-product formation. Arch Immunol Ther Exp (Warsz) 2006;54(5):357–62.

67. Wautier JL, Schmidt AM. Protein glycation: a firm link to endothelial cell dysfunction. Circ Res 2004;95(3):233–8.

68. Wilkes DS. Primary graft dysfunction: it's all the rage. Am J Respir Crit Care Med 2009;180(10):915–6.

69. Pelaez A, Force SD, Gal AA, et al. Receptor for advanced glycation end products in donor lungs is associated with primary graft dysfunction after lung transplantation. Am J Transplant 2010;10(4):900–7.

70. Salama M, Andrukhova O, Hoda MA, et al. Concomitant endothelin-1 overexpression in lung transplant donors and recipients predicts primary graft dysfunction. Am J Transplant 2010;10(3):628–36.

71. Shargall Y, Guenther G, Ahya VN, et al. Report of the ISHLT Working Group on Primary Lung Graft Dysfunction part VI: treatment. J Heart Lung Transplant 2005;24(10):1489–500.

72. Meade MO, Granton JT, Matte-Martyn A, et al. A randomized trial of inhaled nitric oxide to prevent ischemia-reperfusion injury after lung transplantation. Am J Respir Crit Care Med 2003;167(11):1483–9.

73. Botha P, Jeyakanthan M, Rao JN, et al. Inhaled nitric oxide for modulation of ischemia-reperfusion injury in lung transplantation. J Heart Lung Transplant 2007;26(11):1199–205.

74. Moreno I, Vicente R, Mir A, et al. Effects of inhaled nitric oxide on primary graft dysfunction in lung transplantation. Transplant Proc 2009;41(6):2210–2.

75. Inci I, Erne B, Arni S, et al. Prevention of primary graft dysfunction in lung transplantation by N-acetylcysteine after prolonged cold ischemia. J Heart Lung Transplant 2010;29:1293–301.

76. Hirayama S, Cypel M, Sato M, et al. Activated protein C in ischemia-reperfusion injury after experimental lung transplantation. J Heart Lung Transplant 2009;28(11):1180–4.

77. Currey J, Pilcher DV, Davies A, et al. Implementation of a management guideline aimed at minimizing the severity of primary graft dysfunction after lung transplant. J Thorac Cardiovasc Surg 2010;139(1):154–61.

78. Adatia I, Lillehei C, Arnold JH, et al. Inhaled nitric oxide in the treatment of postoperative graft dysfunction after lung transplantation. Ann Thorac Surg 1994;57(5):1311–8.

79. Date H, Triantafillou AN, Trulock EP, et al. Inhaled nitric oxide reduces human lung allograft dysfunction. J Thorac Cardiovasc Surg 1996;111(5):913–9.

80. Macdonald P, Mundy J, Rogers P, et al. Successful treatment of life-threatening acute reperfusion injury after lung transplantation with inhaled nitric oxide. J Thorac Cardiovasc Surg 1995;110(3):861–3.

81. Garat C, Jayr C, Eddahibi S, et al. Effects of inhaled nitric oxide or inhibition of endogenous nitric oxide formation on hyperoxic lung injury. Am J Respir Crit Care Med 1997;155(6):1957–64.

82. Meyers BF, Sundt TM 3rd, Henry S, et al. Selective use of extracorporeal membrane oxygenation is warranted after lung transplantation. J Thorac Cardiovasc Surg 2000;120(1):20–6.

83. Smedira NG, Moazami N, Golding CM, et al. Clinical experience with 202 adults receiving extracorporeal membrane oxygenation for cardiac failure: survival at five years. J Thorac Cardiovasc Surg 2001;122(1):92–102.

84. Bermudez CA, Adusumilli PS, McCurry KR, et al. Extracorporeal membrane oxygenation for primary graft dysfunction after lung transplantation: long-term survival. Ann Thorac Surg 2009;87(3):854–60.

85. Kuntz CL, Hadjiliadis D, Ahya VN, et al. Risk factors for early primary graft dysfunction after lung transplantation: a registry study. Clin Transplant 2009;23(6):819–30.

86. Fisher AJ, Donnelly SC, Hirani N, et al. Elevated levels of interleukin-8 in donor lungs is associated with early graft failure after lung transplantation. Am J Respir Crit Care Med 2001;163(1):259–65.

87. De Perrot M, Sekine Y, Fischer S, et al. Interleukin-8 release during early reperfusion predicts graft function in human lung transplantation. Am J Respir Crit Care Med 2002;165(2):211–5.

88. Kaneda H, Waddell TK, de Perrot M, et al. Pre-implantation multiple cytokine mRNA expression analysis of donor lung grafts predicts survival after lung transplantation in humans. Am J Transplant 2006;6(3):544–51.

89. Krenn K, Klepetko W, Taghavi S, et al. Recipient vascular endothelial growth factor serum levels predict primary lung graft dysfunction. Am J Transplant 2007;7(3):700–6.

90. Christie JD, Robinson N, Ware LB, et al. Association of protein C and type 1 plasminogen activator inhibitor with primary graft dysfunction. Am J Respir Crit Care Med 2007;175(1):69–74.

91. Herrington CS, Prekker ME, Arrington AK, et al. A randomized, placebo-controlled trial of aprotinin to reduce primary graft dysfunction following lung transplantation. Clin Transplant 2011;25(1):90–6.

92. Marasco SF, Pilcher D, Oto T, et al. Aprotinin in lung transplantation is associated with an increased incidence of primary graft dysfunction. Eur J Cardiothorac Surg 2010;37(2):420–5.

93. Zamora MR, Davis RD, Keshavjee SH, et al. Complement inhibition attenuates human lung transplant reperfusion injury: a multicenter trial. Chest 1999;116(1 Suppl):46S.

94. Wittwer T, Grote M, Oppelt P, et al. Impact of PAF antagonist BN 52021 (Ginkolide B) on post-ischemic graft function in clinical lung transplantation. J Heart Lung Transplant 2001;20(3):358–63.

Acute Allograft Rejection: Cellular and Humoral Processes

Tereza Martinu, MD[a],*, Elizabeth N. Pavlisko, MD[b], Dong-Feng Chen, PhD[c], Scott M. Palmer, MD, MHS[d]

KEYWORDS
- Lung transplantation • Acute rejection • Humoral rejection
- Antibody-mediated rejection • Histocompatibility

Acute allograft rejection remains a prevalent and serious problem in lung transplantation, with an incidence of 36% in the first year after transplant according to the latest report from the registry of the International Society for Heart and Lung Transplantation (ISHLT).[1] Although acute lung rejection in itself is rarely fatal, its indirect consequences have considerable adverse effects on transplant outcomes. Treatment of acute rejection with increased immunosuppression increases the risk for many post-transplant infections. Furthermore, despite treatment, cellular rejection and humoral rejection constitute the major risk factors for bronchiolitis obliterans syndrome (BOS). BOS is a condition of progressive airflow obstruction thought to reflect a manifestation of chronic lung transplant rejection. Most post-transplant deaths beyond the first year occur directly or indirectly as a result of BOS.[2]

Compared with other solid organs, the lung appears to be at particularly high risk for rejection. Although the reasons are not entirely clear, increased lung vulnerability to early ischemic injury, recurrent infections, and constant environmental exposures might contribute to the high rates of lung rejection. In this article, the authors present the immunologic basis for acute lung allograft rejection, describing the clinical and pathologic features of acute cellular perivascular (A-grade) rejection and acute cellular airway (B-grade) rejection also known as lymphocytic bronchiolitis (**Figs. 1** and **2**). In addition, the authors discuss the emerging understanding of the importance of humoral rejection in lung transplantation, focusing on the role of anti-HLA antibodies, which can be present before or develop de novo after transplantation (see **Figs. 1** and **2**). Current strategies will be highlighted for the

The authors had financial support from National Institutes of Health (5 KL2 RR024127-03, 1P50-HL084917-01, 1 K24 HL91140-01A2).

Financial disclosures/conflicts of interest: The authors have nothing to disclose.

[a] Lung and Heart-Lung Transplant Program, Division of Pulmonary and Critical Care, Department of Medicine, Duke University Medical Center, 106 Research Drive, Building MSRB2, Suite 2073-2 (Box 103000), Durham, NC 27710, USA

[b] Division of Thoracic Pathology, Department of Pathology, Duke University Medical Center, Duke South, Green Zone, Room 3120, Durham, NC 27710, USA

[c] Department of Pathology, Clinical Transplantation Immunology Laboratory, Duke University Medical Center, DUMC 3712, RP III, RM 116, Durham, NC 27710, USA

[d] Lung and Heart-Lung Transplant Program, Division of Pulmonary and Critical Care, Department of Medicine, Duke University Medical Center, 106 Research Drive, Building MSRB2, Suite 2073 (Box 103002), Durham, NC 27710 USA

* Corresponding author.

E-mail address: tereza.martinu@duke.edu

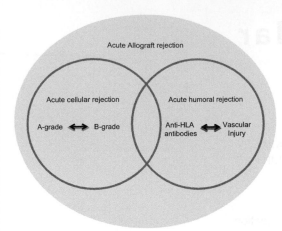

Fig. 1. Venn diagram representing the relationship between acute cellular rejection (grade A and grade B) and humoral rejection manifest by presence of anti-HLA antibodies or histologic findings.

prevention and treatment of both cellular and humoral allograft rejection.

MECHANISMS OF ACUTE REJECTION

In the absence of immunosuppression, the transplant recipient develops a robust response to the allograft, predominantly driven by T-cell recognition of foreign major histocompatibility complex (MHC) proteins, called human leukocyte antigens (HLA) in humans. Foreign MHC, expressed on transplanted tissue cells, is first presented directly to recipient T-cells by donor dendritic cells in the graft (direct pathway). As donor antigen presenting cells (APCs) die out or are destroyed, recipient dendritic cells process and present alloantigens to recipient T-cells (indirect pathway).[3]

HLA genes are located on the short arm of human chromosome 6 and are traditionally divided into two classes based on historic differentiation. The classical HLA class 1 genes include A, B, and Cw loci, which are expressed on most nucleated cells. The classical HLA class 2 genes include DR, DQ, and DP genes, which are expressed constitutively on B-cells, monocytes, dendritic cells, and other APCs, but can be upregulated on various other cells under inflammatory conditions. The extraordinary diversity of HLA polymorphisms creates a considerable barrier to transplantation, as the donor organ is quickly recognized as nonself on the basis of HLA differences with the recipient.[3]

The common pathway of acute cellular rejection involves the recruitment and activation of recipient lymphocytes (predominantly effector T-cells) to the lung allograft, which can result in allograft injury and loss of function.[3] Consequently, successful outcomes after lung transplantation did not

become a possibility until the widespread introduction into clinical practice of the calcineurin inhibitor cyclosporine, which permits a highly effective blockade of T-cell activation and proliferation.[4,5] However, in spite of intensive T-cell suppressive strategies, lung transplant patients continue to experience high rates of rejection. This process of allorecognition is likely augmented by local innate immune activation through endogenous tissue injury and exogenous infection. Innate immune activation can promote alloantigen presentation, costimulation, and T-cell activation.

Humoral responses following lung transplantation have only recently been appreciated due to the advent of modern highly sensitive solid-phase antibody detection techniques. It is now clear that some patients present for transplantation with preformed anti-HLA antibodies, which are usually acquired through prior pregnancy, transfusions, or transplantation. Immune stimulation by prior infections or autoimmunity might contribute to the development of antibodies to allo-MHC in those patients with no identifiable risk factors. These pre-existing antibodies can react with donor antigens, leading to immediate graft loss (hyperacute rejection) or accelerated humoral rejection and BOS.[6] In addition, some lung transplant recipients appear to mount a humoral response to the allograft after transplantation. Most evidence suggests that this humoral response occurs to donor MHC antigens, although other endothelial or epithelial antigens expressed in the lung may become antibody targets as well. T-cells activated through indirect presentation provide help for B-cell memory, antibody class switching, and affinity maturation in the presence of appropriate cytokines and costimulatory factors. Acute and chronic humoral rejection have been well described in renal transplantation.[6] Furthermore, histologic features of antibody-mediated rejection can be found on lung biopsy in the absence of measurable anti-HLA antibodies.[7]

The precise immune mechanisms and their complex interactions leading to stimulation of cellular or humoral immunity and ultimately to lung rejection remain to be fully elucidated. Nevertheless, acute cellular rejection, acute humoral rejection resulting in vascular injury, and the presence of anti-HLA antibodies are processes that overlap clinically and may potentiate each other (see **Fig. 1**).

ACUTE CELLULAR REJECTION
Clinical Presentation and Diagnosis

Acute lung allograft rejection can be asymptomatic at the time of pathologic diagnosis. When present,

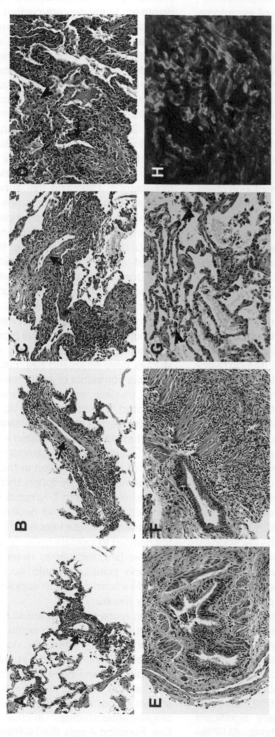

Fig. 2. Examples of acute lung allograft rejection pathology. (*A–D*) Grade A acute cellular rejection; arrows indicate vessel lumina. (*A*) Grade A1 acute rejection with rare perivascular lymphocytes, H&E. (*B*) Grade A2 acute rejection with a prominent perivascular mononuclear infiltrate, H&E. (*C*) Grade A3 acute rejection with extensive perivascular infiltrate extending into interstitial spaces, H&E. (*D*) Grade A4 acute rejection with a diffuse mononuclear infiltrate with lung injury, including fibrinous exudate (*arrowhead*), H&E. (*E*) Grade B1R (low-grade) lymphocytic bronchiolitis with small numbers of bronchiolar mononuclear cells, H&E. (*F*) Grade B2R (high-grade) lymphocytic bronchiolitis with dense bronchiolar mononuclear infiltrate and epithelial involvement, H&E. (*G*) Neutrophilic capillaritis consistent with humoral rejection (*arrowheads* indicate neutrophils), H&E, with (*H*) associated immunofluorescence on frozen lung tissue, demonstrating ring-shaped profiles of C4d staining in alveolar septal capillaries, Immunofluorescent staining. All images are at 200× magnification.

symptoms range from dyspnea, cough, or sputum production to acute respiratory distress, with physical findings that may include fever, hypoxia, and adventitious sounds on lung auscultation.[8] Because of the nonspecific nature of symptoms and signs, emphasis should be placed on objective data, mainly pulmonary function testing, in identifying patients at risk for rejection. Spirometry has been found to have a sensitivity of greater than 60% for detecting infection or rejection grade A2 and higher, but it cannot differentiate between the two.[9] Radiographic imaging of lung transplant patients is useful in identifying specific causes of symptoms or decreased pulmonary function, such as focal infections or neoplasms. Findings of ground glass opacities, septal thickening, volume loss, and pleural effusions on high-resolution chest computed tomography (CT) scans suggest acute rejection. Although early small studies attempted to demonstrate the usefulness of chest radiographs and chest CT scans in the diagnosis of rejection, more recent data show very low sensitivity for acute rejection (as low as 35%) and no discriminatory value between rejection and other processes.[10,11] Given the poor specificity of pulmonary function tests and radiographic studies, the authors discourage empiric treatment of rejection and recommend histopathologic analysis of lung tissue to diagnose and grade acute lung rejection. The incidence of acute rejection is highest within the first year after transplant, arguing for a high clinical suspicion during this time period.

Bronchoscopy, with bronchoalveolar lavage (BAL) and transbronchial biopsies, is the most important diagnostic modality for acute allograft rejection and should be considered in any lung transplant recipient with allograft dysfunction. It allows acute rejection to be distinguished from other potential etiologies of allograft dysfunction such as airway stenosis or infection. Most transbronchial biopsies are performed in the lower lobes, a practice that seems reasonable in light of data showing that different lung lobes have similar rejection grades and that if rejection is present, the grade is usually worse in the lower lobes as compared with the upper lobes.[12] The Lung Rejection Study Group (LRSG) now recommends 5 pieces of well-expanded alveolated lung parenchyma to provide adequate sensitivity to diagnose rejection.[13] Adverse events reported with bronchoscopy in lung transplant recipients are relatively low and include transient hypoxemia (10.5%), bleeding greater than 100 mL (4%), clinically significant pneumothorax (0.6–2.5%), arrhythmia (0.57%–4%), possibly postprocedural pneumonia (8%), and ventilation support (0.32%), but no reported mortality.[14–17]

While there is widespread agreement on the benefit of clinically-directed bronchoscopy in lung transplantation, the role of surveillance bronchoscopy in asymptomatic patients remains disputed. Many centers perform scheduled bronchoscopies at about 1 month, 3 months, 6 months, and annually after transplant, in addition to the clinically-indicated and post-rejection follow-up bronchoscopies.[18] The rationale includes the occurrence of clinically silent acute rejection, inadequate surrogate markers for acute rejection, and the relatively low risks of the bronchoscopy procedure. Grade A2 and higher acute rejection has been found in up to 18% to 39% of asymptomatic patients,[14,19,20] with occasional presence of late-onset acute rejection beyond 1 year after transplant.[21] Disputing this approach, one group showed that 3-year outcomes in patients who underwent only clinically-indicated bronchoscopies were comparable to outcomes in patients who underwent surveillance bronchoscopies,[15] as well as to the ISHLT database outcomes.[22] A randomized trial would be helpful to determine the benefit of surveillance bronchoscopies in lung transplant recipients.

In an attempt to obviate the need for surveillance biopsies, many reports have focused on less invasive surrogates of acute lung rejection. Multiple studies have assessed BAL cells and proteins as possible correlates of acute rejection, but many of these studies were small and have not been replicated.[23] Acute rejection has been associated with elevated CD8 T-cells, activated CD4 T-cells,[24] activated NK cells,[25] elevated interleukin (IL)-17,[26] IL-15,[27] and interferon-gamma in the BAL.[28] A pilot study of gene expression in the BAL fluid of lung transplant recipients found that gene expression signatures related to T-lymphocyte function, cytotoxic CD8 activity, and neutrophil degranulation correlate with acute rejection.[29] Additional studies are needed to validate these findings and establish whether BAL microarray determinations of acute rejection signature could be cost-effective and provide information that supplements or replaces biopsy results.

Even more attractive are studies of noninvasive means of diagnosing acute rejection without bronchoscopy. Although no effective serum biomarkers are currently in use in clinical lung transplant, many have been studied, and some, such as the hepatocyte growth factor, have been shown to correlate with acute rejection in small single-center studies.[30] In 2002, the Cylex Immune Cell Function Assay (ImmuKnow; Cylex, Incorporated, Columbia, MA, USA) was approved by the US Food and Drug Administration to measure global immune function in solid organ transplant recipients. This assay measures the in vitro production of adenosine triphosphate (ATP) by the patient's peripheral blood CD4 T-cells in response to stimulation by phytohemagglutinin-L. Several studies in kidney, liver, heart, and small bowel allograft recipients have demonstrated that low ATP levels (≤ 225 ng/mL) correlate with infection, while high levels (≥ 525 ng/mL) are associated with rejection.[31] Two studies that evaluated this assay in lung transplant recipients demonstrated that low ATP levels correlated with infection,[32,33] but association with acute rejection was not assessed. Preliminary data published in abstract form showed that 87% of lung rejection episodes occurred in the setting of low-to-moderate ATP levels.[34] Additionally, exhaled breath analysis studies have shown some promising results. Exhaled nitric oxide (NO) has been correlated with lymphocytic bronchiolitis[35] and acute rejection,[36] and, in a study of inert gas single-breath washout, the slope of alveolar plateau for Helium (S_{He}) had a sensitivity of 68% for acute rejection.[9] In summary, no surrogate markers have been sufficiently validated as a means to reproducibly identify patients with acute rejection with adequate specificity, and none supplant direct histopathological examination of lung tissue. Nevertheless, further studies in this arena will likely provide valuable information about underlying mechanisms of rejection and better explain clinical heterogeneity of the disease.

Histology and Cellular Infiltration of Acute Lung Rejection

The histologic appearance of acute lung allograft rejection and the grading rules for acute cellular rejection (A-grade), airway inflammation (B-grade), chronic airway rejection or bronchiolitis obliterans (C-grade), and chronic vascular rejection or accelerated graft vascular sclerosis (D-grade) are outlined in the Working Formulation published by the Lung Rejection Study Group (LRSG) of the ISHLT.[13] The grading scheme and its key features are summarized in **Table 1**, and illustrative images from the authors' institution are shown in **Fig. 2**.

Table 1
Pathologic grading of lung rejection

Category of Rejection	Grade	Severity	Histologic Appearance
Grade A: acute rejection	0	None	Normal lung
	1	Minimal	Inconspicuous small mononuclear perivascular infiltrates
	2	Mild	More frequent, more obvious, perivascular infiltrates; eosinophils may be present
	3	Moderate	Dense perivascular infiltrates, extension into interstitial space, can involve endothelialitis, eosinophils, and neutrophils
	4	Severe	Diffuse perivascular, interstitial, & air-space infiltrates with lung injury. Neutrophils may be present.
Grade B: airway inflammation	0	None	No evidence of bronchiolar inflammation
	1R	Low grade	Infrequent, scattered, or single-layer mononuclear cells in bronchiolar submucosa
	2R	High grade	Larger infiltrates of larger and activated lymphocytes in bronchiolar submucosa; can involve eosinophils and plasmacytoid cells
	X	Ungradable	No bronchiolar tissue available
Grade C: chronic airway rejection—obliterative bronchiolitis	0	Absent	If present describes intraluminal airway obliteration with fibrous connective tissue
	1	Present	
Grade D: chronic vascular rejection—accelerated graft vascular sclerosis		No grading	Fibrointimal thickening of arteries and poorly cellular hyaline sclerosis of veins; usually requires open lung biopsy for diagnosis

Abbreviation: R, revised.

Data from Stewart S, Fishbein MC, Snell GI, et al. Revision of the 1996 working formulation for the standardization of nomenclature in the diagnosis of lung rejection. J Heart Lung Transplant 2007;26(12):1229–42.

The typical A-grade acute cellular rejection of the lung allograft manifests as perivascular mononuclear inflammatory cell infiltrates with or without interstitial mononuclear cells. Most of these mononuclear cells are T-cells, with a preponderance of CD8 T-cells,[37] although a few studies have described increased populations of B-cells or eosinophils.[13,38,39] Increasing thickness of the mononuclear cell cuff around vessels with increasing mononuclear invasion into the interstitial and alveolar spaces determines the A-grade (see **Table 1** and **Fig. 2**A–D). While the intra-reader agreement for acute rejection has been found to be good (kappa 0.65–0.795),[40,41] the inter-reader reliability of this grading scheme has ranged from good to suboptimal (kappa as high as 0.73 and as low as 0.47).[40–42] Confounding features, such as concurrent infection or alveolar damage early after transplant, may additionally blur the picture and contribute to the inter-reader pathologist discordance.[42] In general, the LRSG recommends grading rejection only after the exclusion of infection.

The B-grade airway mononuclear inflammation is clearly part of the spectrum of acute cellular rejection (see **Fig. 2**E, F), but grading remains inconsistent due to frequent lack of airway tissue on biopsies, susceptibility to tissue artifacts, and confounding by concurrent infections. Because of low inter-reader reliability of the prior 5-grade (0–4) grading schema for B-grade rejection,[40,41] the LRSG has simplified the B-grading to 3 grades (0–2) (see **Table 1**).[13] This nomenclature is to be used for grading noncartilaginous small airways only after rigorous exclusion of infection.

Clinical Significance of Acute Rejection

Multiple studies have demonstrated that acute rejection is the major risk factor for the development of chronic airflow obstruction: a single episode of acute rejection as well as increased frequency and severity of acute rejection increase the risk for BOS.[2,43] An area of controversy has been the significance of minimal acute rejection (A1) or of a solitary perivascular infiltrate. In the early years of lung transplantation, A1 rejection was usually discounted and not treated. Studies have since found that minimal acute rejection (grade A1) increases the risk of subsequent higher-grade rejections (grade ≥A2)[44,45] and of subsequent BOS[46] and that an untreated solitary perivascular monocytic infiltrate may lead to worsening acute rejection.[47] Furthermore, based on multiple studies, grade B lymphocytic bronchiolitis is now also known to be an important risk factor for BOS[48] and death, independent of acute vascular rejection.[2,48] Although lymphocytic inflammation is frequently seen on endobronchial biopsies of large cartilaginous airways, its clinical and prognostic significance remain unclear, and there is no demonstrated link between lymphocytic inflammation seen on endobronchial biopsies and lymphocytic bronchiolitis or bronchitis seen on transbronchial biopsies.[49–52] Although eosinophils,[53] B-cells,[38] and mast cells[54] have been identified in acute rejection biopsies and have been correlated with worse prognosis, their exact clinical significance remains unclear.

Risk Factors for Acute Rejection

While many risk factors for acute lung allograft rejection have been studied, this article will focus on those that have been found to be significant and categorize them as allorecognition-related, immunosuppression-related, recipient-related, and infectious.

Allorecognition-related risk factors

It is generally thought that the intensity of the host alloimmune response is related to recipient recognition of differences with the donor antigens and that this process drives acute lung allograft rejection. Consistent with this idea, several single-center studies have shown that an increasing degree of HLA mismatch, especially at the HLA-DR, HLA-B, and HLA-A loci, increases the risk of acute rejection.[55–57] Additionally, the ISHLT registry data show a correlation between HLA matching and gender-matching and 5-year survival.[1] Although not very well understood, multiorgan transplantation is generally believed to provide an immunologic advantage and lead to lower rates of rejection due to dampening of allorecognition through a high burden of foreign HLA antigens. Decreased rejection has been shown for grafted kidney, liver, and heart in combined heart–kidney, liver–kidney, and heart–lung transplant recipients,[58,59] although this benefit does not seem to translate into prolonged graft or recipient survival. The data regarding lung rejection in the presence of a second organ remain inconclusive.[1,59–61]

Immunosuppression-related risk factors

While it is clear that adequate immunosuppression is necessary for lung allograft maintenance, the optimal regimen has not been defined. Standard immune suppression includes a calcineurin inhibitor, a cell-cycle inhibitor, and a corticosteroid. Several studies suggest that there may be lower incidence of acute rejection with tacrolimus as opposed to cyclosporine.[62,63] One randomized double-blind trial showed decreased rejection with everolimus as opposed to azathioprine.[64]

The self-reported ISHLT registry data support the idea of decreased acute rejection episodes with tacrolimus and MMF as compared with cyclosporine and azathioprine.[1] Surprisingly very few studies have directly examined the link between levels of immunosuppression and acute rejection. High titers of Epstein-Barr virus (EBV) in peripheral blood, a surrogate marker of a high overall level of immunosuppression, have been found to correlate with lower incidence of acute rejection.[65] Furthermore, one episode of early high-grade acute rejection appears predictive of additional acute rejection episodes within the first year after lung transplant, suggesting that more aggressive immunosuppression should be used in these patients.[45]

Recipient-related risk factors

Genetic polymorphisms have also been considered as potential independent risk factors for rejection.[66] A genotype leading to increased IL-10 production may protect against acute rejection,[67] while a multidrug resistance genotype (MDR1 C3435T) appears to predispose to treatment-resistant acute rejection,[68] and a copy number variation in the CCL4L chemokine gene is associated with susceptibility to acute rejection.[69] Additionally, the idea has been developed that genetic variation in innate pattern recognition receptors modulates the development of acute rejection after lung transplantation. In this regard, the authors have found reduced acute rejection in association with a variant in toll-like receptor 4 (TLR4) that blunts the innate immune response, and increased rejection with a CD14 variant that augments the innate response.[70,71] Although these studies suggest that polymorphic variants outside of the HLA region also influence the risk for acute rejection, larger multicenter efforts are needed to fully validate these findings and also test for gene–gene and gene–environment interactions among relevant polymorphisms.

Collectively these genetic studies provide considerable support for the overall hypothesis that the constant interplay between the environment and pulmonary innate immunity modulates adaptive alloimmunity after lung transplantation. Consistent with this paradigm, gastroesophageal reflux disease also has been associated with increased rates of acute rejection.[72] Furthermore, as will be discussed, rejection has been appreciated following a number of respiratory infections.

The effect of age on acute rejection appears to be bimodal, with lowest incidence of acute rejection in infancy (younger than age 2)[73] and increased risk during childhood as compared with adulthood.[74] The incidence of acute rejection in older lung transplant recipients (age 65 or higher) appears to be similar to that of younger adults,[75] while their rate of infections appears higher, potentially contributing to increased mortality.[76] However, more studies are needed to determine the true effect of age on rejection before a strategy of reduced immunosuppression can be advocated in older recipients.

Infectious risk factors

Infectious etiologies have been given a lot of attention as potentiators of adaptive immunity in solid organ transplantation. Viral infections have long been thought to modulate the immune system and heighten alloreactivity. Indeed, a high incidence of acute rejection has been found in lung transplant recipients following community-acquired respiratory tract infections with rhinovirus, parainfluenza virus, influenza virus, human metapneumovirus, coronavirus, and respiratory syncytial virus (RSV),[77–80] although respiratory viruses do not appear to be associated with acute rejection during the acute phase of infection.[81] Studies on the role of other herpes viruses and polyoma viruses are being conducted, with no evidence of association with acute rejection to date.[82–84] Studies directly linking cytomegalovirus (CMV) infection or CMV prophylaxis strategies with acute rejection have been inconsistent,[2] and a recent randomized trial of CMV prophylaxis did not identify a correlation between CMV incidence and acute rejection rates.[85] In one study, bacterial infection with *Chlamydia pneumoniae* was linked to the development of acute rejection and BOS.[86]

Treatment of Acute Lung Rejection

Treatment of acute lung allograft rejection consists of increased immunosuppression. There has been clear consensus that grade A2 and higher-grade rejection episodes require treatment. However, in light of recent evidence that grade A1 rejection and lymphocytic bronchiolitis are major risk factors for BOS, treatment seems prudent for those entities as well. The mainstays of treatment for acute lung rejection are pulse steroids. Several studies from the 1990s showed successful resolution or improvement of acute rejection after high-dose steroid treatment.[38,87] There are no data to clearly guide dosing of the pulse steroids; a standard dose is 500 mg of methylprednisolone intravenously,[4] although centers use doses that range from 125 mg up to 1000 mg per day. Duration of treatment also varies but typically includes at least 3 doses, followed by an oral prednisone taper.

Response to steroids is variable, but early post-transplant rejection seems to respond better than late rejection.[88] A major challenge in lung transplantation has been the treatment of persistent or recurrent rejection. A repeat course of corticosteroids is one option. Several studies support switching from cyclosporine to tacrolimus for treatment of persistent acute rejection.[89,90] Many centers use alternative immunosuppressive agents such as polyclonal antithymocyte globulin (ATG), anti-IL-2 receptor (IL2R) antagonists, or muromonab-CD3 (OKT3).[91] A recent report demonstrated the utility of alemtuzumab, an anti-CD52 monoclonal antibody, in the treatment of refractory acute rejection in a small cohort of patients who previously failed treatment with ATG.[39] Other therapies that have been considered include inhaled cyclosporine,[92,93] extracorporeal photopheresis,[94] and total lymphoid irradiation.[95]

The relationship between acute rejection, its current treatments, and the eventual occurrence of BOS is an area of considerable interest. Although acute rejection appears to be a major risk factor for BOS, it remains unclear how its treatment impacts long-term allograft function and patient survival.

HUMORAL REJECTION

Antibody-mediated allograft rejection is an increasingly recognized entity in lung transplantation. Early observations were based on the phenomenon of hyperacute rejection, where pre-existent donor-specific antibodies led to complement activation and rapid graft loss. With the advent of improved crossmatching before transplant, the incidence of hyperacute rejection in all organs has decreased. However, acute or chronic antibody-mediated lung rejection is an emerging and controversial subject. With the development of improved antibody detection and identification techniques, allograft-specific antibodies have been implicated in both acute and chronic kidney as well as heart rejection, and recent data have expanded the concept to lung transplantation.

The mechanisms by which antibody promotes lung allograft injury remain poorly understood. Antibody binding to allo-MHC or other endothelial or epithelial targets in the lung could lead to activation of the complement cascade with complement deposits leading to endothelial cell injury, production of pro-inflammatory and fibroblast-stimulating molecules, recruitment of inflammatory cells, and increased gene expression and subsequent proliferation,[6,96] potentially contributing to the generation of obliterative airway lesions.

This section will discuss emerging issues in humoral lung rejection, including humoral sensitization both before and after lung transplantation, as well as pathologic features of humoral rejection, which can occur with or without the presence of detectable antibodies in the serum.

Detection of anti-HLA Antibodies

The original methodology for HLA serologic typing, antibody screening and identification, and direct crossmatching was the complement-dependent cytotoxicity (CDC) assay. The assay is based on the specific reactivity between serum antibody and cell surface antigen that activates complement, causing cell death, which can be identified under the microscope using vital dyes for cell staining.

The CDC assay has now been replaced at most institutions with the more sensitive and specific solid-phase technologies that use a solid matrix coated with purified HLA antigens obtained from either cell lines or recombinant technology. These assays have the ability to detect both complement-fixing antibodies and noncomplement-fixing antibodies. Screening for antibodies is usually achieved by flow cytometry using a panel of 30 populations of beads coated with HLA antigens extracted from 30 individual donors (**Fig. 3**). This assay determines the panel reactive antibody (PRA), which is the percentage of beads or lymphocytes from the given panel that are recognized by patient's anti-HLA antibodies. Once a patient's PRA is determined to be positive, the actual HLA specificity of a recipient's anti-HLA antibodies is determined using a single antigen bead assay with beads coated with recombinant HLA single antigens.[97] The most recently developed solid-phase methodology for single-antigen detection is the Luminex single-antigen bead array assay (Luminex Corporation, Austin, TX, USA), which can simultaneously detect a maximum of 100 different colored beads in suspension with a different HLA antigen bound to each colored bead (**Fig. 4**).

In spite of these technological advances, antibodies may still be present at a level of detection below the sensitivity of the methodology or against antigens not represented by the screening reagents. However, it is believed that antibodies that remain undetected by current methods are mostly weak antibodies and may be clinically irrelevant. Nevertheless, the most definitive compatibility test remains the real-time crossmatch of the recipient serum with the potential donor cells. Flow crossmatch, whereby actual donor cells are incubated with recipient serum and bound antibodies are then tagged with secondary fluorescent anti-immunoglobulin (Ig)G antibodies, has been proven to be up to 10 to 250 times more sensitive than a CDC crossmatch.[98]

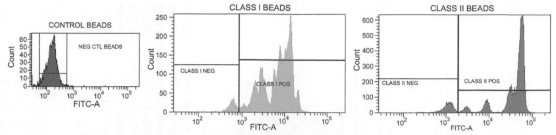

Fig. 3. Flow cytometric antibody screening for measurement of panel reactive antibody (PRA). FlowPRA beads are coated with purified HLA antigens. After incubation with patient serum and subsequent staining with FITC-labeled antihuman immunoglobulin (Ig)G, FlowPRA beads were analyzed on a flow cytometer. Beads with antibody binding have greater fluorescence intensity as represented by the rightward channel shift compared with the negative control. A percentage value of PRA is calculated based on the area of peak shifted. This patient demonstrated a PRA of 95% for HLA class 1 and a PRA of 94% for HLA class 2. The multiple peaks in the positive flow histogram are due to different bead populations emitting fluorescence of different intensity. The negative control was generated using uncoated beads. FITC, fluorescein isothiocyanate.

Pre-transplant Considerations for Sensitized Patients

One of the major goals in donor selection is to avoid HLA antigens, against which the potential recipient has preformed antibodies. About 10% to 15% of lung transplant recipients are presensitized to HLA antigens.[99] Antibody-detection technologies identify unacceptable donor antigens that should be avoided at the time of transplant. When a donor becomes available, information about the donor HLA antigens and the recipient antibodies is compared, constituting a virtual crossmatch and allowing for the real-time prospective crossmatch to be waived. This virtual cross-match approach has significantly shortened the waiting time for presensitized recipients, and correlates highly with cross-match results performed at the time of transplant.[100,101] A high number of anti-HLA antibodies can significantly decrease the donor pool and increase waiting time for a lung transplant candidate. In these instances, interventions to remove or decrease the production of these antibodies may be considered before transplantation.

Post-transplant Considerations in Sensitized Recipients

Even though unacceptable antigens are avoided during the virtual crossmatch, patients with positive pre-transplant PRA (ie, circulating anti-HLA antibodies) are at higher risk for post-transplant complications. Their post-transplant PRA can remain stable or increase via generation of either donor-specific or nondonor-specific anti-HLA antibodies. Similarly, patients who had negative PRA screening tests before transplant can develop de novo nondonor-specific or donor-specific anti-HLA antibodies after transplant. Using modern sensitive antibody detection techniques, recent studies have consistently demonstrated increased incidence of acute rejection,[102] persistent rejection, increased BOS,[103] and worse overall survival[104] in patients with anti-HLA antibodies. This effect is apparent with both pre-transplant HLA sensitization as well as with the development of de novo donor-specific anti-HLA antibodies after transplantation.[103]

The importance of donor specificity and target antigens in humoral rejection is not well understood. The risk of poor outcome may be heightened in the setting of donor-specific antibodies and positive retrospective crossmatches.[104] However, patients with positive PRA, with negative crossmatches and without specificity to mismatched donor HLA antigens also have been found to be at increased risk for poor outcome. On the one hand, nondonor-specific antibodies that are present might cross-react with the donor HLA, or antibodies specific to donor HLA might be rapidly absorbed in the lung allograft precluding their detection in the sera. Alternatively, other non-HLA antibodies could contribute to graft injury. For example, de novo autoimmunity after lung transplantation against type V collagen[105] and K-alpha1 tubulin expressed on airway epithelial cells have been shown to predispose to BOS.[106] Another study demonstrated the presence of anti-endothelial antibody directed against donor antigens in the absence of anti-HLA antibodies.[7]

It remains unclear exactly how often post-transplant PRAs should be measured and to what extent humoral rejection occurs among lung transplant recipients. Additional research is needed to more precisely define the significance

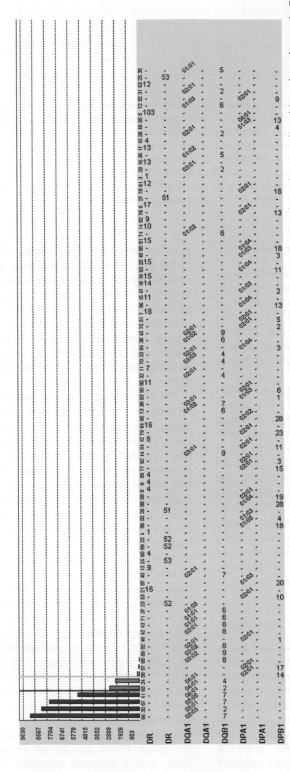

Fig. 4. Standard Luminex single antigen (SA) bead assay results for detection of specific anti-HLA antibodies. SA bead numbers are listed in red on the x-axis. Each SA bead is coated with multiple copies of a single recombinant HLA antigen. The mean fluorescence intensity (MFI), which represents the strength of antibody binding to the beads, is plotted on the y-axis: the color of the bar represents the score of the antibody reactivity strength. The specific HLA antigens tested are listed in the gray chart below the graph. For this patient, positive antibody reactivities were assigned to the 6 beads DQB1*03:01/DQA1*05:03, DQB1*02:01/DQA1*05:01, DQB1*03:01/DQA1*05:05, DQB1*03:01/DQA1*06:01, DQB1*02:01/DQA1*04:01, and DQB1*04:01/DQA1*04:01 based on the cutoff established in the laboratory. Therefore, the patient has specific antibodies against HLA DQA 1 chains encoded by DQA1 alleles DQA1*05:03, DQA1*05:01, DQA1*05:05, DQA1*06:01, and DQA1*04:01. The presence of antibodies against DQB1 chains encoded by alleles DQB1*03:01, DQB1*02:01, and DQB1*04:01 can be excluded based on the negative reactivities with other beads, which also carry the DQB1 chains/antigens encoded by these alleles.

of antibody to donor HLA, to third-party HLA, or to self-antigens after lung transplantation.

Pathologic and Clinical Patterns of Humoral Lung Rejection

Although uncommon due to the use of cross-match screening, hyperacute rejection, caused by pre-existing recipient antibodies against donor HLA antigens, has been described. Hyperacute rejection usually occurs within hours of transplantation and manifests with acute pulmonary decompensation, profound hypoxemia, diffuse pulmonary edema, and alveolar hemorrhage. Such patients may respond to aggressive antihumoral therapy, but mortality is high.[107]

More recently, the concept of acute (distinct from hyperacute) humoral rejection, occurring later (weeks to years) in the post-transplant course, has evolved. However, the notion of a specific histopathological syndrome associated with acute humoral rejection remains controversial. Post-transplant vascular injury with pulmonary capillaritis has been described as an atypical form of rejection that may be resistant to steroids but in several cases responsive to plasmapheresis, suggesting that it may represent an antibody-mediated process. The clinical presentation of this form of pulmonary capillaritis typically includes dyspnea, hypoxemia, and pulmonary infiltrates on chest radiograph, mimicking acute cellular rejection.[108] Frank hemoptysis, reflecting underlying diffuse alveolar hemorrhage, has been described in a subset of recipients with antibody-mediated capillaritis and should prompt consideration of this entity.[108,109]

More recent studies have attempted to evaluate immunoglobulin and complement deposits in the subendothelial space as possible manifestations of antibody-mediated rejection. Septal capillary deposits of immunoglobulins and complement products such as C1q, C3d, C4d (see **Fig. 2**H), and C5b-9, as well as elevation of C4d in the BAL, have been described in association with circulating anti-HLA antibodies.[110,111] Similar pathologic findings have also been identified in the setting of treatment-resistant cellular rejection,[112] decreased pulmonary function tests, or BOS.[113,114] However, other studies have not found evidence of antibody deposits or complement activation in the setting of allograft rejection or vascular injury.[115–117] Others have demonstrated that C3d and C4d staining can occur in lung transplant patients with nonalloimmune lung injury such as infection and primary graft dysfunction with no evidence of anti-HLA antibodies, although this staining does appear to be an independent risk factor for BOS.[114] Differences in staining techniques between laboratories and subjective interpretation of results by pathologists may further explain some of the inconsistencies in the published data.

The LRSG report on the working formulation for the diagnosis of lung rejection remains very cautious in defining the pathologic appearance of humoral rejection. The consensus is that capillary injury can be detected on lung allograft biopsies (see **Fig. 2**G), although it can be a nonspecific finding. Findings of small vessel injury with intimitis or endothelialitis along with immunohistochemical demonstration of complement deposition should raise the suspicion for acute humoral rejection.[13] Although such pathologic findings have been reported without evidence of circulating anti-HLA antibodies and visa versa, the presence in one patient of both circulating anti-HLA antibodies and characteristic pathologic findings should be seen as strong evidence for acute humoral rejection.

Prevention and Therapy for Antibody-Mediated Rejection

Plasmapheresis is the mainstay for antibody removal from the circulation and has been shown to lead to clinical improvement in lung transplant recipients with pulmonary capillaritis unresponsive to steroids.[108] However, it is usually reserved for severe cases of suspected humoral rejection, given its relatively invasive and cumbersome nature. Intravenous immunoglobulin (IVIG) is one of the most common therapies used to decrease antibody-mediated immunity, with a relatively low adverse effect profile. IVIG causes B-cell apoptosis, reduces B-cell numbers, blocks binding of donor-reactive antibodies, and may inhibit complement activation. The peri-transplant use of IVIG and plasmapheresis at the authors' institution in presensitized patients led to elimination of antibodies in 6 of 7 patients with class I anti-HLA antibodies and 1 of 3 patients with class II anti-HLA antibodies. As a group, those presensitized patients who received this regimen demonstrated a significant decrease in acute rejection episodes and a trend toward greater freedom from BOS compared with a cohort of presensitized patients who did not receive desensitization therapy.[99] Rituximab, an anti-CD20 monoclonal antibody that causes B-cell depletion, has been proven effective in the treatment of presensitized renal transplant recipients in conjunction with IVIG.[6,118] In a recent study of 61 lung transplant recipients with newly acquired post-transplant donor-specific antibodies, a regimen of IVIG combined with rituximab (44 patients) or administered alone (17 patients) led to clearing of antibodies in 62%.[119] Notably, freedom from BOS and survival were better in the group of patients who cleared their donor-specific antibodies than those with persistent antibodies. Bortezomib, a selective inhibitor of the 26S proteosome that causes plasma cell apoptosis, is a new therapy that appears useful in the reversal of alloantibody-mediated rejection in renal transplant recipients.[120] Its use in lung transplantation has been described in one case report.[121]

Despite new highly sensitive measures to screen for anti-HLA antibodies and evidence that such antibodies are detrimental to the allograft, optimal monitoring, treatment parameters for humoral rejection, and the benefits of pre-emptive strategies to deplete these antibodies remain uncertain. Further studies are needed to determine whether IVIG, plasmapheresis, rituximab, or bortezomib alter the risk for chronic allograft dysfunction in sensitized patients.

SUMMARY

Acute cellular rejection affects greater than one-third of lung transplant recipients. Alloreactive T-lymphocytes, responding directly or indirectly to donor antigen, constitute the basis of lung allograft rejection, as diagnosed by well-established histopathological criteria that reflect the severity of perivascular or peribronchial inflammation in the lung allograft. Recent evidence supports a more complex immune response to the allograft with involvement of humoral mechanisms, characterized by circulating antibody to donor HLA and specific patterns of lung injury, occurring in parallel with T-cell-based rejection. Emerging evidence further suggests that the interaction between recipient genetics, immunosuppression therapies, and allograft environmental exposures, including pulmonary infection, contributes to high rejection rates after lung transplantation. A greater understanding of the heterogeneous mechanisms of lung rejection is critical to developing effective therapies that target the precise pathophysiology of the disease and ultimately improve long-term lung transplant outcomes.

REFERENCES

1. Christie JD, Edwards LB, Kucheryavaya AY, et al. The Registry of the International Society for Heart and Lung Transplantation: twenty-seventh official adult lung and heart–lung transplant report—2010. J Heart Lung Transplant 2010;29(10): 1104–18.

2. Sharples LD, McNeil K, Stewart S, et al. Risk factors for bronchiolitis obliterans: a systematic review of recent publications. J Heart Lung Transplant 2002;21(2):271–81.

3. Snyder LD, Palmer SM. Immune mechanisms of lung allograft rejection. Semin Respir Crit Care Med 2006;27(5):534–43.

4. Lau CL, Palmer SM, D'Amico TA, et al. Lung transplantation at Duke University Medical Center. Clin Transpl 1998;327–40.

5. Sarahrudi K, Carretta A, Wisser W, et al. The value of switching from cyclosporine to tacrolimus in the treatment of refractory acute rejection and obliterative bronchiolitis after lung transplantation. Transpl Int 2002;15(1):24–8.

6. Colvin RB, Smith RN. Antibody-mediated organ–allograft rejection. Nat Rev Immunol 2005;5(10): 807–17.

7. Magro CM, Klinger DM, Adams PW, et al. Evidence that humoral allograft rejection in lung transplant patients is not histocompatibility antigen-related. Am J Transplant 2003;3(10):1264–72.

8. De Vito Dabbs A, Hoffman LA, Iacono AT, et al. Are symptom reports useful for differentiating between acute rejection and pulmonary infection after lung transplantation? Heart Lung 2004;33(6):372–80.

9. Van Muylem A, Melot C, Antoine M, et al. Role of pulmonary function in the detection of allograft dysfunction after heart–lung transplantation. Thorax 1997;52(7):643–7.

10. Gotway MB, Dawn SK, Sellami D, et al. Acute rejection following lung transplantation: limitations in accuracy of thin-section CT for diagnosis. Radiology 2001;221(1):207–12.

11. Ng YL, Paul N, Patsios D, et al. Imaging of lung transplantation: review. AJR Am J Roentgenol 2009;192(Suppl 3):S1–13 [quiz: S14–9].

12. Hasegawa T, Iacono AT, Yousem SA. The anatomic distribution of acute cellular rejection in the allograft lung. Ann Thorac Surg 2000;69(5):1529–31.

13. Stewart S, Fishbein MC, Snell GI, et al. Revision of the 1996 working formulation for the standardization of nomenclature in the diagnosis of lung rejection. J Heart Lung Transplant 2007;26(12): 1229–42.

14. McWilliams TJ, Williams TJ, Whitford HM, et al. Surveillance bronchoscopy in lung transplant recipients: risk versus benefit. J Heart Lung Transplant 2008;27(11):1203–9.

15. Valentine VG, Gupta MR, Weill D, et al. Single-institution study evaluating the utility of surveillance bronchoscopy after lung transplantation. J Heart Lung Transplant 2009;28(1):14–20.

16. Hopkins PM, Aboyoun CL, Chhajed PN, et al. Prospective analysis of 1235 transbronchial lung biopsies in lung transplant recipients. J Heart Lung Transplant 2002;21(10):1062–7.

17. Chan CC, Abi-Saleh WJ, Arroliga AC, et al. Diagnostic yield and therapeutic impact of flexible bronchoscopy in lung transplant recipients. J Heart Lung Transplant 1996;15(2):196–205.

18. Kukafka DS, O'Brien GM, Furukawa S, et al. Surveillance bronchoscopy in lung transplant recipients. Chest 1997;111(2):377–81.

19. Guilinger RA, Paradis IL, Dauber JH, et al. The importance of bronchoscopy with transbronchial biopsy and bronchoalveolar lavage in the management of lung transplant recipients. Am J Respir Crit Care Med 1995;152:2037–43.

20. Trulock EP, Ettinger NA, Brunt EM, et al. The role of transbronchial lung biopsy in the treatment of lung transplant recipients. An analysis of 200 consecutive procedures. Chest 1992;102(4):1049–54.

21. Chakinala MM, Ritter J, Gage BF, et al. Yield of surveillance bronchoscopy for acute rejection and lymphocytic bronchitis/bronchiolitis after lung transplantation. J Heart Lung Transplant 2004; 23(12):1396–404.

22. Valentine VG, Taylor DE, Dhillon GS, et al. Success of lung transplantation without surveillance bronchoscopy. J Heart Lung Transplant 2002;21(3): 319–26.

23. Reynaud-Gaubert M, Thomas P, Gregoire R, et al. Clinical utility of bronchoalveolar lavage cell phenotype analyses in the postoperative monitoring of lung transplant recipients. Eur J Cardiothorac Surg 2002;21(1):60–6.

24. Gregson AL, Hoji A, Saggar R, et al. Bronchoalveolar immunologic profile of acute human lung transplant allograft rejection. Transplantation 2008; 85(7):1056–9.

25. Meehan AC, Sullivan LC, Mifsud NA, et al. Natural killer cell activation in the lung allograft early post-transplantation. Transplantation 2010; 89(6):756–63.

26. Vanaudenaerde BM, Dupont LJ, Wuyts WA, et al. The role of interleukin-17 during acute rejection after lung transplantation. Eur Respir J 2006; 27(4):779–87.

27. Bhorade SM, Yu A, Vigneswaran WT, et al. Elevation of interleukin-15 protein expression in bronchoalveolar fluid in acute lung allograft rejection. Chest 2007;131(2):533–8.

28. Ross DJ, Moudgil A, Bagga A, et al. Lung allograft dysfunction correlates with gamma-interferon gene expression in bronchoalveolar lavage. J Heart Lung Transplant 1999;18(7):627–36.

29. Patil J, Lande JD, Li N, et al. Bronchoalveolar lavage cell gene expression in acute lung rejection: development of a diagnostic classifier. Transplantation 2008;85(2):224–31.

30. Aharinejad S, Taghavi S, Klepetko W, et al. Prediction of lung-transplant rejection by hepatocyte growth factor. Lancet 2004;363(9420):1503–8.

31. Kowalski RJ, Post DR, Mannon RB, et al. Assessing relative risks of infection and rejection: a meta-analysis using an immune function assay. Transplantation 2006;82(5):663–8.

32. Bhorade SM, Janata K, Vigneswaran WT, et al. Cylex ImmuKnow assay levels are lower in lung transplant recipients with infection. J Heart Lung Transplant 2008;27(9):990–4.

33. Husain S, Raza K, Pilewski JM, et al. Experience with immune monitoring in lung transplant recipients: correlation of low immune function with infection. Transplantation 2009;87(12):1852–7.

34. Huang Y, Nizami Nazih Zuhdi I. Correlation of Cylex ImmuKnow assay with lung allograft biopsy. J Heart Lung Transplant 2007;26(2):S175.

35. De Soyza A, Fisher AJ, Small T, et al. Inhaled corticosteroids and the treatment of lymphocytic bronchiolitis following lung transplantation. Am J Respir Crit Care Med 2001;164(7):1209–12.

36. Silkoff PE, Caramori M, Tremblay L, et al. Exhaled nitric oxide in human lung transplantation. A noninvasive marker of acute rejection. Am J Respir Crit Care Med 1998;157:1822–8.

37. Tavora F, Drachenberg C, Iacono A, et al. Quantitation of T lymphocytes in post-transplant transbronchial biopsies. Hum Pathol 2009;40(4):505–15.

38. Yousem SA, Martin T, Paradis IL, et al. Can immunohistological analysis of transbronchial biopsy specimens predict responder status in early acute rejection of lung allografts? Hum Pathol 1994;25(5): 525–9.

39. Reams BD, Musselwhite LW, Zaas DW, et al. Alemtuzumab in the treatment of refractory acute rejection and bronchiolitis obliterans syndrome after human lung transplantation. Am J Transplant 2007;7(12):2802–8.

40. Chakinala MM, Ritter J, Gage BF, et al. Reliability for grading acute rejection and airway inflammation after lung transplantation. J Heart Lung Transplant 2005;24(6):652–7.

41. Stephenson A, Flint J, English J, et al. Interpretation of transbronchial lung biopsies from lung transplant recipients: inter- and intraobserver agreement. Can Respir J 2005;12(2):75–7.

42. Colombat M, Groussard O, Lautrette A, et al. Analysis of the different histologic lesions observed in transbronchial biopsy for the diagnosis of acute rejection. Clinicopathologic correlations during the first 6 months after lung transplantation. Hum Pathol 2005;36(4):387–94.

43. Burton CM, Iversen M, Carlsen J, et al. Acute cellular rejection is a risk factor for bronchiolitis obliterans syndrome independent of post-transplant baseline FEV1. J Heart Lung Transplant 2009; 28(9):888–93.

44. Burton CM, Iversen M, Scheike T, et al. Minimal acute cellular rejection remains prevalent up to 2

years after lung transplantation: a retrospective analysis of 2697 transbronchial biopsies. Transplantation 2008;85(4):547–53.

45. DeVito Dabbs A, Hoffman LA, Iacono AT, et al. Pattern and predictors of early rejection after lung transplantation. Am J Crit Care 2003;12(6): 497–507.

46. Hachem RR, Khalifah AP, Chakinala MM, et al. The significance of a single episode of minimal acute rejection after lung transplantation. Transplantation 2005;80(10):1406–13.

47. Kim DW, Dacic S, Iacono A, et al. Significance of a solitary perivascular mononuclear infiltrate in lung allograft recipients with mild acute cellular rejection. J Heart Lung Transplant 2005;24(2): 152–5.

48. Glanville AR, Aboyoun CL, Havryk A, et al. Severity of lymphocytic bronchiolitis predicts long-term outcome after lung transplantation. Am J Respir Crit Care Med 2008;177(9):1033–40.

49. Husain AN, Siddiqui MT, Montoya A, et al. Postlung transplant biopsies: an 8-year Loyola experience. Mod Pathol 1996;9(2):126–32.

50. Irani S, Gaspert A, Vogt P, et al. Inflammation patterns in allogeneic and autologous airway tissue of lung transplant recipients. Am J Transplant 2005; 5(10):2456–63.

51. Ward C, Snell GI, Orsida B, et al. Airway versus transbronchial biopsy and BAL in lung transplant recipients: different but complementary. Eur Respir J 1997;10(12):2876–80.

52. Xu X, Golden JA, Dolganov G, et al. Transcript signatures of lymphocytic bronchitis in lung allograft biopsy specimens. J Heart Lung Transplant 2005;24(8):1055–66.

53. Scholma J, Slebos DJ, Boezen HM, et al. Eosinophilic granulocytes and interleukin-6 level in bronchoalveolar lavage fluid are associated with the development of obliterative bronchiolitis after lung transplantation. Am J Respir Crit Care Med 2000; 162(6):2221–5.

54. Yousem SA. The potential role of mast cells in lung allograft rejection. Hum Pathol 1997;28(2):179–82.

55. Schulman LL, Weinberg AD, McGregor C, et al. Mismatches at the HLA-DR and HLA-B loci are risk factors for acute rejection after lung transplantation. Am J Respir Crit Care Med 1998; 157:1833–7.

56. Quantz MA, Bennett LE, Meyer DM, et al. Does human leukocyte antigen matching influence the outcome of lung transplantation? An analysis of 3,549 lung transplantations. J Heart Lung Transplant 2000;19(5):473–9.

57. Wisser W, Wekerle T, Zlabinger G, et al. Influence of human leukocyte antigen matching on long-term outcome after lung transplantation. J Heart Lung Transplant 1996;15(12):1209–16.

58. Ruiz R, Kunitake H, Wilkinson AH, et al. Long-term analysis of combined liver and kidney transplantation at a single center. Arch Surg 2006;141(8): 735–41 [discussion: 741–732].

59. Pinderski LJ, Kirklin JK, McGiffin D, et al. Multiorgan transplantation: is there a protective effect against acute and chronic rejection? J Heart Lung Transplant 2005;24(11):1828–33.

60. Keenan RJ, Bruzzone P, Paradis IL, et al. Similarity of pulmonary rejection patterns among heart–lung and double-lung transplant recipients. Transplantation 1991;51(1):176–80.

61. Moffatt-Bruce SD, Karamichalis J, Robbins RC, et al. Are heart–lung transplant recipients protected from developing bronchiolitis obliterans syndrome? Ann Thorac Surg 2006;81(1):286–91 [discussion: 291].

62. Treede H, Klepetko W, Reichenspurner H, et al. Tacrolimus versus cyclosporine after lung transplantation: a prospective, open, randomized two-center trial comparing two different immunosuppressive protocols. J Heart Lung Transplant 2001;20(5): 511–7.

63. Hachem RR, Yusen RD, Chakinala MM, et al. A randomized controlled trial of tacrolimus versus cyclosporine after lung transplantation. J Heart Lung Transplant 2007;26(10):1012–8.

64. Snell GI, Valentine VG, Vitulo P, et al. Everolimus versus azathioprine in maintenance lung transplant recipients: an international, randomized, double-blind clinical trial. Am J Transplant 2006; 6(1):169–77.

65. Ahya VN, Douglas LP, Andreadis C, et al. Association between elevated whole blood Epstein-Barr virus (EBV)-encoded RNA EBV polymerase chain reaction and reduced incidence of acute lung allograft rejection. J Heart Lung Transplant 2007;26(8):839–44.

66. Girnita DM, Webber SA, Zeevi A. Clinical impact of cytokine and growth factor genetic polymorphisms in thoracic organ transplantation. Clin Lab Med 2008;28(3):423–40.

67. Zheng HX, Burckart GJ, McCurry K, et al. Interleukin-10 production genotype protects against acute persistent rejection after lung transplantation. J Heart Lung Transplant 2004;23(5):541–6.

68. Zheng HX, Zeevi A, McCurry K, et al. The impact of pharmacogenomic factors on acute persistent rejection in adult lung transplant patients. Transpl Immunol 2005;14(1):37–42.

69. Colobran R, Casamitjana N, Roman A, et al. Copy number variation in the CCL4L gene is associated with susceptibility to acute rejection in lung transplantation. Genes Immun 2009;10(3):254–9.

70. Palmer SM, Burch LH, Trindade AJ, et al. Innate immunity influences long-term outcomes after human lung transplant. Am J Respir Crit Care Med 2005;171(7):780–5.

71. Palmer SM, Klimecki W, Yu L, et al. Genetic regulation of rejection and survival following human lung transplantation by the innate immune receptor CD14. Am J Transplant 2007;7(3):693–9.

72. Shah N, Force SD, Mitchell PO, et al. Gastroesophageal reflux disease is associated with an increased rate of acute rejection in lung transplant allografts. Transplant Proc 2010;42(7):2702–6.

73. Ibrahim JE, Sweet SC, Flippin M, et al. Rejection is reduced in thoracic organ recipients when transplanted in the first year of life. J Heart Lung Transplant 2002;21(3):311–8.

74. Scott JP, Whitehead B, de Leval M, et al. Paediatric incidence of acute rejection and obliterative bronchiolitis: a comparison with adults. Transpl Int 1994;7(Suppl 1):S404–6.

75. Mahidhara R, Bastani S, Ross DJ, et al. Lung transplantation in older patients? J Thorac Cardiovasc Surg 2008;135(2):412–20.

76. Gutierrez C, Al-Faifi S, Chaparro C, et al. The effect of recipient's age on lung transplant outcome. Am J Transplant 2007;7(5):1271–7.

77. Kumar D, Husain S, Chen MH, et al. A prospective molecular surveillance study evaluating the clinical impact of community-acquired respiratory viruses in lung transplant recipients. Transplantation 2010;89(8):1028–33.

78. Kumar D, Erdman D, Keshavjee S, et al. Clinical impact of community-acquired respiratory viruses on bronchiolitis obliterans after lung transplant. Am J Transplant 2005;5(8):2031–6.

79. Vilchez RA, Dauber J, McCurry K, et al. Parainfluenza virus infection in adult lung transplant recipients: an emergent clinical syndrome with implications on allograft function. Am J Transplant 2003;3(2):116–20.

80. Garantziotis S, Howell DN, McAdams HP, et al. Influenza pneumonia in lung transplant recipients: clinical features and association with bronchiolitis obliterans syndrome. Chest 2001;119(4):1277–80.

81. Soccal PM, Aubert JD, Bridevaux PO, et al. Upper and lower respiratory tract viral infections and acute graft rejection in lung transplant recipients. Clin Infect Dis 2010;51(2):163–70.

82. Costa C, Delsedime L, Solidoro P, et al. Herpesviruses detection by quantitative real-time polymerase chain reaction in bronchoalveolar lavage and transbronchial biopsy in lung transplant: viral infections and histopathological correlation. Transplant Proc 2010;42(4):1270–4.

83. Bergallo M, Costa C, Terlizzi ME, et al. Quantitative detection of the new polyomaviruses KI, WU and Merkel cell virus in transbronchial biopsies from lung transplant recipients. J Clin Pathol 2010; 63(8):722–5.

84. Astegiano S, Bergallo M, Solidoro P, et al. Prevalence and clinical impact of polyomaviruses KI and WU in lung transplant recipients. Transplant Proc 2010;42(4):1275–8.

85. Palmer SM, Limaye AP, Banks M, et al. Extended valganciclovir prophylaxis to prevent cytomegalovirus after lung transplantation: a randomized, controlled trial. Ann Intern Med 2010;152(12):761–9.

86. Glanville AR, Gencay M, Tamm M, et al. Chlamydia pneumoniae infection after lung transplantation. J Heart Lung Transplant 2005;24(2):131–6.

87. Clelland C, Higenbottam T, Stewart S, et al. Bronchoalveolar lavage and transbronchial lung biopsy during acute rejection and infection in heart-lung transplant patients. Studies of cell counts, lymphocyte phenotypes, and expression of HLA-DR and interleukin-2 receptor. Am Rev Respir Dis 1993; 147:1386–92.

88. Fuehner T, Simon A, Dierich M, et al. Indicators for steroid response in biopsy proven acute graft rejection after lung transplantation. Respir Med 2009;103(8):1114–21.

89. Vitulo P, Oggionni T, Cascina A, et al. Efficacy of tacrolimus rescue therapy in refractory acute rejection after lung transplantation. J Heart Lung Transplant 2002;21(4):435–9.

90. Sarahrudi K, Estenne M, Corris P, et al. International experience with conversion from cyclosporine to tacrolimus for acute and chronic lung allograft rejection. J Thorac Cardiovasc Surg 2004;127(4):1126–32.

91. Shennib H, Massard G, Reynaud M, et al. Efficacy of OKT3 therapy for acute rejection in isolated lung transplantation. J Heart Lung Transplant 1994; 13(3):514–9.

92. Keenan RJ, Iacono A, Dauber JH, et al. Treatment of refractory acute allograft rejection with aerosolized cyclosporine in lung transplant recipients. J Thorac Cardiovasc Surg 1997;113(2):335–40 [discussion: 340–331].

93. Iacono A, Dauber J, Keenan R, et al. Interleukin 6 and interferon-gamma gene expression in lung transplant recipients with refractory acute cellular rejection: implications for monitoring and inhibition by treatment with aerosolized cyclosporine. Transplantation 1997;64(2):263–9.

94. Dall'Amico R, Murer L. Extracorporeal photochemotherapy: a new therapeutic approach for allograft rejection. Transfus Apher Sci 2002;26(3):197–204.

95. Valentine VG, Robbins RC, Wehner JH, et al. Total lymphoid irradiation for refractory acute rejection in heart–lung and lung allografts. Chest 1996; 109(5):1184–9.

96. Jaramillo A, Smith CR, Maruyama T, et al. Anti-HLA class I antibody binding to airway epithelial cells induces production of fibrogenic growth factors

and apoptotic cell death: a possible mechanism for bronchiolitis obliterans syndrome. Hum Immunol 2003;64(5):521–9.

97. Pei R, Lee JH, Shih NJ, et al. Single human leukocyte antigen flow cytometry beads for accurate identification of human leukocyte antigen antibody specificities. Transplantation 2003;75(1):43–9.

98. McKenna RM, Takemoto SK, Terasaki PI. Anti-HLA antibodies after solid organ transplantation. Transplantation 2000;69(3):319–26.

99. Appel JZ 3rd, Hartwig MG, Davis RD, et al. Utility of peritransplant and rescue intravenous immunoglobulin and extracorporeal immunoadsorption in lung transplant recipients sensitized to HLA antigens. Hum Immunol 2005;66(4):378–86.

100. Appel JZ 3rd, Hartwig MG, Cantu E 3rd, et al. Role of flow cytometry to define unacceptable HLA antigens in lung transplant recipients with HLA-specific antibodies. Transplantation 2006; 81(7):1049–57.

101. Taylor CJ, Smith SI, Morgan CH, et al. Selective omission of the donor cross-match before renal transplantation: efficacy, safety, and effects on cold storage time. Transplantation 2000;69(5): 719–23.

102. Girnita AL, McCurry KR, Iacono AT, et al. HLA-specific antibodies are associated with high-grade and persistent–recurrent lung allograft acute rejection. J Heart Lung Transplant 2004; 23(10):1135–41.

103. Palmer SM, Davis RD, Hadjiliadis D, et al. Development of an antibody specific to major histocompatibility antigens detectable by flow cytometry after lung transplant is associated with bronchiolitis obliterans syndrome. Transplantation 2002;74(6): 799–804.

104. Hadjiliadis D, Chaparro C, Reinsmoen NL, et al. Pre-transplant panel reactive antibody in lung transplant recipients is associated with significantly worse post-transplant survival in a multicenter study. J Heart Lung Transplant 2005;24(Suppl 7): S249–54.

105. Burlingham WJ, Love RB, Jankowska-Gan E, et al. IL-17-dependent cellular immunity to collagen type V predisposes to obliterative bronchiolitis in human lung transplants. J Clin Invest 2007;117(11):3498–506.

106. Goers TA, Ramachandran S, Aloush A, et al. De novo production of K-alpha1 tubulin-specific antibodies: role in chronic lung allograft rejection. J Immunol 2008;180(7):4487–94.

107. Masson E, Stern M, Chabod J, et al. Hyperacute rejection after lung transplantation caused by undetected low-titer anti-HLA antibodies. J Heart Lung Transplant 2007;26(6):642–5.

108. Astor TL, Weill D, Cool C, et al. Pulmonary capillaritis in lung transplant recipients: treatment and effect on allograft function. J Heart Lung Transplant 2005;24(12):2091–7.

109. Badesch DB, Zamora M, Fullerton D, et al. Pulmonary capillaritis: a possible histologic form of acute pulmonary allograft rejection. J Heart Lung Transplant 1998;17(4):415–22.

110. Ionescu DN, Girnita AL, Zeevi A, et al. C4d deposition in lung allografts is associated with circulating anti-HLA alloantibody. Transpl Immunol 2005; 15(1):63–8.

111. Miller GG, Destarac L, Zeevi A, et al. Acute humoral rejection of human lung allografts and elevation of C4d in bronchoalveolar lavage fluid. Am J Transplant 2004;4(8):1323–30.

112. Girnita AL, McCurry KR, Yousem SA, et al. Antibody-mediated rejection in lung transplantation: case reports. Clin Transpl 2006;508–10.

113. Magro CM, Abbas AE, Seilstad K, et al. C3d and the septal microvasculature as a predictor of chronic lung allograft dysfunction. Hum Immunol 2006;67:274–83.

114. Westall GP, Snell GI, McLean C, et al. C3d and C4d deposition early after lung transplantation. J Heart Lung Transplant 2008;27(7):722–8.

115. Saint Martin GA, Reddy VB, Garrity ER, et al. Humoral (antibody-mediated) rejection in lung transplantation. J Heart Lung Transplant 1996; 15(12):1217–22.

116. Wallace WD, Reed EF, Ross D, et al. C4d staining of pulmonary allograft biopsies: an immunoperoxidase study. J Heart Lung Transplant 2005;24(10): 1565–70.

117. Magro CM, Deng A, Pope-Harman A, et al. Humorally mediated post-transplantation septal capillary injury syndrome as a common form of pulmonary allograft rejection: a hypothesis. Transplantation 2002;74(9):1273–80.

118. Vo AA, Lukovsky M, Toyoda M, et al. Rituximab and intravenous immune globulin for desensitization during renal transplantation. N Engl J Med 2008; 359(3):242–51.

119. Hachem RR, Yusen RD, Meyers BF, et al. Anti-human leukocyte antigen antibodies and preemptive antibody-directed therapy after lung transplantation. J Heart Lung Transplant 2010;29(9):973–80.

120. Lemy A, Toungouz M, Abramowicz D. Bortezomib: a new player in pre- and post-transplant desensitization? Nephrol Dial Transplant 2010;25(11): 3480–9.

121. Neumann J, Tarrasconi H, Bortolotto A, et al. Acute humoral rejection in a lung recipient: reversion with bortezomib. Transplantation 2010;89(1): 125–6.

Chronic Allograft Dysfunction

Christiane Knoop, MD, PhD*, Marc Estenne, MD, PhD

KEYWORDS

- Lung transplantation • Chronic lung allograft dysfunction
- Bronchiolitis obliterans • Bronchiolitis obliterans syndrome
- Neutrophilic reversible allograft/airways dysfunction
- Macrolides

Bronchiolitis obliterans (BO) in the context of lung transplantation was first described in 1984 at Stanford University in a patient who developed progressive airflow obstruction after heart-lung transplantation.[1] Lung biopsies revealed intraluminal polyps of fibromyxoid granulation tissue, which tended to obliterate the lumen of terminal bronchioles, and dense submucosal eosinophilic fibrous scars (**Fig. 1**). Since this early report, BO has been recognized as the major complication and the leading cause of death after lung transplantation.[2]

Because the small airway lesions have a patchy distribution, they can hardly be demonstrated by transbronchial lung biopsies (TBBs), which have a low sensitivity (28%) and specificity (75%).[3] As a result, in order to establish the diagnosis of BO without the need for open lung biopsy, the International Society for Heart and Lung Transplantation (ISHLT) proposed in 1993 a clinical definition based on pulmonary function criteria. The term, bronchiolitis obliterans syndrome (BOS), was coined to identify patients with a progressive and irreversible decline in forced expiratory volume in one second (FEV_1). In the initial classification, BOS was divided into 4 stages based on the degree of loss in FEV_1 compared with the best postoperative value. In the updated classification proposed in 2002, a potential BOS (BOS 0-p) stage—defined by a decline in FEV_1 or in midexpiratory flow rates (FEF_{25-75})—was added to detect early but potentially important changes in pulmonary function (**Table 1**).[4] Several conditions

needed to be satisfied for a patient to be classified in the staging system: (1) the functional loss had to be present for at least 3 weeks to exclude an acute, reversible process; (2) the loss had to include a decrease in both FEV_1 and FEV_1/vital capacity ratio (ie, patients with a loss in FEV_1 in the context of a restrictive ventilatory defect are not considered as having BOS), and (3) confounding conditions that may produce a decrease in FEV_1 (eg, infection, acute rejection, anastomotic complications, disease recurrence, and progression of native lung hyperinflation in patients with single-lung transplantation [SLT] for emphysema) needed to be excluded.

Transplant centers worldwide have adopted this staging system as a descriptor of chronic lung allograft dysfunction. This proved useful because it provided a common language to classify patients and compare results between programs. Several limitations, however, have become apparent in recent years. First, many patients who have confounding conditions cannot be staged for BOS. Second, as the experience with lung transplantation accrued, an increasing number of patients presented with forms of chronic allograft dysfunction that did not comprise all the characteristic features of BOS. Several types of chronic allograft dysfunction, which differ from BOS, were identified in the past years. These include (1) a reversible phenotype characterized by airway neutrophilia and functional improvement with azithromycin (AZM), (2) a phenotype characterized by a restrictive ventilatory impairment associated with upper

Department of Chest Medicine, Erasme University Hospital, Université Libre de Bruxelles, 808 Route de Lennik, B-1070 Brussels, Belgium
* Corresponding author. Chest Service, Erasme University Hospital, 808 Route de Lennik, B-1070 Brussels, Belgium.
E-mail address: christiane.knoop@erasme.ulb.ac.be

Clin Chest Med 32 (2011) 311–326
doi:10.1016/j.ccm.2011.02.009
0272-5231/11/$ – see front matter © 2011 Elsevier Inc. All rights reserved.

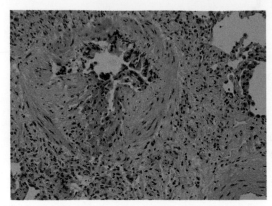

Fig. 1. Histological picture of post-transplant BO. The lumen of the bronchiole is almost totally occluded by fibromyxoid granulation tissue.

lobe fibrosis or persistent parenchymal or pleural abnormalities, (3) exudative or follicular bronchiolitis, and (4) large airway stenosis/malacia. This review deals primarily with classical BOS, which has been more extensively studied, but other recently described presentations of chronic allograft dysfunction also are addressed.

THE CLINICAL SPECTRUM OF CHRONIC ALLOGRAFT DYSFUNCTION
Classical BOS

In the registry report of the ISHLT published in 2010,[2] freedom from BOS in a cohort of 12,058 patients followed between April 1994 and June 2009 was 89.7% at 1 year, 67.4% at 3 years, 51.2% at 5 years, and 24.8% at 10 years after surgery. These percentages represent a clear decrease in the prevalence of the complication compared with earlier series. Yet BOS remains by far the most significant long-term complication and the leading cause of late death after lung transplantation, accounting for 20% to 30% of all deaths after the third postoperative year.[2]

BOS may affect all lung transplant recipients irrespective of donor and recipient characteristics, type of transplantation, and pretransplant disease. The clinical presentation of BOS is heterogeneous.[5] The type of presentation, the time from transplantation to onset, and the rate of progression are all variable between patients (**Fig. 2**). BOS may present as an acute illness and imitate a respiratory infection,[5] but in most patients it starts as an asymptomatic process that produces an insidious decline in lung function. In approximately 20% of patients, BOS develops within 2 years of transplantation (early-onset BOS), but the vast majority of patients develop the complication at a later point in time.[2,6] Some patients present with a substantial loss of lung function and are already in BOS stage 2 or 3 (high-grade onset) at presentation whereas others show a slow decline over time.[6] In a study by Jackson and colleagues[5] 56% of 204 patients who developed BOS showed a sudden drop in FEV_1, whereas 18% presented with a smooth linear decline; time to BOS onset was longer in the latter group. Acute rejection during the first 6 months was significantly associated with acute onset of BOS. Auscultation of the lungs is often normal, but squeaks and coarse crackles may be heard. High-resolution CT may reveal air trapping (**Fig. 3**) and bronchiectasis,[7,8] without significant parenchymal infiltrate. As the disease progresses, permanent airway colonization with pathogens, such as *Pseudomonas aeruginosa* and *Aspergillus fumigatus*, frequently develops. Survival at 5 years after diagnosis ranges from 26% to 43%,[6,9–11] and survival at 5 years after transplantation is 20% to 40% lower in patients with, compared to patients without, BOS.[11] There is also evidence that the number of respiratory infections and the aggressiveness with which they are treated have an impact on BOS progression.[9] In addition to representing a major obstacle to long-term survival,

Table 1
Bronchiolitis obliterans syndrome classification system

	1993 Classification	2002 Classification	
	FEV_1 80% or more of baseline	FEV_1 >90% of baseline *and* FEF_{25-75} >75% of baseline	BOS 0
		FEV_1 81% to 90% of baseline *and/or* FEF_{25-75} = or <75% of baseline	BOS 0-p
BOS 1	FEV_1 66% to 80% of baseline	FEV_1 66% to 80% of baseline	BOS 1
BOS 2	FEV_1 51% to 65% of baseline	FEV_1 51% to 65% of baseline	BOS 2
BOS 3	FEV_1 50% or less of baseline	FEV_1 50% or less of baseline	BOS 3

Data from Estenne M, Maurer JR, Boehler A, et al. Bronchiolitis obliterans syndrome 2001: an update of the diagnostic criteria. J Heart Lung Transplant 2002;21:297–310.

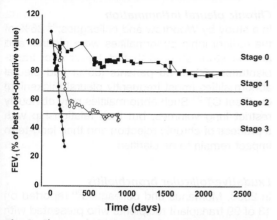

Fig. 2. Changes in FEV_1 over time elapsed since transplantation in 3 patients with BOS. Stages refer to the BOS classification, and horizontal lines indicate transitions between stages 0 and 1, stages 1 and 2, and stages 2 and 3. The figure illustrates the highly variable pattern of functional evolution between patients affected by BOS. (*From* Estenne M, Maurer JR, Boehler A, et al. Bronchiolitis obliterans syndrome 2001: an update of the diagnostic criteria. J Heart Lung Transplant 2002;21:297–310; with permission.)

BOS causes significant morbidity and loss of health-related quality of life.[12]

BOS is used as a surrogate marker of BO but does not equal BO. Therefore, as expected for any functional marker, a drop in FEV_1 is likely to have a low specificity for the diagnosis of BO (this is why exclusionary criteria were added to the definition of BOS). This lack of specificity is difficult to assess because a gold standard is

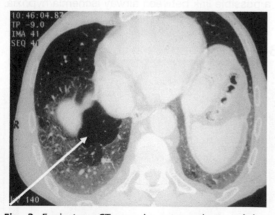

Fig. 3. Expiratory CT scan in a transplant recipient with BOS. The arrow indicates lobules with low attenuation, a sign of the presence of air trapping. (*From* Bankier AA, Muylem AV, Knoop C, et al. BOS in heart-lung transplant recipients: diagnosis with expiratory CT. Radiology 2001;218:533–9; with permission.)

rarely available. Yet in a study of lungs explanted at the time of retransplantation for BOS,[13] pathology examination always showed at least some degree of BO, but a wide range of other pathologic processes of potential clinical significance was also evident in half of the specimens.

Other Forms of Chronic Allograft Dysfunction

In contrast to classical BOS, which is characterized by a progressive, irreversible airflow obstruction and few, if any, parenchymal or pleural abnormalities, recently described new phenotypes of chronic allograft dysfunction may include one or more of the following features: partial reversibility of airway obstruction, restrictive ventilatory impairment, parenchymal/pleural abnormalities, and large airway stenosis/malacia.

Neutrophilic reversible allograft/airways dysfunction

Because it is well known that macrolide antibiotics are effective in treating airway diseases which, like BOS, are associated with neutrophilic inflammation (eg, panbronchiolitis and cystic fibrosis), Gerhardt and colleagues[14] performed an open trial with AZM in lung transplant recipients. In this study, AZM (250 mg 3 times a week) was added to the current immunosuppressive treatment in 6 patients with BOS; 5 patients responded with a mean improvement in the FEV_1 of 21.6% after 14 weeks. One patient even had a complete restoration of FEV_1 to peak post-transplant values. This landmark study was followed by at least 6 studies,[15–20] of which 4 confirmed the results published by Gerhardt and colleagues.[14] One study by Benden and colleagues[21] also reported a positive effect of clarithromycin on FEV_1. Taking these publications together, approximately 35% of all patients in different BOS stages responded to macrolide treatment by a mean increase in FEV_1 of approximately 14%. Furthermore, a higher bronchoalveolar lavage (BAL) fluid neutrophilia was associated with a greater likelihood of functional response.[18] Based on these observations, Verleden and colleagues[22] suggested that BOS might be dichotomized into an AZM-responsive phenotype characterized by airway neutrophilia and functional improvement with AZM (the so-called neutrophilic reversible allograft/airways dysfunction [NRAD]), and an AZM-unresponsive phenotype, which corresponds to the classical, fibroproliferative form of BO. These two phenotypes might have different pathophysiology, clinical presentation, and prognosis; for example, NRAD might start earlier after transplantation and progress slower than fibroproliferative BOS; and crackles, increased sputum production, bronchiectasis, and mucus plugging might be more prominent in the former than in the latter.

Upper lobe fibrosis

In 2005, a joint retrospective study by the Toronto General Hospital and the Duke University Hospital identified 13 of 686 lung transplant recipients who developed upper lobe fibrosis.[23] Radiographic changes started initially as nonspecific interstitial markings in the upper lobes and slowly progressed to honeycombing, traction bronchiectasis, and volume loss (**Fig. 4**). Most patients had a restrictive ventilatory defect, with some eventually developing concomitant airflow obstruction. Open lung biopsy specimens revealed dense interstitial fibrosis, with occasional features of BO, acute fibrinous and organizing pneumonia, bronchiolitis obliterans organizing pneumonia, and aspiration. The rate of progression of clinical symptoms ranged from slow to rapid but, overall, the condition had a poor prognosis. The prevalence and cause of this form of chronic allograft dysfunction are still unclear.

Recently, Woodrow and colleagues[24] reported on lung transplant recipients who had a decline in lung function associated with persistent parenchymal (alveolar, nodular, ground-glass, or interstitial) abnormalities on chest CT—not specifically involving the upper lobes (**Fig. 5**). No precise cause was found for the parenchymal infiltrates and the patients showed a functional deterioration over time that paralleled the course of patients with classical BOS. A similar proportion of patients (approximately 50%) had a restrictive ventilatory defect in the group with, and in the group without, parenchymal infiltrates.

Chronic pleural inflammation

In a study by Woodrow and colleagues,[24] 36% of the radiographic abnormalities were pleural, and another study showed that at 1 year after transplantation, 50 of 58 patients (86%) had pleural abnormalities (most frequently pleural thickening) on chest CT.[25] Such abnormalities may obviously restrict lung volumes, but their relationship with a process of chronic rejection and their long-term impact remain to be clarified.

Exudative/follicular bronchiolitis

In 2008, McManus and colleagues[26] reported on 13 of 99 transplant recipients who presented with exudative bronchiolitis, which appeared on high-resolution CT as a tree-in-bud pattern (centrilobular nodules and branching lines). This condition was associated with early infection post-transplant and a history of *Aspergillus* infection. Neutrophil count in bronchial washing was increased and most patients improved clinically and radiologically with AZM. Yet, exudative bronchiolitis increased markedly the likelihood of developing BOS. Recently, Vos and colleagues[27] described a patient who developed follicular bronchiolitis characterized by abundant peribronchiolar lymphoid follicles; this condition was also associated with the development of BOS.

Large airway stenosis/malacia

A recent article by Akindipe and colleagues[28] reported on 5 patients who had to be retransplanted for severe recurrent airway narrowing. In all patients, allograft lung pathology revealed evidence of BO. This observation suggests a possible link between airway ischemia/hypoxia,

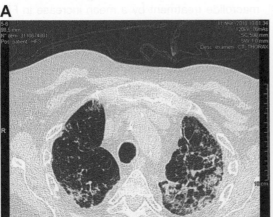
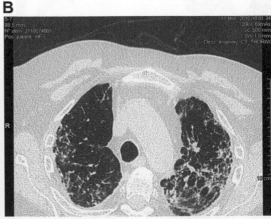

Fig. 4. CT scans obtained at two different levels (*A* and *B*) in a lung transplant recipient showing the peculiar pattern of upper lobe fibrosis. Culture for infectious agents of BAL specimens were repeatedly negative in these zones and transbronchial biopsies showed nonspecific inflammation and fibrotic changes.

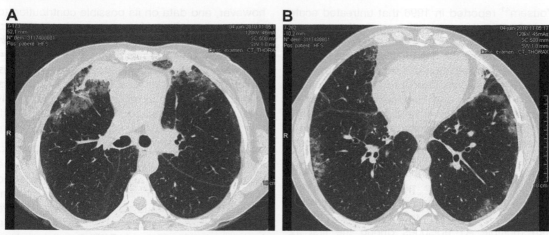

Fig. 5. This patient with CF had been transplanted for 10 years when she developed an acute, rapidly progressive, and completely therapy-resistant drop in lung function. CT scan of the lungs repeatedly showed peripheral infiltrates in the upper (A) but also lower (B) lung zones. BAL showed prominent neutrophilia but also—even if to a lesser extent—eosinophilia. No infectious agents could be incriminated; in particular, there were no diagnostic criteria for invasive pulmonary aspergillosis. She, eventually, could undergo redo-double lung transplantation. The explanted lungs showed zones of nonspecific interstitial fibrosis with pneumocyte hyperplasia and fibroblast proliferation in the areas of the parenchymal abnormalities, and advanced BO lesions in other lung regions.

large airway stenosis/malacia, and the development of BO.

PATHOGENESIS AND RISK FACTORS
Pathogenesis

In the earlier days of lung transplantation, BOS/BO was believed to be equivalent to chronic allograft rejection (ie, a process caused by an alloimmune reaction). The lung is uniquely exposed to the environment, however, and thus to recurrent nonalloimmune insults, such as infections, inhalation of toxic fumes, or gastroesophageal reflux. Furthermore, recent studies suggest a possible role of autoantibodies developed against specific epithelial proteins and of airway hypoxia in the pathogenesis of BOS/BO. The current view is that these insults, acting alone or in combination, upregulate dendritic cells in the airway epithelium, leading to epithelial damage and inflammation with production of chemokines and cytokines by airway epithelium and smooth muscle cells, macrophages, and neutrophils. Activated neutrophils further increase epithelial damage via the production of reactive oxygen species and metalloproteinases. After the initial inflammatory phase, a fibroproliferative phase occurs, driven by growth factors and leading to proliferation of smooth muscle cells and myofibroblasts. This process eventually results in aberrant collagen deposition, excessive fibroproliferation, and small airway obliteration. BO would thus represent a final common pathway lesion secondary to multiple, repetitive insults to the airway epithelium.[29,30]

Alloimmune Risk Factors

Ninety-five percent of patients receive grafts with 3 or more HLA mismatches. Using the Collaborative Transplant Study database, 5-year graft outcome according to HLA mismatch was examined in 8020 lung transplants performed during 1989 through 2009. Graft survival rates showed a stepwise decrease as the combined number of HLA-A+B+DR mismatches increased from 1 to 6, with a high number of HLA mismatches having an unfavorable impact on survival.[31] Because of the average high number of mismatches, studies to examine the effect of HLA mismatching on the incidence of acute rejection have proved difficult and their results have been inconsistent. Most of them have, however, identified some negative impact of HLA mismatching.[32,33] Multivariate logistic regression analyses of data on 3549 adult lung transplant recipients retrieved from the United Network for Organ Sharing/ISHLT registry demonstrated an association between mismatching at the HLA-A locus (but not at the HLA-B or HLA-DR loci) and acute rejection episodes requiring hospital admission.[34] Several studies have confirmed that the development of anti-HLA class I and class II antibodies after surgery is associated with a risk for acute rejection and BOS.[35–39] Binding of these antibodies to airway epithelial cells may induce epithelial injury and proliferation.[40]

Acute vascular rejection histology graded greater than or equal to A2 has been identified in many studies as a statistical risk factor for BOS.

Yousem[41] reported in 1996 that untreated acute vascular rejection grade A2 leads to the development of BOS in 50% of patients. Several studies have shown that the risk of BOS increases when acute vascular rejection is histologically severe or persistent or recurs after treatment (studies reviewed by Knoop and Estenne[42]). The impact of minimal acute rejection (grade A1) on the development of BOS, however, has been long neglected. Recently, in a study by Hopkins and colleagues[43] less than10% of grade A1 rejections were associated with clinical symptoms but 34% of the asymptomatic patients progressed to higher-grade acute rejection or lymphocytic bronchiolitis (LB) within 3 months. In this report also, patients with multiple A1 episodes during the first 12 months post-transplant had a significantly higher risk of developing BOS, and this occurred earlier than in patients with 1 or less grade A1 episode.[43] Khalifa and colleagues[44] retrospectively examined data from 228 lung transplant patients followed over a 7-year period and confirmed that grade A1 rejection is a distinct risk factor for BOS. Hachem and colleagues[45] from the same group determined that even a single episode of A1 rejection, without recurrence or subsequent progression to a higher rejection grade, was a significant risk factor for the development of BOS. Treatment of grade A1 rejection with diverse approaches in order to augment the net immunosuppression decreased the risk for subsequent progression to BOS stage 1.[44]

LB in the absence of acute vascular rejection may also predate BOS.[46,47] Glanville and colleagues[48] retrospectively assessed data from 1770 TBB specimens obtained from 341 patients over a period of 10 years and showed that the cumulative incidence of BOS was significantly associated with the severity of LB. Another retrospective analysis of 2697 TBB specimens obtained from nearly 300 consecutive patients followed during the first 2 postoperative years at the University of Copenhagen showed that the cumulative incidences of LB ($\geq$ B2) were 33%, 53%, 62%, and 68% at 1 month, 3 months, 6 months, and 12 months, respectively. Approximately 25% and 50% of patients had a second episode graded B2 or higher within 3 months and 2 years of transplantation, respectively. In this study, LB during the first 2 years was independently associated with the frequency and/or severity of acute rejection, and LB grade B2 or higher was associated with an increased risk of BO.[49]

The concept of acute or chronic antibody-mediated rejection is still controversial after lung transplantation.[50] There are now well documented reports that this type of rejection exists,[51]

however, and data on its possible contribution to chronic allograft dysfunction are beginning to appear.[52] The observation that patients developing HLA antibodies fare less well than those who do not and the novel data on self-antibodies directed against epithelial antigens in patients with BOS/BO (discussed later) lend some credibility to this hypothesis.

Autoimmune Risk Factors

Recently, the development of autoimmune processes directed against epithelial-specific proteins has been incriminated in the development of BOS/BO. In one study, collagen type V-reactive CD4+ T cells were associated with a nearly 10-fold increase in the risk of BOS in clinical lung transplantation.[53] In another study, anti-K–α1 tubulin antibodies were present in a significant number of patients with BOS.[54] Anti-K–α1 tubulin circulating antibodies may induce profibrotic growth factors from airway epithelial cell lines, thus providing evidence that autoimmunity—like alloimmunity—may induce fibrosis.[55] Conversely, it has also been shown that alloimmune responses in the lung can promote the development of collagen type V and K–α1-tubulin autoimmunity.[56] Thus, the picture has become more complex: alloimmunity, autoimmunity, and the innate immune system (discussed later) may all trigger allograft airway fibrosis, and these processes are moreover likely intertwined.[57]

Other Risk Factors

As discussed previously, the association between acute rejection and BOS has been reported for both early and late rejection episodes. Yet many patients with acute rejection do not develop BOS, and some patients with BOS have never experienced acute rejection. One possible explanation is that the use of intense induction and maintenance immunosuppression and of aggressive treatment of rejection might uncouple the association between acute rejection and BOS. Another potential explanation, however, is that BOS/BO might be triggered by nonalloimmune–dependent factors. These may directly injure the airways—as is the case for gastric aspiration—and/or augment the alloimmune response via activation of the innate immune system, as is the case for respiratory bacterial and viral infections.[58]

Bacterial colonization of the graft was formerly believed to be the consequence of BOS/BO. It has been recently reported, however, that bacterial colonization, notably with *Pseudomonas aeruginosa*, might be one of the possible alloimmune-independent risk factors for BOS/OB.

In a study by Botha and colleagues,[59] including 155 lung transplant recipients, the development of allograft colonization with *Pseudomonas* was strongly associated with the development of BOS within 2 years of transplant (23.4% and 7.7% in those colonized and not colonized, respectively). The isolation of *Pseudomonas* predated the diagnosis of BOS in more than 75% of affected patients by a median exceeding 200 days. Similar findings have been reported for *Aspergillus* colonization.[60] Valentine and colleagues[61] analyzed the role of bacterial and fungal respiratory tract infections in the development of BOS in a single-center study comprising 161 lung recipients who had survived at least 180 days. Multivariate analysis indicated that gram-negative, gram-positive, and fungal pneumonias were associated with the development of BOS. Gram-positive pneumonia and fungal pneumonia in the first 100 days conferred hazard ratios of 3.8 and 2.1, respectively. They concluded that early recognition and treatment of these pathogens might improve long-term outcomes.

Kumar and colleagues[62] screened serial surveillance and diagnostic BAL specimens obtained from 93 lung transplant recipients over 3 years for community-acquired respiratory viral infections (CARVIs) using sensitive molecular methods that simultaneously detected 19 respiratory viral types/subtypes. Respiratory viruses—rhinovirus, parainfluenza virus 1 to 4, coronavirus, influenza, metapneumovirus, and respiratory syncytial virus—were isolated in 48 of 93 (51.6%) patients in at least one BAL sample. Biopsy-proven acute rejection ($\geq$ A2) or decline in FEV_1 greater than or equal to 20% occurred in 33.3% of CARVI-positive patients (within 3 months of CARVI) compared with only 6.7% of CARVI-negative patients. No significant difference was seen in the incidence of acute rejection between symptomatic and asymptomatic patients. Biopsy-proved BO was diagnosed in 10 of 16 (62.5%) patients within 1 year of infection, indicating that symptomatic or asymptomatic viral infection may trigger acute rejection and/or BOS/BO. In contrast, Gottlieb and colleagues[63] found that only symptomatic CARVI increases the risk of BOS. *Chlamydia pneumoniae*[64,65] and human herpesvirus 6 respiratory infections[66] are also known to increase the risk of BOS.

CMV mismatching (ie, seronegative recipients receiving organs from seropositive donors) and CMV pneumonitis have been associated with BOS in several series, but others found only a marginal or no relationship at all. These differences might be accounted for, at least in part, by the different strategies used to match recipients with regard to CMV status and to prevent and treat CMV illness over the decades. Valentine and colleagues[61] reported that CMV pneumonitis within the first 100 days conferred a hazard ratio of 3.1 to develop BOS. The same group reported on their experience with ganciclovir (GCV) prophylaxis in 130 patients surviving at least 100 days. CMV pneumonitis occurred in 16%, 8%, 17%, and 19% of patients in the D+R+, D−R+, D+R− and D−R− groups, respectively. Ninety patients received indefinite GCV prophylaxis whereas 40 patients discontinued the prophylaxis (STOP). Cumulative incidences of CMV pneumonitis in the indefinite GCV prophylaxis and STOP groups at 5 years were 2% and 57%, respectively. In the STOP cohort, 15 of 40 patients developed CMV pneumonitis after GCV was stopped, and 10 of these developed BOS. The risk of CMV pneumonitis in the STOP cohort was significantly higher when GCV prophylaxis was discontinued within the first year. BOS-free survival and survival were, however, similar across groups.[67] On the contrary, Tamm and colleagues[68] showed in their series that CMV pneumonitis, when treated with GCV, is not a risk factor for BOS and does not affect survival.

Gastroesophageal reflux disease (GERD) is thought to be a risk factor for the development or progression of BOS/OB. GERD is observed in approximately half of all lung transplant patients.[69] The prevalence of delayed gastric emptying is also high.[69] In addition, these patients have an impaired cough reflex because of lung denervation and have altered mucociliary clearance. Taken together, these factors increase the likelihood of aspiration and subsequent airway injury. Pepsin[70] and bile acids[71] can be readily found in the BAL fluid of many lung transplant recipients, which confirms the frequent occurrence of gastric aspiration. The finding of increased bile acids in BAL fluid (a marker of nonacidic reflux) correlates with the presence of BOS/BO.[70,71] Exposure of the airway epithelium to bile acids may predispose to colonization with *Pseudomonas aeruginosa* and airway neutrophilia. Because of concern that GERD increases the risk of BOS, the general trend has been to propose a surgical solution, namely gastric fundoplication, to all recipients presenting with significant GERD. Supportive evidence for this strategy is derived from retrospective studies in which gastric fundoplication within 3 months after transplant was associated with greater freedom from BOS and increased survival.[72] Another study from the same center showed that fundoplication improved lung function in many patients with established BOS.[73] Before adopting this radical approach for every single lung transplant recipient, however, it is important to be aware that (1) the best way to diagnose GERD in lung transplant recipients—pH monitoring versus impedance monitoring—is at present controversial; (2) GERD—as well as the cough reflex—may improve over time; (3) fundoplication may have serious side effects (eg, significant weight loss, which can be of importance in recipients with significant malnutrition); (4) the protective function of the surgical sleeve may wane over time; (5) the precise indications, timing, and choice of fundoplication technique are yet to be defined; and (6) the overall impact on lung function and survival are unknown because there are no controlled studies to date.[74]

Allograft ischemia may arise during the period of warm ischemia during explantation, because of the absence of bronchial arterial reanastomosis at implantation, or through small airway microvascular damage at later time points.[75] In a study of 334 lung transplant recipients of whom 65 developed primary graft dysfunction (which is a severe form of ischemia/reperfusion lung injury), this complication was an independent risk factor for BOS.[76] Allograft ischemia might result in hypoxic inflammatory conditions leading to vascular remodeling and angiogenesis, which may in turn be a potent stimulus for airway fibrosis.[77,78] By gaining a better understanding of the complex interaction between airway ischemia, vascular remodeling and angiogenesis-mediated airway fibroproliferation, it might become increasingly possible to rationally design therapies that can halt conditions of maladaptive fibrosis[79] and, possibly, decrease the risk of BOS/BO.

The role of other risk factors for BOS, such as graft ischemic time, donor-recipient gender or size mismatch, and type of surgical procedure, is currently controversial.

The Role of Neutrophils

It is widely accepted that BOS/BO involves a neutrophilic airway inflammation, although this feature is lacking in a substantial proportion of patients. Recent studies (summarized by Verleden and colleagues[22]) have shown that interleukin (IL)-17 may have an important role in the development of BOS/BO. IL-17 is a potent indirect neutrophil-attracting chemokine through its ability to induce IL-8 secretion from different cell types in the airways. IL-17 is increased in the airways of patients with BOS/BO and induces production of IL-8 by airway smooth muscle and epithelial cells, which, in turn, promotes airway neutrophilia. The IL-17/IL-8 axis may be triggered by both alloimmune and autoimmune mechanisms, airway

bacterial colonization, and GERD,[22] but the reasons why BOS is accompanied by airway neutrophilia in some patients and not in others remain unclear. The effect of AZM on this inflammatory process is likely primarily accounted for by its ability to inhibit the IL-17/IL-8 pathway; other potential mechanisms include a positive effect of AZM on GERD (AZM is a known agonist of motilin) as well as its inhibitory effect on bacterial growth.

Open Questions and Controversial Issues

It is important to stress that BOS and the newly described phenotypes of chronic allograft dysfunction are syndromes defined by clinical criteria, changes in pulmonary function, radiographic features, and analysis of BAL cellularity, alone or in combination. These entities are merely descriptive and do not sort by specific pathogenic pathways, risk factors, pathology, or prognosis. Patients may have more than one phenotype at a time or over time, and different pathogenic pathways and pathology may coexist (discussed previously). More work is required to understand the clinical relevance and pathogenesis of each entity as well as the mechanisms by which the different risk factors produce one phenotype or another.

For the time being, we still have to work with the current definition of BOS (ie, a progressive and irreversible airflow obstruction due to a loss of small airway function attributed to BO) although the difficulties associated with a staging system based on a retrospective diagnosis and exclusionary criteria are acknowledged. BOS should probably no longer be presumed to reflect specifically a process of chronic rejection because nonalloimmune insults likely often contribute to the development of the small airway lesions. Finally, whether or not NRAD should be considered a subtype of BOS or a distinct entity is currently debated in the transplant community (discussed later).

DIAGNOSIS

To the extent that current therapies work to stop or slow down the progression of BOS, they do so mostly by an anti-inflammatory, not an antifibrotic, effect. Therefore, they are more likely to be effective in the early stage of the disease. For this reason, various parameters have been evaluated as early biomarkers of BOS.

Lung Function

Spirometry is appealing as an early marker because it is widely available, noninvasive, reproducible, and relatively inexpensive. Two studies have assessed the predictive value of BOS stage 0-p for the diagnosis of BOS stage 1. In the study by Hachem and colleagues,[80] which included 203 adult bilateral lung transplant (BLT) recipients, the FEV_1 criterion had a sensitivity, specificity, positive predictive value, and negative predictive value of 74%, 86%, 79%, and 82%, respectively; corresponding values for the modified FEF_{25-75} criterion (computed using baseline values obtained at the time of the two highest FEV_1 measurements) were 66%, 88%, 81%, and 76%, respectively. In the 197 SLT recipients studied by Lama and colleagues,[81] the FEV_1 criterion was also predictive of BOS 1; its predictive value was superior to that of the FEF_{25-75} criterion and was superior in patients with underlying restrictive as opposed to obstructive physiology.

Exhaled Biomarkers

Distribution of ventilation

The slope of the alveolar plateau of the single-breath washout test reflects the homogeneity of ventilation distribution and increases as ventilation becomes more heterogeneous. The single-breath test can be performed using an inspiration of pure oxygen and measuring the concentration of

nitrogen during expiration; a gas mixture containing inert gases (for example helium) can also be used during inspiration, and the concentration of these gases be measured during expiration. Two prospective studies have assessed the usefulness of the single-breath test for the early detection of BOS in BLT recipients. In these studies, nitrogen slope became abnormal 178[82] and 151[83] days before the criterion for BOS 1 was met. The positive predictive value of the test was 70% to 80% and the negative predictive value approximately 100%. Furthermore, 2 studies by Estenne and colleagues[82] and Van Muylem and colleagues[84] showed that helium slope is an even earlier marker than nitrogen slope (**Fig. 6**).

Two recent studies in recipients of SLT for emphysema or fibrosis suggested that when performed in lateral decubitus, the single-breath test may also provide information on ventilation distribution in the graft in this patient population.[85,86]

Exhaled gases

Exhaled nitric oxide (eNO) is a well-recognized biomarker of airway inflammation. In stable lung transplant recipients and patients with BOS, eNO reflects the expression of bronchial epithelial

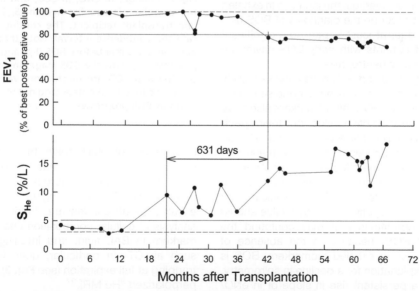

Fig. 6. In patients presenting BOS, the slope of the alveolar plateau for helium increases as ventilation becomes more heterogeneous and this early marker of BOS becomes abnormal before spirometric criteria for BOS 1 are fulfilled. This figure shows changes in FEV_1 and in the slope of the alveolar plateau for helium obtained during a single-breath washout test (S_{He}) in one heart-lung transplant recipient. In the upper panel, the dashed line corresponds to 100% of the two best postoperative values and the continuous line indicates a 20% decrease (BOS stage 1). In the lower panel, the dashed line corresponds to the average of the two lowest postoperative values, and the continuous line is the upper limit of the 97.5% CI computed from data obtained in 10 stable transplant patients. Note that a significant change in S_{He} is observed 631 days before the 20% drop in FEV_1. (*From* Van Muylem A, Knoop C, Estenne M. Early detection of chronic pulmonary allograft dysfunction by exhaled biomarkers. Am J Respir Crit Care Med 2007;175:731–6; with permission.)

inducible NO synthase and positively correlates with airway neutrophilia.[87-90] Carbon monoxide (CO) is produced endogenously by the stress protein heme oxygenase, which is increased in a variety of oxidant/inflammatory-mediated injuries. In BO lesions, heme oxygenase staining correlates with myeloperoxidase expression (reflecting oxidant load) and with neutrophilic infiltration of the bronchial wall. Heme oxygenase degrades heme with the production of iron, biliverdin, and CO. Therefore, both eNO[87-89] and exhaled CO (eCO)[90] may reflect airway neutrophilia and, hence, be used as surrogate markers of BOS.

Four studies have shown that eNO is increased in patients with BOS compared with patients without BOS,[89,91-93] independent of the type of surgical procedure. The potential contribution of serial eNO measurements to the early detection of BOS, however, was difficult to assess from these studies. In a recent study of 65 recipients of bilateral grafts who were followed for approximately 1250 days, Van Muylem and colleagues[84] found that eNO and eCO only transiently increased in BOS 0-p and then returned to baseline as BOS progressed (Fig. 7). The sensitivity of exhaled gases for the diagnosis of BOS 0-p was only 50% to 60%, but it increased to approximately 80% when values of eNO and eCO were combined; yet, on average, the increase in exhaled gases did not precede the diagnosis of BOS 0-p. This may be due, at least in part, to a significant proportion of patients with early BOS having no increase in airway neutrophilia.

In summary, eNO and eCO have a fair sensitivity and nitrogen or helium slope has a good sensitivity for the detection of BOS. All biomarkers also have a high negative predictive value, but their specificity and positive predictive value are much lower. The low specificity reflects that these markers—like the FEV_1—may be affected by complications other than BOS (eg, acute rejection, lymphocytic bronchiolitis, and infection). From a clinical point of view, the high negative predictive value should help detect conditions that may confound the diagnosis of BOS, because in the absence of a significant rise in exhaled biomarkers, BOS is an unlikely explanation for a decline in spirometry. Conversely, a persistent rise in slope or in eNO/eCO should be interpreted as a warning signal and prompt close monitoring of a patient's lung function and clinical condition.

Other Markers

Several other surrogate markers of BOS have been proposed, but their clinical utility is limited by one or more of the following factors: they are

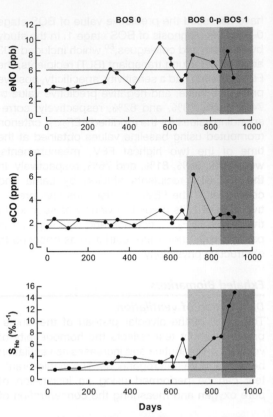

Fig. 7. Changes in eNO, in eCO, and in the slope of the alveolar plateau for helium (S_{He}) over time in one transplant recipient. The continuous lines indicate the confidence interval. Note that values of S_{He} become abnormal before BOS 0-p, and then increase progressively with the BOS stage; in contrast, values of eNO and eCO are much more variable between successive measurements and do not show a consistent trend as BOS progresses.

invasive or potentially toxic, they are expensive, they are not widely available, or their predictive value has not been appropriately tested or is controversial. These surrogate markers include exhaled breath condensate,[94] induced sputum,[95] analysis of cellular composition and inflammatory markers in BAL fluid, and imaging techniques, such as CT—in particular, quantification of air trapping at full expiration (see Fig. 3),[7,8,96] and hyperpolarized ^{3}He MRI.[97]

TREATMENT
Optimization and/or Change in Immunosuppressive Regimen

All interventions that target risk factors and may prevent the development of BOS are valuable because therapy is often ineffective when BOS is established. In this context, optimization of the immunosuppressive regimen to prevent the occurrence of acute rejection is a critical issue (discussed previously). Several studies have looked at the effects of increasing the net level of immunosuppression (eg, by using high-dose methylprednisolone, cytolytic therapy, or methotrexate) and/or changing the maintenance regimen (eg, by shifting from cyclosporine A to tacrolimus or from azathioprine to mycophenolate mofetil, or by adding inhaled cyclosporine A) in patients with established BOS (reviewed by Knoop and Estenne[42]). In some patients, these modalities have been shown to stabilize lung function or decrease the rate of decline of FEV_1 for short periods of time. The small number of patients studied, the mostly retrospective design of these studies, the lack of adequate control group, and the relatively short follow-up time, however, make it difficult to assess the effectiveness of these treatments. No single strategy has proved more successful than another. In addition, augmented immunosuppression increases the risk of toxicity and predisposes to intercurrent bronchopulmonary infections, which must be factored into the risk-benefit analysis as they may promote the progression of BOS (discussed previously).

Macrolides

As discussed previously, several studies with a follow-up of 12 to 40 weeks have shown that macrolide treatment improves FEV_1 in approximately one-third of patients in different BOS stages. Two studies[20,98] have assessed the long-term effect of AZM. The study by Gottlieb and colleagues included 81 patients with a median follow-up of 1.3 years[20] and the study by Vos and colleagues[98] included 108 patients treated for a median time of 612 days. An initial response (defined as a 10% or more increase in FEV_1) was observed in 30% to 40% of the patients, but 30% to 40% of these subsequently relapsed. By multivariate analysis, initial response to AZM and earlier post-transplant time of initiation of treatment were protective factors for disease progression or relapse; in contrast, the level of BAL neutrophilia had no predictive value. These longitudinal data thus show that AZM provides a sustained functional improvement in the long-term in only a small minority of patients with BOS (approximately 10%–15%). This observation suggests, therefore, that in most patients (even those with the NRAD phenotype), BOS is a condition that worsens with time.

Despite this relatively modest effect of AZM on lung function, 3 studies in patients with BOS have shown that this treatment is associated with a significant reduction in the risk of death.[20,98,99] In studies by Gottlieb and colleagues[20] and by Vos and colleagues,[98] responders had significantly better overall survival compared with nonresponders; as expected, the difference between groups was more pronounced when only responders with a sustained response were taken into account.

Using AZM for the prevention of BOS (ie, when patients are still in BOS stage 0) may have an even greater clinical impact than using it as a treatment. In a recent prospective randomized trial of AZM (40 patients) versus placebo (43 patients), Vos and colleagues[100] initiated treatment at discharge and followed the patients for 2 years. BOS occurred less in patients receiving AZM (12.5%) than placebo (44.2%), and BOS-free survival was better with AZM. Patients receiving AZM demonstrated better FEV_1, lower BAL neutrophilia, and less systemic inflammation. There was no difference in survival between groups, but this may be due to the short follow-up time.

Statins

In a large retrospective study published in 2003, Johnson and colleagues[101] found that patients who received statins during the first year after transplantation for treatment of hypercholesterolemia were at less risk of developing BOS than patients who were not treated. In addition, patients receiving statins were less likely to develop severe BOS and had better survival. Unfortunately, there have been no subsequent reports to confirm these observations nor have there been controlled studies. In vitro, it has been demonstrated that simvastatin attenuates the release of airway neutrophilic and remodeling mediators from primary bronchial epithelial cells from stable lung transplant patients and inhibits their up-regulation by transforming growth factor β and IL-17.[102] In practice, many lung transplant programs systematically prescribe a statin in order to exploit this immunomodulatory effect even if the true clinical benefit is still hypothetical.

Total Lymphoid Irradiation

Fisher and colleagues[103] summarized their experience with total lymphoid irradiation in 37 patients treated for progressive BOS. In the 27 recipients who completed more than 80% of the treatment, the rate of decline in FEV_1 decreased from 122.7 mL/mo pre–total lymphoid irradiation to 25.1 mL/mo post–total lymphoid irradiation. Patients with a greater rate of functional decline before treatment were more likely to respond.

Results of these studies are promising, but in the absence of adequately powered randomized control trials, they should be regarded as providing suggestive, rather than convincing, evidence.

Photospheresis

Two recent single-center reports document experience with extracorporeal photopheresis in the treatment of BOS. Benden and colleagues[104] reported on a series of 12 patients with various stages of BOS; rate of decline in FEV_1 was 112 mL/mo before photopheresis and 12 mL/mo after completion of 12 cycles. No complications related to therapy were recorded in this study. In a larger study of 60 patients with BOS, Morrell and colleagues[105] documented a similarly dramatic reduction in rate of decline in FEV_1 from 116 mL/mo prior to treatment to 28.9 mL/mo during the 6 months after initiation of photopheresis. Eight patients experienced catheter-related bacteremias, one patient had a catheter-associated thrombus, and one patient experienced transient hypotension during a treatment. The mechanisms by which photopheresis exerts immunomodulatory and anti-inflammatory effects remain poorly understood. In the absence of randomized trials, it is premature to endorse photopheresis as a definitive therapy for BOS.

Retransplantation

In 1998, Novick and colleagues[106] reported results of 230 retransplants performed at 47 centers worldwide, 63% of which were performed for BOS. The report indicated that early survival after retransplantation was reduced compared with first transplants, but results of retransplants performed for BOS were not different than those done for other indications. In addition, recurrent BOS was observed in a frequency similar to that seen after first transplants. Subsequently, three single-center reports have confirmed this observation. Brugière and colleagues[107] reported on long-term outcome in 15 single-lung retransplantations for BOS. The median time between primary lung transplantation and retransplantation was 31 months (range, 12 to 39 months). Actuarial survival rates at 1 year, 2 years, and 5 years after retransplantation were 60%, 53%, and 45%, respectively. Ten patients died during long-term follow-up, 6 of them from infection (60%). The retained graft was the initial site of the fatal infection in 4 of these patients. Two other patients experienced disabling chronic purulent expectoration arising from the old graft. Lung retransplantation thus offered a viable therapeutic option for selected SLT recipients with BOS, but given the morbidity and mortality

related to the retained graft, the team now favors replacement of the primary graft when retransplantation is considered.[107] Strueber and colleagues[108] reported on 54 redo-transplants among 614 lung transplantation procedures performed at their institution. Retransplantation for BOS achieved 1-year and 5-year survival rates of 78% and 62%, respectively, which were not different from those observed after first-time lung transplantations. Recipients had a similar incidence of BOS after retransplantation for BOS versus after a first procedure. The same group published similar results for 7 retransplantations performed in children.[109] At present, 1% to 2% of lung transplantations performed yearly worldwide are retransplantations.[2] In assessing these procedures, medical issues and the issue of equitable use of scarce resources need be addressed.

SUMMARY

Chronic allograft dysfunction, especially BOS/BO, remains the major obstacle to long-term survival after lung transplantation. Major advances in understanding the risk factors and pathogenic mechanisms leading to irreversible small airway lesions have been made and new options for the prevention and treatment of BOS/BO are available. There is no doubt that the coming years will further improve our ability to cope with this devastating complication of lung transplantation.

REFERENCES

1. Burke CM, Theodore J, Dawkins KD, et al. Post-transplant obliterative bronchiolitis and other late lung sequelae in human heart-lung transplantation. Chest 1984;86:824–9.
2. Christie JD, Edwards LB, Kucheryavaya AY, et al. The Registry of the International Society for Heart and Lung Transplantation: twenty-seventh official adult lung and heart-lung transplant report—2010. J Heart Lung Transplant 2010;29:1004–18.
3. Glanville AR. Bronchoscopic monitoring after lung transplantation. Semin Respir Crit Care Med 2010;31:208–21.
4. Estenne M, Maurer JR, Boehler A, et al. Bronchiolitis obliterans syndrome 2001: an update of the diagnostic criteria. J Heart Lung Transplant 2002;21:297–310.
5. Jackson CH, Sharples LD, McNeil K, et al. Acute and chronic onset of bronchiolitis obliterans syndrome (BOS): are they different entities? J Heart Lung Transplant 2002;21:658–66.
6. Finlen Copeland CA, Snyder LD, Zaas DW, et al. Survival after bronchiolitis obliterans syndrome

among bilateral lung transplant recipients. Am J Respir Crit Care Med 2010;182:784–9.

7. Bankier AA, Muylem AV, Knoop C, et al. BOS in heart-lung transplant recipients: diagnosis with expiratory CT. Radiology 2001;218:533–9.

8. de Jong PA, Dodd JD, Coxson HO, et al. Bronchiolitis obliterans following lung transplantation: early detection using computed tomographic scanning. Thorax 2006;61:799–804.

9. Heng D, Sharples LD, McNeil K, et al. Bronchiolitis obliterans syndrome: incidence, natural history, prognosis, and risk factors. J Heart Lung Transplant 1998;17:1255–63.

10. Bando K, Paradis IL, Similo S, et al. Obliterative bronchiolitis after lung and heart-lung transplantation. An analysis of risk factors and management. J Thorac Cardiovasc Surg 1995;110:4–13.

11. Valentine VG, Robbins RC, Berry GJ, et al. Actuarial survival of heart-lung and bilateral sequential lung transplant recipients with obliterative bronchiolitis. J Heart Lung Transplant 1996;15:371–83.

12. van den Berg JW, Geertsma A, van de Bij W, et al. Bronchiolitis obliterans syndrome after lung transplantation and health-related quality of life. Am J Respir Crit Care Med 2000;161:1937–41.

13. Martinu T, Howell DN, Davis RD, et al. Pathologic correlates of bronchiolitis obliterans syndrome in pulmonary retransplant recipients. Chest 2006; 129:1016–23.

14. Gerhardt SG, McDyer JF, Girgis RE, et al. Maintenance azithromycin therapy for bronchiolitis obliterans syndrome: results of a pilot study. Am J Respir Crit Care Med 2003;168:121–5.

15. Verleden GM, Dupont LJ. Azithromycin therapy for patients with bronchiolitis obliterans syndrome after lung transplantation. Transplantation 2004; 77:1465–7.

16. Yates B, Murphy DM, Forrest IA, et al. Azithromycin reverses airflow obstruction in established bronchiolitis obliterans syndrome. Am J Respir Crit Care Med 2005;172:772–5.

17. Shitrit D, Bendayan D, Gidon S, et al. Long-term azithromycin use for treatment of bronchiolitis obliterans syndrome in lung transplant recipients. J Heart Lung Transplant 2005;24:1440–3.

18. Verleden GM, Vanaudenaerde BM, Dupont LJ, et al. Azithromycin reduces airway neutrophilia and IL-8 in patients with bronchiolitis obliterans syndrome. Am J Respir Crit Care Med 2006;174:566–70.

19. Porhownik NR, Batobara W, Kepron W, et al. Effect of maintenance azithromycin on established bronchiolitis obliterans syndrome in lung transplnat patients. Can Respir J 2008;15:199–202.

20. Gottlieb J, Szangolies J, Koehnlein T, et al. Long-term azithromycin for bronchiolitis obliterans syndrome after lung transplantation. Transplantation 2008;85:36–41.

21. Benden C, Boehler A. Long-term clarithromycin therapy in the management of lung transplant recipients. Transplantation 2009;87:1538–40.

22. Verleden GM, Vos R, De Vleeschauwer SI, et al. Obliterative bronchiolitis following lung transplantation: from old to new concepts? Transpl Int 2009; 22:771–9.

23. Pakhale SS, Hadjiliadis D, Howell DN, et al. Upper lobe fibrosis: a novel manifestation of chronic allograft dysfunction in lung transplantation. J Heart Lung Transplant 2005;24:1260–8.

24. Woodrow JP, Shlobin OA, Barnett SD, et al. Comparison of bronchiolitis obliterans syndrome to other forms of chronic lung allograft dysfunction after lung transplantation. J Heart Lung Transplant 2010;29:1159–64.

25. Ferrer J, Roldan J, Roman A, et al. Acute and chronic pleural complications in lung transplantation. J Heart Lung Transplant 2003;22:1217–25.

26. McManus TE, Milne DG, Whyte KF, et al. Exudative bronchiolitis after lung transplantation. J Heart Lung Transplant 2008;27:276–81.

27. Vos R, Vanaudenaerde BM, De Vleeschauwer SI, et al. Follicular bronchiolitis: a rare cause of bronchiolitis obliterans syndrome after lung transplantation: a case report. Am J Transplant 2009;9: 644–50.

28. Akindipe O, Fernandez-Bussy S, Jantz M, et al. Obliterative bronchiolitis in lung allografts removed at retransplant for intractable airway problems. Respirology 2009;14:601–5.

29. Halloran PF, Homik J, Goes N, et al. The "injury response": a concept linking nonspecific injury, acute rejection, and long-term transplant outcomes. Transplant Proc 1997;29:79–81.

30. Egan JJ. Obliterative bronchiolitis after lung transplantation: a repetitive multiple injury airway disease. Am J Respir Crit Care Med 2004;170: 931–2.

31. Opelz G, Süsal C, Ruhenstroth A, et al. Impact of HLA compatibility on lung transplant survival and evidence for an HLA restriction phenomenon: a collaborative transplant study report. Transplantation 2010;90:912–7.

32. Keogh A, Kaan A, Doran T, et al. HLA mismatching and outcome in heart, heart-lung and single lung transplantation. J Heart Lung Transplant 1995;14: 444–51.

33. Schulman LL, Weinberg AD, McGregor C, et al. Mismatches at the HLA-DR and HLA-B loci are risk factors for acute rejection after lung transplantation. Am J Respir Crit Care Med 1998;157:1833–7.

34. Quantz MA, Bennett LE, Meyer DM, et al. Does human leukocyte antigen matching influence the outcome of lung transplantation? An analysis of 3,549 lung transplantations. J Heart Lung Transplant 2000;19:473–9.

35. Girnita AL, McCurry KR, Iacono AT, et al. HLA-specific antibodies are associated with high-grade and persistent-recurrent lung allograft acute rejection. J Heart Lung Transplant 2004;23:1135–41.

36. Girnita AL, Duquesnoy R, Yousem SA, et al. HLA-specific antibodies are risk factors for lymphocytic bronchiolitis and chronic lung allograft dysfunction. Am J Transplant 2005;5:131–8.

37. Jaramillo A, Smith MA, Phelan D, et al. Development of ELISA-detected anti-HLA antibodies precedes the development of bronchiolitis obliterans syndrome and correlates with progressive decline in pulmonary function after lung transplantation. Transplantation 1999;67:1155–6.

38. Palmer SM, Davis RD, Hadjiliadis D, et al. Development of an antibody specific to major histocompatibility antigens detectable by flow cytometry after lung transplant is associated with bronchiolitis obliterans syndrome. Transplantation 2002;74:799–804.

39. Girnita AL, McCurry KR, Zeevi A. Increased lung allograft failure in patients with HLA-specific antibody. Clin Transpl 2007;231–9.

40. Jaramillo A, Smith CR, Maruyama T, et al. Anti-HLA class I antibody binding to airway epithelial cells induces production of fibrogenic growth factors and apoptotic cell death: a possible mechanism for bronchiolitis obliterans syndrome. Hum Immunol 2003;64:521–9.

41. Yousem SA. Significance of clinically silent untreated mild acute cellular rejection in lung allograft recipients. Hum Pathol 1996;27:269–73.

42. Knoop C, Estenne M. Acute and chronic rejection after lung transplantation. Semin Respir Crit Care Med 2006;27:521–33.

43. Hopkins PM, Aboyoun CL, Chhajed PN, et al. Association of minimal rejection in lung transplant recipients with obliterative bronchiolitis. Am J Respir Crit Care Med 2004;170:1022–6.

44. Khalifah AP, Hachem RR, Chakinala MM, et al. Minimal acute rejection after lung transplantation: a risk for bronchiolitis obliterans syndrome. Am J Transplant 2005;5:2022–30.

45. Hachem RR, Khalifah AP, Chakinala MM, et al. The significance of a single episode of minimal acute rejection after lung transplantation. Transplantation 2005;80:1406–13.

46. Ross DJ, Marchevsky A, Kramer M, et al. Refractoriness of airflow obstruction associated with isolated lymphocytic bronchiolitis/bronchitis in pulmonary allografts. J Heart Lung Transplant 1997;16:832–8.

47. Husain AN, Siddiqui MT, Holmes EW, et al. Analysis of risk factors for the development of bronchiolitis obliterans syndrome. Am J Respir Crit Care Med 1999;159:829–33.

48. Glanville AR, Aboyoun CL, Havryk A, et al. Severity of lymphocytic bronchiolitis predicts long-term outcome after lung transplantation. Am J Respir Crit Care Med 2008;177:1033–40.

49. Burton CM, Iversen M, Scheike T, et al. Is lymphocytic bronchiolitis a marker of acute rejection? An analysis of 2,697 transbronchial biopsies after lung transplantation. J Heart Lung Transplant 2008;27:1128–34.

50. Glanville AR. Antibody-mediated rejection in lung transplantation: myth or reality? J Heart Lung Transplant 2010;29:395–400.

51. Morrell MR, Patterson GA, Trulock EP, et al. Acute antibody-mediated rejection after lung transplantation. J Heart Lung Transplant 2009;28:96–100.

52. Magro CM, Abbas AE, Seilstad K, et al. C3d and the septal microvasculature as a predictor of chronic lung allograft dysfunction. Hum Immunol 2006;67:274–83.

53. Burlingham WJ, Love RB, Jankowska-Gan E, et al. IL-17-dependent cellular immunity to collagen type V predisposes to obliterative bronchiolitis in human lung transplants. J Clin Invest 2007;117:3498–506.

54. Goers TA, Ramachandran S, Aloush A, et al. De novo production of K-alpha1 tubulin-specific antibodies: role in chronic lung allograft rejection. Hum Immunol 2008;180:4487–94.

55. Tiriveedhi V, Angaswamy N, Weber J, et al. Lipid raft facilitated ligation of K-alpha1-tubulin by specific antibodies on epithelial cells: role in pathogenesis of chronic rejection following human lung transplantation. Biochem Biophys Res Commun 2010;399:251–5.

56. Nath DS, Basha HI, Mohanakumar T. Antihuman leukocyte antigen antibody-induced autoimmunity: role in chronic rejection. Curr Opin Organ Transplant 2010;15:16–20.

57. Shilling RA, Wilkes DS. Immunobiology of chronic lung allograft dysfunction: new insights from the bench and beyond. Am J Transplant 2009;9:1714–8.

58. Kastelijn EA, van Moorsel CH, Rijkers GT, et al. Polymorphisms in innate immunity genes associated with development of bronchiolitis obliterans after lung transplantation. J Heart Lung Transplant 2010;29:665–71.

59. Botha P, Archer L, Anderson RL, et al. Pseudomonas aeruginosa colonization of the allograft after lung transplantation and the risk of bronchiolitis obliterans syndrome. Transplantation 2008;85:771–4.

60. Weigt SS, Elashoff RM, Huang C, et al. Aspergillus colonization of the lung allograft is a risk factor for bronchiolitis obliterans syndrome. Am J Transplant 2009;9:1903–11.

61. Valentine VG, Gupta MR, Walker JE Jr, et al. Effect of etiology and timing of respiratory tract infections on development of bronchiolitis obliterans syndrome. J Heart Lung Transplant 2009;28:163–9.

62. Kumar D, Husain S, Chen MH, et al. A prospective molecular surveillance study evaluating the clinical impact of community-acquired respiratory viruses in lung transplant recipients. Transplantation 2010;89:1028–33.

63. Gottlieb J, Schulz TF, Welte T, et al. Community-acquired respiratory viral infections in lung transplant recipients: a single season cohort study. Transplantation 2009;87:1530–7.

64. Glanville AR, Gencay M, Tamm M, et al. Chlamydia pneumoniae infection after lung transplantation. J Heart Lung Transplant 2005;24:131–6.

65. Kotsimbos TC, Snell GI, Levvey B, et al. Chlamydia pneumoniae serology in donors and recipients and the risk of bronchiolitis obliterans syndrome after lung transplantation. Transplantation 2005;79: 269–75.

66. Neurohr C, Huppmann P, Leuchte H, et al. Human herpesvirus 6 in bronchalveolar lavage fluid after lung transplantation: a risk factor for bronchiolitis obliterans syndrome? Am J Transplant 2005;5: 2982–91.

67. Valentine VG, Weill D, Gupta MR, et al. Ganciclovir for cytomegalovirus: a call for indefinite prophylaxis in lung transplantation. J Heart Lung Transplant 2008;27:875–81.

68. Tamm M, Aboyoun CL, Chhajed PN, et al. Treated cytomegalovirus pneumonia is not associated with bronchiolitis obliterans syndrome. Am J Respir Crit Care Med 2004;170:1120–3.

69. Davis CS, Shankaran V, Kovacs EJ, et al. Gastro-esophageal reflux disease after lung transplantation: pathophysiology and implications for treatment. Surgery 2010;148:737–44.

70. Blondeau K, Mertens V, Vanaudenaerde BA, et al. Gastro-oesophageal reflux and gastric aspiration in lung transplant patients with or without chronic rejection. Eur Respir J 2008;31:707–13.

71. D'Ovidio F, Mura M, Tsang M, et al. Bile acid aspiration and the development of bronchiolitis obliterans after lung transplantation. J Thorac Cardiovasc Surg 2005;129:1144–52.

72. Cantu E 3rd, Appel JZ 3rd, Hartwig MG, et al. Early fundoplication prevents chronic allograft dysfunction in patients with gastroesophageal reflux disease. Ann Thorac Surg 2004;78:1142–51.

73. Davis RD Jr, Lau CL, Eubanks S, et al. Improved lung allograft function after fundoplication in patients with gastroesophageal reflux disease undergoing lung transplantation. J Thorac Cardiovasc Surg 2003;125:533–42.

74. Robertson AG, Ward C, Pearson JP, et al. Lung transplantation, gastroesophageal reflux, and fundoplication. Ann Thorac Surg 2010;89:653–60.

75. Snell GI, Westall GP. The contribution of airway ischemia and vascular remodelling to the pathophysiology of bronchiolitis obliterans syndrome and chronic lung allograft dysfunction. Curr Opin Organ Transplant 2010;15:558–62.

76. Daud SA, Yusen RD, Meyers BF, et al. Impact of immediate primary lung allograft dysfunction on bronchiolitis obliterans syndrome. Am J Respir Crit Care Med 2007;175:507–13.

77. Belperio JA, Keane MP, Burdik MD, et al. Role of CXCR2/CXCR2 ligands in vascular remodelling during bronchiolitis obliterans syndrome. J Clin Invest 2005;115:1150–62.

78. Douglas IS, Nicolls MR. Chemokine-mediated angiogenesis: an essential link in the evolution of airway fibrosis? J Clin Invest 2005;115:1133–6.

79. Dhillon GS, Zamora MR, Roos JE, et al. Lung transplant airway hypoxia: a diathesis to fibrosis? Am J Respir Crit Care Med 2010;182:230–6.

80. Hachem RR, Chakinala MM, Yusen RD, et al. The predictive value of bronchiolitis obliterans syndrome stage 0-p. Am J Respir Crit Care Med 2004;169:468–72.

81. Lama IN, Murray S, Mumford JA, et al. Prognostic value of bronchiolitis obliterans syndrome stage 0-p in single-lung transplant recipients. Am J Respir Crit Care Med 2005;172:379–83.

82. Estenne M, Van Muylem A, Knoop C, et al. Detection of obliterative bronchiolitis by indexes of ventilation distribution. Am J Respir Crit Care Med 2000; 162:1047–51.

83. Reynaud-Gaubert M, Thomas P, Badier M, et al. Early detection of airway involvement in obliterative bronchiolitis after lung transplantation. Functional and bronchoalveolar lavage cell findings. Am J Respir Crit Care Med 2000;161:1924–9.

84. Van Muylem A, Knoop C, Estenne M. Early detection of chronic pulmonary allograft dysfunction by exhaled biomarkers. Am J Respir Crit Care Med 2007;175:731–6.

85. Van Muylem A, Scillia P, Knoop C, et al. Single-breath test in lateral decubitus reflects function of single lungs grafted for emphysema. J Appl Physiol 2006;100:834–8.

86. Van Muylem A, Gevenois PA, Kallinger E, et al. Single-breath test in lateral decubitus reflects function of single lungs grafted for interstitial lung disease. J Appl Physiol 2008;104:224–9.

87. Gabbay E, Haydn Walters E, Orsida B, et al. In stable lung transplant recipients, exhaled nitric oxide levels positively correlate with airway neutrophilia and bronchial epithelial iNOS. Am J Respir Crit Care Med 1999;160:2093–9.

88. Gabbay E, Walters EH, Orsida B, et al. Post-lung transplant bronchiolitis obliterans syndrome (BOS) is characterized by increased exhaled nitric oxide levels and epithelial inducible nitric oxide synthase. Am J Respir Crit Care Med 2000;162:2182–7.

89. Zheng L, Whitford HM, Orsida B, et al. The dynamics and associations of airway neutrophilia

post lung transplantation. Am J Transplant 2006;6: 599–608.

90. Vos R, Cordemans C, Vanaudenaerde BM, et al. Exhaled carbon monoxide as a noninvasive marker of airway neutrophilia after lung transplantation. Transplantation 2009;87:1579–83.

91. Fisher AJ, Gabbay E, Small T, et al. Cross sectional study of exhaled nitric oxide levels following lung transplantation. Thorax 1998;53:454–8.

92. Verleden GM, Dupont LJ, Van Raemdonck DE, et al. Accuracy of exhaled nitric oxide measurements for the diagnosis of bronchiolitis obliterans syndrome after lung transplantation. Transplantation 2004;78:730–3.

93. Brugiere O, Thabut G, Mal H, et al. Exhaled NO may predict the decline in lung function in bronchiolitis obliterans syndrome. Eur Respir J 2005; 25:813–9.

94. Dupont LJ, Dewandeleer Y, Vanaudenaerde BM, et al. The pH of exhaled breath condensate of patients with allograft rejection after lung transplantation. Am J Transplant 2006;6:1486–92.

95. Allen DJ, Fildes JE, Yonan N, et al. Changes in induced sputum in the presence of bronchiolitis obliterans syndrome and correlation with spirometry in single and bilateral lung transplant recipients. J Heart Lung Transplant 2005;24:88–91.

96. Bankier AA, Van Muylem A, Scillia P, et al. Air trapping in heart-lung transplant recipients: variability of anatomic distribution and extent at sequential expiratory thin-section CT. Radiology 2003;229: 737–42.

97. Gast KK, Zaporozhan J, Ley S, et al. (3)He-MRI in follow-up of lung transplant recipients. Eur Radiol 2004;14:78–85.

98. Vos R, Vanaudenaerde BM, Ottevaere A, et al. Long-term azithromycin therapy for bronchiolitis obliterans syndrome: divide and conquer? J Heart Lung transplant 2010;29:1358–68.

99. Jain R, Hachem RR, Morrell MR, et al. Azithromycin is associated with increased survival in lung transplant recipients with bronchiolitis obliterans syndrome. J Heart Lung Transplant 2010;29:531–7.

100. Vos R, Vanaudenaerde BM, Verleden SE, et al. A randomized placebo-controlled trial of azithromycin to prevent bronchiolitis obliterans syndrome after lung transplantation. Eur Respir J 2011;37: 164–72.

101. Johnson BA, Iacono AT, Zeevi A, et al. Statin use is associated with improved function and survival of lung allografts. Am J Respir Crit Care Med 2003; 167:1271–8.

102. Murphy DM, Forrest IA, Corris PA, et al. Simvastatin attenuates release of neutrophilic and remodeling factors from primary bronchial epithelial cells derived from stable lung transplant recipients. Am J Physiol Lung Cell Mol Physiol 2008;294: L592–9.

103. Fisher AJ, Rutherford RM, Bozzino J, et al. The safety and efficacy of total lymphoid irradiation in progressive bronchiolitis obliterans syndrome after lung transplantation. Am J Transplant 2005; 5:537–43.

104. Benden C, Speich R, Wanger C, et al. Extracorporeal photopheresis after lung transplantation: a 10-year single-center experience. Transplantation 2008;86:1625–7.

105. Morrell MR, Despotis GJ, Lublin DM, et al. The efficacy of photopheresis for bronchiolitis obliterans syndrome after lung transplantation. J Heart Lung Transplant 2010;29:424–31.

106. Novick RJ, Stitt LW, Al-Kattan K, et al. Pulmonary retransplantation: predictors of graft function and survival in 230 patients. Pulmonary Retransplant Registry. Ann Thorac Surg 1998;65:227–34.

107. Brugière O, Thabut G, Castier Y, et al. Lung retransplantation for bronchiolitis obliterans syndrome: long-term follow-up in a series of 15 recipients. Chest 2003;123:1832–7.

108. Strueber M, Fischer S, Gottlieb J, et al. Long-term outcome after pulmonary retransplantation. J Thorac Cardiovasc Surg 2006;132:407–12.

109. Müller C, Görler H, Ballmann M, et al. Pulmonary retransplantation in paediatric patients: a justified therapeutic option? A single-centre experience. Eur J Cardiothorac Surg 2011;39:201–5.

Common Infections in the Lung Transplant Recipient

Karen D. Sims, MD, PhD[a], Emily A. Blumberg, MD[b],*

KEYWORDS

- Lung transplant • Infection • Respiratory virus
- Mycobacteria • Fungal infection
- Gram-negative bacterial infection • Prophylaxis

Despite more than a quarter century of experience in lung transplantation, marked by advances in surgical techniques, immunosuppressive medications and prophylaxis strategies, survival among lung transplant recipients lags behind most other solid-organ transplant (SOT) recipients.[1] In part, this situation may be attributed to infection-related complications, which continue to be a major source of morbidity and mortality in these patients.[2–4] The lung allograft is unique in that it remains in constant exposure to the environment and potential respiratory pathogens. The nature of the transplant procedure adversely affects normal host defenses, including impairment of cough mechanics and mucociliary clearance. Additional contributors include the risk of cross-contamination of the transplanted lung by the native lung in single-lung-transplant patients, and the reduction of immune system function because of the high immunosuppression requirements in lung transplantation. By implementing a careful strategy of pretransplant screening of recipients and donors, pretransplantation and posttransplantation vaccination, antimicrobial prophylaxis, and microbial surveillance techniques, the incidence and severity of infectious complications after transplantation can be minimized. This review is an overview of some of the more common but increasingly challenging infections after lung transplantation, and provides guidance on current prevention and treatment strategies.

RECIPIENT PRETRANSPLANT SCREENING AND PREVENTION

The prevention of infectious complications after SOT is paramount, and careful pretransplant evaluation for risks from infectious diseases should be conducted in all potential recipients. Comprehensive recommendations for the evaluation of SOT candidates and all other aspects of transplant-related infectious diseases have been recently summarized in guidelines from the American Society of Transplantation (AST) Infectious Diseases Community of Practice.[5] Consultation with a specialist in infectious diseases in transplant should always be considered as part of the pretransplantation evaluation. A careful medical, social, and travel history should be performed to ascertain any potential exposures to problem pathogens (such as endemic mycoses or parasitic infections) so that appropriate risk stratification can occur, including consideration of specific posttransplantation prophylaxis. Vaccine histories should be reviewed, with careful attention paid to completion of childhood vaccination series (ie, measles/mumps/rubella), history of infection with pathogens such as varicella (chicken pox), and maintenance of adult vaccination schedules.[6] In many cases, the patient's primary disease process may render him or her functionally immunosuppressed, so initiation of missed or delayed vaccine series should begin as early in the transplant evaluation as possible, especially for live attenuated vaccines such as varicella vaccine (Varivax Merck,

[a] Discovery Medicine, Virology, Bristol-Myers Squibb, PO Box 5400, Princeton, NJ 08543-5400, USA
[b] Division of Infectious Diseases, University of Pennsylvania Medical Center, University of Pennsylvania School of Medicine, 3 Silverstein Pavilion, Suite E, 3400 Spruce Street, Philadelphia, PA 19104, USA
* Corresponding author.
E-mail address: blumbere@mail.med.upenn.edu

Clin Chest Med 32 (2011) 327–341
doi:10.1016/j.ccm.2011.02.010
0272-5231/11/$ – see front matter © 2011 Elsevier Inc. All rights reserved.

West Point, PA, USA), which are currently contraindicated after SOT. If vaccination must be delayed until after transplant, most centers defer administration until 3 to 6 months after transplantation or until baseline immunosuppression levels are achieved. The vaccine status of household contacts and family members should also be assessed for the optimal protection of the transplant recipient, and should be up to date before transplantation, if possible. Current recommendations for routine adult vaccines are summarized in **Table 1**.[6]

All transplant candidates should be screened for the presence of antibodies to CMV, varicella-zoster virus, Epstein-Barr virus, hepatitis B virus, hepatitis C virus, and human immunodeficiency virus to assess both suitability for transplantation and for appropriate risk stratification for prophylaxis (and vaccination when applicable) and monitoring after transplantation.[5] Screening for tuberculosis (TB) should be performed in all transplant candidates, with either purified-protein derivative (or Mantoux) skin testing or an interferon γ release assay such as the Quantiferon TB Gold (Cellestis, Valencia, CA, USA) test.[7] Tuberculin-test–positive patients should be evaluated for active TB; latent TB treatment (preferably with 9 months of isoniazid) is recommended for all transplant candidates if they have not received previous therapy. In lung transplantation in particular, pretransplant screening for highly resistant bacterial and fungal airway colonizers may be considered to help guide peritransplantation antimicrobial prophylaxis.

During the posttransplant period, the risk for particular infections varies depending on the time since the transplant surgery (**Fig. 1**). For example, the risks of surgical complications and nosocomial infections are highest in the first 30 days, whereas the risk of reactivation of latent, opportunistic infections is highest early (when the net state of immunosuppression is at its peak) and then declines with reduction of immunosuppression to maintenance levels.[8] Similarly, the risk of community-acquired infections increases with exposure of the transplant recipient to the outpatient setting. Keeping this timeline in mind, as well as remaining cognizant of the individual patient's pretransplant risk factors and exposures, can aid the clinician in formulating a more focused differential diagnosis for infectious complications that arise in the recipient.

VIRUSES
CMV

CMV remains a significant problem after lung transplantation despite advances in viral diagnostics, prophylaxis, and treatment strategies. A recent prospective multicenter cohort study by the Resistra group showed that despite 3 months of CMV-directed viral prophylaxis, 10% of postlung transplant pneumonias reported were caused by CMV.[9] Lung transplant recipients have the highest risk of developing CMV disease among all SOT recipients, although the risk of CMV has decreased over time.[10] This situation is likely because of the combination of the large CMV viral load that is transmitted via a CMV-positive lung allograft relative to other types of allografts and the more

Table 1
Routine adult vaccines in transplantation[a]

Vaccine	Before Transplant	After Transplant	Frequency
Hepatitis A	Y	Y	Follow titers
Hepatitis B[b]	Y	Y	Follow titers
Human papilloma virus	Y	Y	Unknown
Influenza (including H1N1)[b]	Y	Y	Yearly
Neisseria meningiditis	Y	Y	Unknown
Pertussis/tetanus (Tdap)[b]	Y	Y	Every 10 years
Streptococcus pneumoniae (polysaccharide)[b]	Y	Y	Every 3–5 years or follow titers
Varicella zoster	Y	N	Follow titers

Abbreviations: Y, yes; N, no.
[a] These vaccines should be administered before transplantation to susceptible hosts following standard Advisory Committee on Immunization Practices (ACIP) guidelines for administration, and (with the exception of varicella zoster vaccine) are safe after transplantation.
[b] These vaccines should be considered for all candidates before transplantation with readministration based on standard ACIP guidelines.

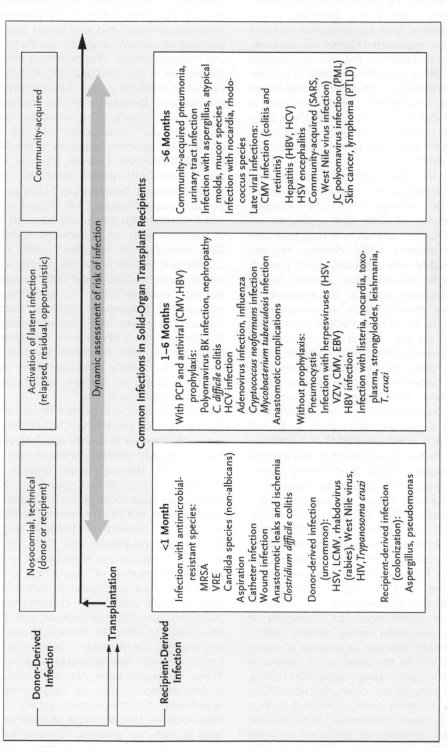

Common Infections in Solid-Organ Transplant Recipients

Donor-Derived Infection

Recipient-Derived Infection

Transplantation

Nosocomial, technical (donor or recipient)

Activation of latent infection (relapsed, residual, opportunistic)

Community-acquired

Dynamic assessment of risk of infection

<1 Month

Infection with antimicrobial-resistant species:
MRSA
VRE
Candida species (non-albicans)

Aspiration
Catheter infection
Wound infection
Anastomotic leaks and ischemia
Clostridium difficile colitis

Donor-derived infection (uncommon):
HSV, LCMV, rhabdovirus (rabies), West Nile virus, HIV, Trypanosoma cruzi

Recipient-derived infection (colonization):
Aspergillus, pseudomonas

1–6 Months

With PCP and antiviral (CMV, HBV) prophylaxis:
Polyomavirus BK infection, nephropathy
C. difficile colitis
HCV infection
Adenovirus infection, influenza
Cryptococcus neoformans infection
Mycobacterium tuberculosis infection
Anastomotic complications

Without prophylaxis:
Pneumocystis
Infection with herpesviruses (HSV, VZV, CMV, EBV)
HBV infection
Infection with listeria, nocardia, toxoplasma, strongyloides, leishmania, T. cruzi

>6 Months

Community-acquired pneumonia, urinary tract infection
Infection with aspergillus, atypical molds, mucor species
Infection with nocardia, rhodococcus species
Late viral infections:
CMV infection (colitis and retinitis)
Hepatitis (HBV, HCV)
HSV encephalitis
Community-acquired (SARS, West Nile virus infection)
JC polyomavirus infection (PML)
Skin cancer, lymphoma (PTLD)

Fig. 1. Timeline of common infections in SOT recipients. (*Reprinted from* Fishman JA. Infection in solid-organ transplant recipients. N Engl J Med 2007;357(25):2606; with permission.)

intensive immunosuppression often required in lung transplant recipients, as well as other common risk factors shared by other organ recipients.[4] These risk factors include the serostatus of the donor and recipient, with a seronegative recipient of a seropositive organ at the highest risk, the presence of allograft rejection, the use of induction immunosuppression, and the presence of concurrent infections (primarily with other viruses). Areas under recent investigation include defects in CMV-specific cell-mediated immunity (CMI), polymorphisms in various components of the innate immune system, and other host factors such as renal dysfunction.[11]

Definitions for CMV infection and disease have been developed for use in both clinical and research settings.[10,12] CMV infection requires evidence of CMV viral replication via an accepted form of laboratory testing (see later discussion), whereas CMV disease requires evidence of CMV viral replication plus attributable symptoms, including fever, malaise, leukopenia, or thrombocytopenia, or evidence of tissue-invasive disease such as pneumonitis, colitis, hepatitis, or retinitis. Recent interest has also focused on the indirect effects of CMV, which include immunomodulatory effects of the virus that increase the risk of developing other opportunistic infections (human herpesvirus 6 [HHV-6], HHV-7, EBV, fungal, and bacterial), EBV-related posttransplant lymphoproliferative disease, and increased risk of both acute and chronic rejection of the allograft.[13] The contribution of CMV to the development of bronchiolitis obliterans syndrome (BOS) is still being investigated, with conflicting results as reported in a recent systematic review and several single-center publications.[14–19] A more recent single-center study by Snyder and colleagues[20] reported a 21% posttransplant incidence of CMV pneumonitis, and found an increased risk of subsequent BOS in both univariate and multivariate analyses (hazard ratio of 1.88 to 2.11 depending on time dependence).

There have been significant advances in CMV-specific diagnostic testing recently, and in many cases CMV infection or disease is initially diagnosed based on the detection of viremia. In the last decade, quantitative nucleic acid testing, primarily via polymerase chain reaction (PCR), has become the most widely accepted method of CMV viral load monitoring. The previous modality, CMV antigenemia detection via pp65 antigen detection in peripheral white blood cells, has fallen out of favor because of its relative insensitivity and labor intensity. However, the lack of standardization of CMV nucleic acid testing platforms and procedures across many laboratories produces significant interlaboratory variability.[21] This situation can make interpretation of viral load results obtained from different laboratories problematic, and also poses problems for establishing uniform viral load cutoffs for positive and negative results. One promising area in CMV diagnostics is the measurement of CMV-specific CMI as a predictor of the development of CMV viremia and disease after the completion of primary prophylaxis. A recent study by Kumar and colleagues[22] used a commercially available CD8+ CMV-specific interferon γ release assay (QuantiFERON-CMV, Cellestis, Valencia, CA, USA) to test serial CMV-specific CMI in SOT recipients during a 3-month posttransplant CMV prophylaxis period. Postprophylaxis CMV disease (within the first 6 months after transplant) occurred in 22.9% of patients with no detectable CMV-specific CMI, versus 5.3% in patients with a positive QuantiFERON-CMV result, suggesting a possible role in predicting late-onset CMV disease. CMV-specific enzyme-linked immunosorbent spot assays and intracellular cytokine staining followed by flow cytometry have also been studied as predictors of CMV viremia and disease, but these assays have not been standardized and may not be readily available at all transplant centers and are not currently recommended for routine patient monitoring.[23]

A 2008 Cochrane Database review of antiviral medications for preventing CMV disease in SOT recipients showed that CMV prophylaxis reduces the risk of CMV infection, disease, and all-cause mortality in heterogeneous groups of SOT recipients.[24] Consensus guidelines for CMV prophylaxis have recently been updated by both the European and North American transplantation societies.[10,23] Screening of potential lung allograft donors and recipients with CMV IgG testing should be performed to allow for risk stratification and implementation of appropriate prophylaxis strategies. There are 2 generally accepted strategies for CMV prophylaxis in solid-organ transplantation: universal prophylaxis (administration of antivirals to all at-risk individuals) and preemptive therapy (administration of antivirals only to individuals with demonstrable viral replication). These strategies have not been compared in a randomized fashion in lung transplantation specifically, but the current expert opinion of both societies favors the use of universal prophylaxis in high-risk patients, including lung transplant recipients. Initial universal prophylaxis strategies used intravenous ganciclovir only, but with the development of the oral prodrug valganciclovir most centers have switched to oral valganciclovir exclusively, or oral valganciclovir after a short course of intravenous ganciclovir immediately after transplantation because similar efficacy has been shown with both medications.[25] Some centers add CMV hyperimmune globulin to universal prophylaxis regimens, but this has not been evaluated in a randomized fashion.[18,26] Significant uncertainty remains regarding the appropriate duration of prophylaxis. Recent trials have suggested that extending prophylaxis to 1 year or longer after transplant may reduce CMV-related complications, but these trials had significant limitations.[15,27] Recently, the first prospective, randomized, placebo-controlled trial comparing short-course (3 months) with long-course (12 months) prophylaxis with valganciclovir in at-risk lung transplant recipients (positive donor or recipient serologic status) was reported by Palmer and colleagues.[28] After completing an initial 3-month course of valganciclovir, patients were randomized to either placebo (short course) or continued prophylaxis (long course) and subsequently followed for the development of CMV disease until month 13 after transplantation. The investigators found 4% of long-course prophylaxis patients developed CMV disease during the trial, versus 32% of short-course patients. No significant differences were found in CMV resistance, adverse events, or acute rejection episodes between the groups during the observation period. Only a subset of study patients was followed for the development of CMV disease beyond the first 13 months after transplant. However, late CMV disease rates were low in both groups (only 3% in long-course and 2% in short-course subjects), suggesting that a longer duration of prophylaxis may not simply delay onset CMV disease but may also reduce the overall incidence.[28] Whether additional studies examining varying durations of prophylaxis between 3 and 12 months or involving longer-term CMV surveillance after prophylaxis will confirm these findings is unknown. Reinitiation of CMV prophylaxis should be considered during the treatment of acute rejection if antilymphocyte antibody therapy or high-dose steroids are used.

Although preemptive approaches may result in reduced drug costs, avoidance of drug-related toxicity, and promotion of CMV-specific CMI via exposure to low-level viral replication, most centers favor universal prophylactic strategies, as do the consensus guidelines. Not only does the preemptive approach require frequent blood work with rapid access and reaction to results, but there is also concern about whether weekly testing might miss the onset of periods of rapid viral replication and thus risk the development of

more severe CMV disease before treatment can be initiated, especially in higher-risk D+/R− and lung transplant recipients in general. It is also unknown whether low-level CMV viral replication may facilitate increased indirect effects of the virus, including rejection. There are limited data regarding the use of preemptive prophylaxis in the lung transplant setting specifically, with no large, randomized trials available. These studies have raised concerns about earlier onset of CMV disease and higher rates of ganciclovir resistance in D+/R− patients receiving preemptive therapy, and highlight the need for further research in this area.[29–31]

Treatment of CMV disease requires a coordinated reduction in maintenance immunosuppression in conjunction with antiviral medication, and is discussed in the recent consensus guidelines.[10,23] For CMV tissue-invasive disease, intravenous ganciclovir at 5 mg/kg every 12 hours (adjusted for renal function) is the preferred treatment, but recent studies have shown that for isolated CMV viremia, CMV syndrome, or mild to moderate CMV disease, oral valganciclovir 900 mg every 12 hours (adjusted for renal function) is noninferior to intravenous ganciclovir in a mixed population of SOT recipients.[32,33] However, caution should be exercised in patients in whom adequate absorption of oral medications is in question (eg, in CMV gastrointestinal disease), or in patients who may not be compliant with oral therapy. Treatment should be continued for a minimum of 2 to 3 weeks and until the cessation of viral replication has been verified and any CMV-attributable symptoms have resolved. Quantitative nucleic acid testing or antigenemia testing should be performed on a weekly basis during treatment to follow virologic response to therapy, and confirmation of resolution of viremia with consecutive negative tests at least 7 days apart is recommended before completion of therapy. Secondary prophylaxis with lower-dose valganciclovir (900 mg daily adjusted for renal function) can be considered for high-risk patients after completion of CMV treatment, especially those in whom reduction of immunosuppression is not possible. The addition of CMV hyperimmune globulin for more severe CMV disease, such as pneumonitis, may be considered. Patients who fail to respond to standard antiviral therapy should be suspected of having ganciclovir-resistant CMV disease and should be evaluated with genotypic resistance testing for mutations in the viral UL97 and UL54 gene products.[10,23] Additional therapy with the more toxic antiviral agents foscarnet or cidofovir may be required in these cases.[34] Infectious diseases consultation should be considered for patients with suspected or documented CMV resistance.

Community-acquired Respiratory Viruses

Community-acquired respiratory viruses (CARVs) are common among lung transplant recipients especially in the ambulatory setting, with a recent prospective study detecting viral pathogens in the bronchoalveolar lavage (BAL) of 53% of lung transplant recipients enrolled during the 3-year study period.[35] These viruses can cause severe lower respiratory tract infections in these patients, resulting in significant morbidity and mortality. Several studies have also suggested that CARV infection is an independent risk factor for both acute and chronic rejection in this population, although this remains controversial.[16,36–39] This group of viruses includes such notable pathogens as influenza A, B, and novel H1N1, respiratory syncytial virus (RSV), adenovirus, parainfluenza, and coronaviruses such as the severe acute respiratory syndrome virus, as well as rhinovirus, enteroviruses, human metapneumovirus, bocavirus, and polyomaviruses such as KI and WU viruses. The diagnosis of respiratory viruses has been aided by the development of PCR-based quantitative nucleic acid testing for most of the known clinically relevant viruses, but there is considerable center-to-center variability in the particular panel of viruses routinely tested. Clinicians should be aware of viruses circulating in the community to ensure that adequate testing is performed. Rapid antigen testing is available for a limited number of CARVs, but their sensitivity in immunocompromised patients is unclear, thus a negative test does not definitively exclude viral infection.[40] Direct fluorescence antibody testing is also available for some CARVs. Appropriate samples for viral diagnostics include nasopharyngeal swabs, aspirates, washes, or BAL specimens; however, assay sensitivity may vary with the sample collected.

Effective antiviral therapies for most CARVs are not available, with the notable exception of influenza virus and perhaps RSV, thus appropriate infection control strategies including hand hygiene and droplet precautions are mandatory to prevent the spread of disease. This finding is especially important in the health care setting, because transplant patients seem to have prolonged viral shedding after infection. Supportive care and reduction of immunosuppression when possible remain the mainstays of CARV treatment. Consensus guidelines for the management of most common CARVs and novel H1N1 influenza have recently been published, and current recommendations for influenza and RSV are briefly summarized in the next sections.[40,41]

Influenza

All transplant recipients and their household contacts should receive yearly influenza vaccination with inactivated influenza vaccine for the prevention of disease. Suspected cases of influenza should be treated ideally within 48 hours of symptom onset, but transplant patients in particular may still receive benefit if therapy is initiated outside this window, and symptomatic patients should be treated regardless of the duration of symptoms.[40,41] Every effort should be made to establish the diagnosis of influenza, including the type, because specific therapy depends on the resistance pattern of the current circulating viruses. In most cases, a neuraminidase inhibitor such as oseltamivir or zanamivir taken twice daily (adjusted for renal function) is recommended for either influenza A or B; alternatively an M2 inhibitor (ie, amantidine or rimantidine) could be considered for influenza A strains. Treatment should be continued for at least 5 to 10 days, and there may be a benefit in extending therapy beyond this period for patients slow to clinically respond or who have evidence of continued viral shedding on repeated testing.[40,41] Unvaccinated patients with a suspected exposure to an individual with influenza should receive prophylaxis with oseltamivir or zanamivir given once daily (adjusted for renal function) for 5 to 10 days after the last known exposure contact. Seasonal or extended prophylaxis is not recommended because of concerns about emerging viral resistance.

RSV

Although RSV is primarily considered a significant pathogen of young children, lung transplant recipients are at risk of developing severe lower respiratory tract infections from RSV. No vaccine is licensed for the prevention of RSV, and antiviral treatment strategies are controversial. Supportive care with the reduction of immunosuppression if possible is universally recommended.[40] The use of ribavirin in transplant recipients remains controversial because of the lack of controlled studies in this population. Aerosolized ribavirin is commonly used in the pediatric population for seasonal RSV bronchiolitis, and limited data suggest a benefit in lower tract disease in the stem cell transplant population.[42] The addition of high-dose steroids and adjunctive antibody-based therapies such as palivizumab, RSV immunoglobulin (Ig), or intravenous immunoglobulin is controversial. Two small case series suggest a role for parenteral or oral ribavirin in lung transplant patients specifically.[43,44]

Both studies treated patients with ribavirin (1 with an oral formulation, 1 with intravenous) plus high-dose oral or parenteral corticosteroids until repeated nasopharyngeal swabs were negative. After a median follow-up of greater than 300 days in both studies, all subjects had full recovery of FEV$_1$ (forced expiratory volume after 1 second) after resolution, and only 1 case of late BOS was identified out of 23 total subjects. The oral ribavirin study reported no adverse events,[44] and the intravenous study reported a mild but reversible hemolytic anemia.[43] Randomized studies are needed to fully assess the usefulness of ribavirin in this population. There is no consensus recommendation for prophylaxis with palivizumab or RSV Ig in transplant recipients.

BACTERIA
Gram-negative Bacterial Infections

Bacterial pathogens remain the most common cause of pneumonia after lung transplantation, with gram-negative bacteria responsible for the bulk of disease.[9,45,46] Of these, *Pseudomonas aeruginosa* is the most commonly isolated species, but other gram-negatives such as *Acinetobacter* spp, Enterobacteriaceae, *Stenotrophomonas* spp, and *Burkholderia* spp are also frequent causes of posttransplant pneumonia. Colonization of the airway before transplantation, especially in patients with cystic fibrosis (CF), is an important consideration for determining both suitability for transplantation and postoperative care, and posttransplant colonization may be an important factor for the development of BOS.

Colonization with most resistant gram-negative bacteria before transplantation does not seem to affect survival after transplant, with the notable exception of certain *Burkholderia* species.[47,48] It is recommended that the resistance patterns of known pretransplant colonizing bacteria be taken into account when peritransplant antimicrobial prophylaxis is used. Historically, patients with CF who were colonized with *B cepacia* before transplant had poorer outcomes than those who were not colonized, leading to the exclusion of these patients from consideration for transplantation. However, recent studies have revealed that 9 genetically distinct species (genomovars) make up the *B cepacia* complex (BCC), with *B cenocepacia* (genomovar III) and *B multivorans* (genomovar II) causing the bulk of disease in patients with CF.[49] This finding has allowed for more precise study of specific BCC genomovars in the context of lung transplantation, and several recent studies have suggested that infection with *B cenocepacia* specifically is a risk factor for poor outcome after

transplantation.[50–52] These studies all found an increased risk of death among patients infected with *B cenocepacia*, whereas those infected with non-*cenocepacia* species did not have significantly worse outcomes than uninfected controls. In addition, in the study by Murray and colleagues,[52] the subset of patients infected with nonepidemic strains of *B cenocepacia* had a higher risk of death compared with transmissible or epidemic strains, which were not significantly different from uninfected patients. These investigators' data also suggested that infection with *B gladioli* before transplantation was associated with an increased risk of death. Taken together, these new data suggest that more specific selection criteria might be established based on the specific BCC genomovar isolated (ie, *B cenocepacia* vs *B multivorans*), the presence of nonepidemic versus epidemic strains of *B cenocepacia*, or the presence of *B gladioli*. This strategy may allow access to transplantation for patients with CF with BCC who are at lower/standard risk for posttransplant complications.

The relevance of positive donor bacterial cultures has been addressed by several recent studies. Historically, the presence of purulent secretions or numerous white blood cells or bacteria on sputum Gram stain precluded consideration of the donor lung for transplantation.[53] A single-center retrospective study by Avlonitis and colleagues[54] suggested longer stay in the intensive care unit, longer duration of mechanical ventilation, and poorer survival in recipients who received a donor lung with a positive Gram stain. However, several recent studies have suggested that a positive donor Gram stain does not lead to poorer posttransplant outcomes if targeted, aggressive antimicrobial prophylaxis is given initially.[45,55,56] Weill and colleagues[55] reported no difference in the incidence of posttransplant pneumonia at 30 days or duration of mechanical ventilation between recipients of donor lungs with positive or negative Gram stains in patients treated with standard postoperative antibiotic prophylaxis (vancomycin plus a third-generation cephalosporin for 7 days). Currently suggested lung donor acceptability criteria state that a positive Gram stain of the donor tracheal aspirate does not preclude lung donation, but the amount of purulent secretions is of probable, but unproven importance.[53]

The association of posttransplantation bacterial colonization and the risk of developing BOS has become more clear in recent years, with several studies suggesting that posttransplantation colonization with gram-negative rods (GNR), particularly *Pseudomonas aeruginosa*, is associated with reduced BOS-free survival.[57–59] Vos and colleagues[57] described a retrospective study of 92 lung transplant recipients in whom colonization by GNR was associated with lower BOS-free survival by univariate analysis, and trended toward statistical significance in multivariable analysis. Gottlieb and colleagues[58] examined a prospective cohort of 59 patients with CF who were colonized with GNR before transplant. These subjects were followed for a median of 966 days, and those subjects who remained chronically colonized with GNR had lower rates of BOS-free survival. Botha and colleagues[59] reported that de novo colonization with P aeruginosa after transplantation was associated with a higher incidence of BOS and a shorter period of BOS-free survival. Why GNR colonization of the airways leads to BOS is still unclear, but the report by Vos and colleagues[60] of an association in lung transplant recipients between P aeruginosa colonization and the presence of bile acid in BAL samples suggests that aspiration may be the underlying mechanism.

Nontuberculous Mycobacteria

The incidence of nontuberculous mycobacterial (NTM) infections in SOT is largely unknown, but several recent reports suggest that it may be an underrecognized cause of posttransplant complications. Two single-center case series from the late 1990s found 9% (22 patients) and 3% (6 patients) of lung transplant patients respectively had an NTM infection over a 12-year to 13-year period in the late 1980s to mid-1990s.[61,62] However, more recent studies suggest an increase in the incidence of NTM infection, particularly Mycobacterium abscessus, and patients with CF may be at particular risk for colonization, if not infection, with this organism.[63] Factors most strongly linked to invasive infection in CF were pretransplant colonization with nontuberculous mycobacteria and isolation of M abscessus in particular.[63]

M abscessus seems to be emerging as a pathogen of special interest in lung transplantation. Multiple case reports and small case series have suggested that M abscessus may result in worse outcomes after transplantation, with several patients experiencing disseminated disease and death as a result of M abscessus infection.[64–68] Although an international survey of lung transplant centers conducted in 2006 found an overall low incidence of M abscessus infection (0.33%), most affected patients had pleuropulmonary infection requiring treatment, and 2 of 17 died as a result of infection.[69] A recent review and several meeting abstracts have focused on the increased recognition of M abscessus in SOT recipients, including

lung recipients, noting increased risk of dissemination and mortality.[70,71]

The effect of other NTM infections has been variable with regard to lung transplant outcomes. Although M avium complex has long been recognized as both a colonizer and cause of pulmonary infection in patients with underlying lung disease, including chronic obstructive pulmonary disease, its effect on lung transplantation is less notable.[72] Similarly, other NTM infections have been reported in lung transplant candidates and recipients, but these organisms have not been commonly described or notable for causing the excessive morbidity and mortality seen with M abscessus. Candidates for lung transplantation should be screened for NTM infections with respiratory cultures if radiographic or clinical findings are suggestive, and considered for treatment before transplantation when possible.

The diagnosis and treatment of NTM infections is summarized in a recent guideline from the American Thoracic Society and the Infectious Diseases Society of America (IDSA).[73] These criteria are applicable to transplant recipients and are reflected in the current AST Infectious Diseases Guidelines.[74] Susceptibility testing should be performed for all clinically relevant isolates because of the evolving resistance patterns of many NTM isolates (eg, M abscessus) and because of potential drug interaction issues (eg, the use of rifamycins in M avium disease). In additional, repeat susceptibility testing should be performed if disease recurs after treatment because of inducible mechanisms of drug resistance in some isolates.

FUNGAL INFECTIONS

Lung transplant recipients are at exceptionally high risk for fungal infections, and recent estimates place the incidence of fungal infection between 15% and 35%, with an overall mortality of 80%.[75,76] Most of these infections are caused by Candida and Aspergillus species, but lung transplant recipients may also be infected with Zygomycetes, Scedosporium, Fusarium, Cryptococcus species, and endemic mycoses such as histoplasmosis and coccidiodomycosis. Pneumocystis jirovecii is uncommon now that universal prophylaxis (most commonly with trimethoprim-sulfamethoxazole) is the standard of care for all lung transplant recipients. It seems that most cases of cryptococcosis and the endemic mycoses are caused by reactivation of latent disease, so a careful pretransplant evaluation is critical to determine a history of disease before transplantation. Some situations of previous or recent disease caused by endemic mycoses may warrant specific antifungal prophylaxis, and current recommendations for SOT recipients have been recently published.[77,78]

Aspergillus

Aspergillus infection can manifest in a variety of ways during the course of lung transplantation, including pretransplant airway colonization, posttransplant tracheobronchitis, invasive pulmonary aspergillosis, and disseminated disease. Working definitions of these entities have been previously published.[79] The incidence of these complications varies depending on the literature cited, but recent literature reviews found airway colonization with *Aspergillus* without disease was most commonly seen (23% of patients), and a minority of patients (less than 10%) developed either tracheobronchitis or invasive aspergillosis (IA).[75,80] Two recent fungal surveillance networks, the PATH alliance registry and TRANSNET (Transplant-Associated Infection Surveillance Network), noted that *Aspergillus* accounted for most fungal infections in SOT patients (44%–59.7%); *Candida* was the second most common fungus seen (approximately 23% in both series).[81,82]

The data regarding the role of pretransplantation *Aspergillus* colonization in the development of posttransplant fungal complications is limited. Helmi and colleagues[83] performed a retrospective single-center study comparing colonization in patients with CF with transplant recipients who did not have CF. Patients with CF were more likely to be colonized with *Aspergillus* and to have tracheobronchial infection after transplantation; nevertheless, IA and disseminated infection did not occur in the patients with CF and was uncommon in recipients who did not have CF. In addition, a literature review comprising studies from 1996 to 1999 found no cases of transplant recipients with CF colonized with *Aspergillus* before transplant progressing to IA.[84] A recent single-center retrospective analysis of mold infections in explanted lungs reported 5% of explants with invasive fungal infections, and pretransplant diagnosis of these infections occurred less than 50% of the time.[85] There was an association of unrecognized pretransplant mold infection with invasive fungal infections after transplant, regardless of voriconazole prophylaxis, and attributable mortality was 29% in these patients.[85] Earlier studies suggested posttransplant *Aspergillus* colonization was associated with an 11-fold higher risk of the development of IA,[86] but a subsequent single-center series combined with a pooled data analysis from the published literature by Mehrad and colleagues[84] suggests that the risk may

be substantially lower. Only 1 of 38 colonized subjects progressed to IA in the single-center series, and only 3 of 97 patients (3%) in the pooled literature review progressed to IA.

The gold standard for the diagnosis of IA remains biopsy with culture, accompanied by compatible clinical and radiographic abnormalities. However, the development of rapid, minimally invasive diagnostic testing modalities for aspergillosis remains an area of urgent clinical need. Galactomannan is a polysaccharide cell wall component of *Aspergillus*, and antigen detection in body fluids can be performed using an enzyme immunoassay technique (Platelia Galactomannan EIA, BioRad Laboratories, Hercules, CA, USA). The galactomannan assay has been studied primarily in the hematopoietic stem cell transplant population, in whom it is currently approved for use as a twice-weekly serum-based screening test for the development of IA. Several studies have assessed its usefulness in the diagnosis of IA infection in lung transplant recipients, with mixed results. Prospective testing of serum specimens had poor sensitivity for IA (30%), and did not detect any cases of *Aspergillus* tracheobronchitis.[87] Testing of BAL was more promising, with sensitivities ranging from 60% to 82% and a specificity of 95% in 2 studies.[88,89] False-positive test results can be seen with the use of β-lactam antibiotics (especially piperacillin-tazobactam, ticarcillin-clavulanate, and amoxicillin), and the test may cross-react in the presence of other molds and endemic fungi. The $(1 \rightarrow 3)$-β-D-glucan assay tests for a cell wall component present in most fungi, thus it is not specific for aspergillosis. The test also has a high false-positive rate in critically ill patients, and does not seem to have better sensitivity than the galactomannan test.[90] PCR-based methods for detection of *Aspergillus* are in development but are not yet standardized for clinical use.[91]

Prophylaxis of fungal infections in lung transplant recipients is widely variable from center to center and there are no large-scale multicenter studies to guide prophylactic choices. Guidelines suggest stratifying patients based on their individual risk factors, including pretransplant colonization with *Aspergillus*, or acquiring colonizing organisms in the first 12 months after transplantation. Other theorized risk factors include early airway ischemia, placement of a bronchial stent, single lung transplantation, hypogammaglobulinemia, CMV infection, use of alemtuzumab or thymoglobulin induction therapies, and acute rejection requiring augmentation of immunosuppression. Both inhaled amphotericin compounds and oral itraconazole and voriconazole prophylaxis strategies have been used, but no randomized controlled trials have assessed these approaches (for a summary of recent study results see Ref.[92]). A recent single-center, retrospective, sequential study compared universal voriconazole prophylaxis for a minimum of 4 months against 4 months of targeted prophylaxis with itraconazole plus or minus inhaled amphotericin in patients with pretransplant or posttransplant *Aspergillus* colonization and reported reduced IA in the voriconazole arm.[93] However, several recent studies have reported unanticipated adverse events in lung transplant patients given prolonged voriconazole therapy for prophylaxis or treatment of IA, including disabling neuromuscular disorders and periostitis resembling hypertrophic osteoarthropathy.[94,95] Because of the numerous drug interactions of azole antifungals with calcineurin inhibitors and mTOR (mammalian target of rapamycin) inhibitors, close attention to the dosing of these immunosuppressive agents is imperative.[96]

Treatment recommendations for *Aspergillus* tracheobronchitis have recently been summarized in 2 guidelines.[97,98] Voriconazole is recommended as first-line therapy for biopsy-confirmed *Aspergillus* tracheobronchitis along with reduction of immunosuppression, with attention paid to drug interactions with calcineurin inhibitors and to potential side effects including hepatotoxicity and visual hallucinations.[97,98] Duration of treatment is typically guided by bronchoscopic surveillance for resolution. Parenteral lipid formulations of amphotericin B deoxycholate remain an alternative in patients who cannot tolerate voriconazole. There has been limited experience using echinocandins (ie, caspofungin) or posaconazole in this setting. Inhaled amphotericin B deoxycholate or lipid formulations of amphotericin have been used in *Aspergillus* tracheobronchitis, but this strategy remains investigational because no standardized approach has been rigorously studied.[97,98] A single case report describing weekly topical instillation of liposomal amphotericin B via bronchoscopy in combination with standard antifungal therapy has also been recently described.[99]

Treatment of IA also relies on voriconazole as a first-line agent, with consideration of parenteral lipid formulations of amphotericin B deoxycholate, echinocandins, posaconazole, or itraconazole as alternatives. Reduction of immunosuppression is again an important component of treatment. Combination therapy with 2 or more agents is not routinely recommended as an initial therapeutic approach because of the lack of evidence for improved outcomes. Recent guidelines also suggest monitoring of voriconazole levels because serum concentrations are highly variable among patient populations, especially in patients with

CF.[98,100] Trough levels between 1 and 5 μg/μL are recommended for optimal efficacy and prevention of toxicity.[101] Surgical intervention, including debridement and resection, may be necessary for life-threatening hemoptysis, lesions in close proximity to the great vessels or pericardium, sinonasal infections, and intracranial lesions.[97] Surgical assessment is also warranted in cases of progressive or refractory disease when optimal antifungal therapy has failed. Duration of treatment is typically guided by clinical and radiographic resolution of attributable abnormalities, with 12 weeks recommended as a minimum course of therapy. The role of immunomodulatory agents such as interferon γ remains investigational, with anecdotal evidence in renal transplant recipients supporting its use.[102] This approach needs to be further studied and validated in a controlled manner before it can be incorporated into clinical practice.

Candida

As noted earlier, *Candida* is the second most common cause of invasive fungal infections in lung transplant recipients. Risk factors for candidal infections in lung transplant recipients are often related to postoperative complications including prolonged stays in the intensive care unit, prolonged indwelling catheters and broad-spectrum antibiotic therapy and parenteral nutrition, as well as heavy growth of *Candida* from the donor lung.[79] Manifestations of candidal disease typically occur in the first 30 days after transplantation, and include bloodstream infections, empyema, mediastinitis, bronchial anastomotic breakdown, and infection of vascular anastomoses with mycotic aneurysm formation. No cases of invasive pulmonary candidiasis have been reported in the adult lung transplant literature, although in 1 pediatric transplantation series 5% of proven pulmonary invasive fungal infections were caused by *Candida* species.[92] Despite relatively good antifungal therapies targeting *Candida* species, the prognosis for patients with most invasive candidal disease (excluding bronchial anastomotic disease) is grim, with mortality greater than 50%.[79] A clinical suspicion of invasive fungal disease in addition to an appropriate positive culture should be the criteria used to begin antifungal therapy.

Culture remains the gold standard for the diagnosis of candidal infections, because other modalities such as β-D-glucan detection and *Candida* mannan antigenemia testing do not yet have sufficient sensitivity or specificity to be useful in the clinical setting.[90] In addition, the identification to the species level for any clinically significant *Candida* isolate is critical. In this regard, several species have intrinsic resistance to certain antifungals, such as *C krusei* resistance to fluconazole, whereas other isolates may have dose-dependent susceptibility, such as *C glabrata* to fluconazole and *C lusitaniae* to amphotericin.[103] Real-time PCR techniques are in development that may aid in the rapid determination of a specific *Candida* species from a clinical specimen, but these assays are currently experimental only.[91] Suggested treatment of invasive candidal infections has been summarized recently in both the 2009 AST guidelines and the 2009 IDSA guidelines.[103,104] Culture data are essential in all cases to determine the identification of the isolate and subsequent susceptibility information. In non-neutropenic patients with mild to moderate illness, no previous significant azole exposure, and at low risk for *C glabrata* infection, high-dose fluconazole may be used initially. However, given the increasing use of azole prophylaxis (both fluconazole and voriconazole) in lung transplant patients and their higher risk level for developing severe illness, many experts recommend empiric therapy with an echinocandin or liposomal amphotericin B (depending on renal tolerability). Ongoing treatment should be adjusted based on susceptibility data. The duration of treatment depends on the extent and severity of disease, and ranges from a minimum of 2 weeks after negative blood cultures for uncomplicated candidemia to prolonged courses of treatment with the potential for life-long suppression for endocarditis or similar conditions.

The treatment of *Candida* species isolated from recipient airway secretions is less straightforward, because *Candida* spp are a common colonizer of the oropharynx, and the incidence of invasive candidal disease in lung transplant recipients colonized with *Candida* spp seems to be rare.[92] Many centers routinely use posttransplant antifungal prophylaxis, but the agent used and the duration of therapy are highly variable, as noted earlier. However, most experts agree that if antifungal prophylaxis is used the agent should target both *Candida* and *Aspergillus* species. In the case of *Candida* tracheobronchitis, a visual inspection of the anastomosis should be performed with both cultures and histologic confirmation. It is critical that cultures be obtained in this setting, because *Aspergillus* is another common cause of necrotizing anastomotic infections, and the choice of antifungal therapy may be different from those commonly used for candidal infections. The choice of therapy should be guided by the culture results, as discussed earlier, and the duration of therapy should be guided by bronchoscopically confirmed resolution of infection.[103]

SUMMARY

Infections continue to be a major source of morbidity and mortality in lung transplant recipients. Careful pretransplant assessments, selection of appropriate prophylactic regimens, and prompt diagnosis and treatment of posttransplant infections may improve posttransplant outcomes. Nevertheless, the unique exposure of the transplanted organ to the external environment and the intensive immunosuppression required to prevent rejection continue to provide unique challenges in the management of infections in lung transplantation.

REFERENCES

1. Christie JD, Edwards LB, Kucheryavaya AY, et al. The Registry of the International Society for Heart and Lung Transplantation: twenty-seventh official adult lung and heart-lung transplant report–2010. J Heart Lung Transplant 2010;29(10):1104–18.
2. Kotloff RM, Ahya VN, Crawford SW. Pulmonary complications of solid organ and hematopoietic stem cell transplantation. Am J Respir Crit Care Med 2004;170(1):22–48.
3. Kotloff RM, Ahya VN. Medical complications of lung transplantation. Eur Respir J 2004;23(2):334–42.
4. Remund KF, Best M, Egan JJ. Infections relevant to lung transplantation. Proc Am Thorac Soc 2009; 6(1):94–100.
5. Fischer SA, Avery RK. Screening of donor and recipient prior to solid organ transplantation. Am J Transplant 2009;9(Suppl 4):S7–18.
6. Danzinger-Isakov L, Kumar D. Guidelines for vaccination of solid organ transplant candidates and recipients. Am J Transplant 2009;9(Suppl 4): S258–62.
7. Subramanian A, Dorman S. Mycobacterium tuberculosis in solid organ transplant recipients. Am J Transplant 2009;9(Suppl 4):S57–62.
8. Fishman JA. Infection in solid-organ transplant recipients. N Engl J Med 2007;357(25):2601–14.
9. Aguilar-Guisado M, Givaldá J, Ussetti P, et al. Pneumonia after lung transplantation in the RESITRA Cohort: a multicenter prospective study. Am J Transplant 2007;7(8):1989–96.
10. Humar A, Snydman D. Cytomegalovirus in solid organ transplant recipients. Am J Transplant 2009;9(Suppl 4):S78–86.
11. Eid AJ, Razonable RR. New developments in the management of cytomegalovirus infection after solid organ transplantation. Drugs 2010;70(8):965–81.
12. Humar A, Michaels M. American Society of Transplantation recommendations for screening, monitoring and reporting of infectious complications in immunosuppression trials in recipients of organ transplantation. Am J Transplant 2006;6(2):262–74.

13. Rubin RH. The pathogenesis and clinical management of cytomegalovirus infection in the organ transplant recipient: the end of the 'silo hypothesis'. Curr Opin Infect Dis 2007;20(4):399–407.

14. Glanville AR, Valentine VG, Aboyoun CL, et al. CMV mismatch is not a risk factor for survival or severe bronchiolitis obliterans syndrome after lung transplantation. Immunol Cell Biol 2004;82(2):A7.

15. Chmiel C, Speich R, Hofer M, et al. Ganciclovir/valganciclovir prophylaxis decreases cytomegalovirus-related events and bronchiolitis obliterans syndrome after lung transplantation. Clin Infect Dis 2008;46(6):831–9.

16. Manuel O, Kumar D, Moussa G, et al. Lack of association between beta-herpesvirus infection and bronchiolitis obliterans syndrome in lung transplant recipients in the era of antiviral prophylaxis. Transplantation 2009;87(5):719–25.

17. Johansson I, Martensson G, Andersson R. Cytomegalovirus and long-term outcome after lung transplantation in Gothenburg, Sweden. Scand J Infect Dis 2010;42(2):129–36.

18. Ruttmann E, Geltner C, Bucher B, et al. Combined CMV prophylaxis improves outcome and reduces the risk for bronchiolitis obliterans syndrome (BOS) after lung transplantation. Transplantation 2006;81(10):1415–20.

19. Tamm M, Aboyoun CL, Chhajed PN, et al. Treated cytomegalovirus pneumonia is not associated with bronchiolitis obliterans syndrome. Am J Respir Crit Care Med 2004;170(10):1120–3.

20. Snyder LD, Finlen-Copeland CA, Turbyfill WJ, et al. Cytomegalovirus pneumonitis is a risk for bronchiolitis obliterans syndrome in lung transplantation. Am J Respir Crit Care Med 2010;181(12):1391–6.

21. Pang XL, Fox JD, Fenton JM, et al. Interlaboratory comparison of cytomegalovirus viral load assays. Am J Transplant 2009;9(2):258–68.

22. Kumar D, Chernenko S, Moussa G, et al. Cell-mediated immunity to predict cytomegalovirus disease in high-risk solid organ transplant recipients. Am J Transplant 2009;9(5):1214–22.

23. Kotton CN, Kumar D, Caliendo AM, et al. International consensus guidelines on the management of cytomegalovirus in solid organ transplantation. Transplantation 2010;89(7):779–95.

24. Hodson EM, Craig JC, Strippoli GF, et al. Antiviral medications for preventing cytomegalovirus disease in solid organ transplant recipients. Cochrane Database Syst Rev 2008;2:CD003774.

25. Zamora MR. Cytomegalovirus and lung transplantation. Am J Transplant 2004;4(8):1219–26.

26. Zamora MR, Nicolls MR, Hodges TN, et al. Following universal prophylaxis with intravenous ganciclovir and cytomegalovirus immune globulin, valganciclovir is safe and effective for prevention of CMV infection following lung transplantation. Am J Transplant 2004;4(10):1635–42.

27. Valentine VG, Weill D, Gupta MR, et al. Ganciclovir for cytomegalovirus: a call for indefinite prophylaxis in lung transplantation. J Heart Lung Transplant 2008;27(8):875–81.

28. Palmer SM, Limaye AP, Banks M, et al. Extended valganciclovir prophylaxis to prevent cytomegalovirus after lung transplantation: a randomized, controlled trial. Ann Intern Med 2010;152(12):761–9.

29. Kelly J, Hurley D, Raghu G. Comparison of the efficacy and cost effectiveness of pre-emptive therapy as directed by CMV antigenemia and prophylaxis with ganciclovir in lung transplant recipients. J Heart Lung Transplant 2000;19(4):355–9.

30. Limaye AP, Raghu G, Koelle DM, et al. High incidence of ganciclovir-resistant cytomegalovirus infection among lung transplant recipients receiving preemptive therapy. J Infect Dis 2002;185(1):20–7.

31. Monforte V, Román A, Gavaldà J, et al. Preemptive therapy with intravenous ganciclovir for the prevention of cytomegalovirus disease in lung transplant recipients. Transplant Proc 2005;37(9):4039–42.

32. Asberg A, Humar A, Rollag H, et al. Oral valganciclovir is noninferior to intravenous ganciclovir for the treatment of cytomegalovirus disease in solid organ transplant recipients. Am J Transplant 2007;7(9):2106–13.

33. Asberg A, Humar A, Jardine AG, et al. Long-term outcomes of CMV disease treatment with valganciclovir versus IV ganciclovir in solid organ transplant recipients. Am J Transplant 2009;9(5):1205–13.

34. Mylonakis E, Kallas WM, Fishman JA. Combination antiviral therapy for ganciclovir-resistant cytomegalovirus infection in solid-organ transplant recipients. Clin Infect Dis 2002;34(10):1337–41.

35. Kumar D, Husain S, Chen MH, et al. A prospective molecular surveillance study evaluating the clinical impact of community-acquired respiratory viruses in lung transplant recipients. Transplantation 2010;89(8):1028–33.

36. Billings JL, Hertz MI, Savik K, et al. Respiratory viruses and chronic rejection in lung transplant recipients. J Heart Lung Transplant 2002;21(5):559–66.

37. Khalifah AP, Hachem RR, Chakinala MM, et al. Respiratory viral infections are a distinct risk for bronchiolitis obliterans syndrome and death. Am J Respir Crit Care Med 2004;170(2):181–7.

38. Kumar D, Erdman D, Keshavjee S, et al. Clinical impact of community-acquired respiratory viruses on bronchiolitis obliterans after lung transplant. Am J Transplant 2005;5(8):2031–6.

39. Milstone AP, Brumble LM, Barnes J, et al. A single-season prospective study of respiratory viral

infections in lung transplant recipients. Eur Respir J 2006;28(1):131–7.

40. Ison MG, Michaels MG. RNA respiratory viral infections in solid organ transplant recipients. Am J Transplant 2009;9(Suppl 4):S166–72.

41. Kumar D, Morris MI, Kotton CN, et al. Guidance on novel influenza A/H1N1 in solid organ transplant recipients. Am J Transplant 2010;10(1):18–25.

42. Boeckh M, Englund J, Li Y, et al. Randomized controlled multicenter trial of aerosolized ribavirin for respiratory syncytial virus upper respiratory tract infection in hematopoietic cell transplant recipients. Clin Infect Dis 2007;44(2):245–9.

43. Glanville AR, Scott AI, Morton JM, et al. Intravenous ribavirin is a safe and cost-effective treatment for respiratory syncytial virus infection after lung transplantation. J Heart Lung Transplant 2005;24(12):2114–9.

44. Pelaez A, Lyon GM, Force SD, et al. Efficacy of oral ribavirin in lung transplant patients with respiratory syncytial virus lower respiratory tract infection. J Heart Lung Transplant 2009;28(1):67–71.

45. Campos S, Caramori M, Teixeira R, et al. Bacterial and fungal pneumonias after lung transplantation. Transplant Proc 2008;40(3):822–4.

46. Valentine VG, Bonvillain RW, Gupta MR, et al. Infections in lung allograft recipients: ganciclovir era. J Heart Lung Transplant 2008;27(5):528–35.

47. Dobbin C, Maley M, Harkness J, et al. The impact of pan-resistant bacterial pathogens on survival after lung transplantation in cystic fibrosis: results from a single large referral centre. J Hosp Infect 2004;56(4):277–82.

48. Hadjiliadis D, Steele MP, Chaparro C, et al. Survival of lung transplant patients with cystic fibrosis harboring panresistant bacteria other than *Burkholderia cepacia*, compared with patients harboring sensitive bacteria. J Heart Lung Transplant 2007;26(8):834–8.

49. Lynch JP 3rd. *Burkholderia cepacia* complex: impact on the cystic fibrosis lung lesion. Semin Respir Crit Care Med 2009;30(5):596–610.

50. Alexander BD, Petzold EW, Reller LB, et al. Survival after lung transplantation of cystic fibrosis patients infected with *Burkholderia cepacia* complex. Am J Transplant 2008;8(5):1025–30.

51. Boussaud V, Guillemain R, Grenet D, et al. Clinical outcome following lung transplantation in patients with cystic fibrosis colonised with *Burkholderia cepacia* complex: results from two French centres. Thorax 2008;63(8):732–7.

52. Murray S, Charbeneau J, Marshall BC, et al. Impact of burkholderia infection on lung transplantation in cystic fibrosis. Am J Respir Crit Care Med 2008; 178(4):363–71.

53. Orens JB, Boehler A, de Perrot M, et al. A review of lung transplant donor acceptability criteria. J Heart Lung Transplant 2003;22(11):1183–200.

54. Avlonitis VS, Krause A, Luzzi L, et al. Bacterial colonization of the donor lower airways is a predictor of poor outcome in lung transplantation. Eur J Cardiothorac Surg 2003;24(4):601–7.

55. Weill D, Dey GC, Hicks RA, et al. A positive donor gram stain does not predict outcome following lung transplantation. J Heart Lung Transplant 2002; 21(5):555–8.

56. Bonde PN, Patel ND, Borja MC, et al. Impact of donor lung organisms on post-lung transplant pneumonia. J Heart Lung Transplant 2006;25(1): 99–105.

57. Vos R, Vanaudenaerde BM, Geudens N, et al. Pseudomonal airway colonisation: risk factor for bronchiolitis obliterans syndrome after lung transplantation? Eur Respir J 2008;31(5):1037–45.

58. Gottlieb J, Mattner F, Weissbrodt H, et al. Impact of graft colonization with gram-negative bacteria after lung transplantation on the development of bronchiolitis obliterans syndrome in recipients with cystic fibrosis. Respir Med 2009;103(5):743–9.

59. Botha P, Archer L, Anderson RL, et al. *Pseudomonas aeruginosa* colonization of the allograft after lung transplantation and the risk of bronchiolitis obliterans syndrome. Transplantation 2008;85(5): 771–4.

60. Vos R, Blondeau K, Vanaudenaerde BM, et al. Airway colonization and gastric aspiration after lung transplantation: do birds of a feather flock together? J Heart Lung Transplant 2008;27(8):843–9.

61. Malouf MA, Glanville AR. The spectrum of mycobacterial infection after lung transplantation. Am J Respir Crit Care Med 1999;160(5 Pt 1):1611–6.

62. Kesten S, Chaparro C. Mycobacterial infections in lung transplant recipients. Chest 1999;115(3):741–5.

63. Chalermskulrat W, Sood N, Neuringer IP, et al. Non-tuberculous mycobacteria in end stage cystic fibrosis: implications for lung transplantation. Thorax 2006;61(6):507–13.

64. Sanguinetti M, Ardito F, Fiscarelli E, et al. Fatal pulmonary infection due to multidrug-resistant *Mycobacterium abscessus* in a patient with cystic fibrosis. J Clin Microbiol 2001;39(2):816–9.

65. Fairhurst RM, Kubak BM, Shpiner RB, et al. *Mycobacterium abscessus* empyema in a lung transplant recipient. J Heart Lung Transplant 2002; 21(3):391–4.

66. Taylor JL, Palmer SM. *Mycobacterium abscessus* chest wall and pulmonary infection in a cystic fibrosis lung transplant recipient. J Heart Lung Transplant 2006;25(8):985–8.

67. Gilljam M, Scherstén H, Silverborn M, et al. Lung transplantation in patients with cystic fibrosis and *Mycobacterium abscessus* infection. J Cyst Fibros 2010;9(4):272–6.

68. Zaidi S, Elidemir O, Heinle JS, et al. *Mycobacterium abscessus* in cystic fibrosis lung transplant

recipients: report of 2 cases and risk for recurrence. Transpl Infect Dis 2009;11(3):243–8.

69. Chernenko SM, Humar A, Hutcheon M, et al. *Mycobacterium abscessus* infections in lung transplant recipients: the international experience. J Heart Lung Transplant 2006;25(12):1447–55.

70. Garrison AP, Morris MI, Doblecki LS, et al. *Mycobacterium abscessus* infection in solid organ transplant recipients: report of three cases and review of the literature. Transpl Infect Dis 2009;11(6):541–8.

71. Longworth SA, Vinnard C, Lee I, et al. Risk factors for non-tuberculous mycobacterial infections in heart and lung transplant recipients. J Heart Lung Transplant 2010;29(2S):S82.

72. Doucette K, Fishman JA. Nontuberculous mycobacterial infection in hematopoietic stem cell and solid organ transplant recipients. Clin Infect Dis 2004;38(10):1428–39.

73. Griffith DE, Aksamit T, Brown-Elliott BA, et al. An official ATS/IDSA statement: diagnosis, treatment, and prevention of nontuberculous mycobacterial diseases. Am J Respir Crit Care Med 2007; 175(4):367–416.

74. Dorman S, Subramanian A. Nontuberculous mycobacteria in solid organ transplant recipients. Am J Transplant 2009;9(Suppl 4):S63–9.

75. Kubak BM. Fungal infection in lung transplantation. Transpl Infect Dis 2002;4(Suppl 3):24–31.

76. Sole A, Salavert M. Fungal infections after lung transplantation. Curr Opin Pulm Med 2009;15(3): 243–53.

77. Proia L, Miller R. Endemic fungal infections in solid organ transplant recipients. Am J Transplant 2009; 9(Suppl 4):S199–207.

78. Singh N, Forrest G. Cryptococcosis in solid organ transplant recipients. Am J Transplant 2009;9(Suppl 4):S192–8.

79. Sole A, Salavert M. Fungal infections after lung transplantation. Transplant Rev (Orlando) 2008; 22(2):89–104.

80. Singh N. Antifungal prophylaxis for solid organ transplant recipients: seeking clarity amidst controversy. Clin Infect Dis 2000;31(2):545–53.

81. Neofytos D, Fishman JA, Horn D, et al. Epidemiology and outcome of invasive fungal infections in solid organ transplant recipients. Transpl Infect Dis 2010;12(3):220–9.

82. Pappas PG, Alexander BD, Andes DR, et al. Invasive fungal infections among organ transplant recipients: results of the Transplant-Associated Infection Surveillance Network (TRANSNET). Clin Infect Dis 2010; 50(8):1101–11.

83. Helmi M, Lover RB, Welter D, et al. *Aspergillus* infection in lung transplant recipients with cystic fibrosis: risk factors and outcomes comparison to other types of transplant recipients. Chest 2003; 123(3):800–8.

84. Mehrad B, Paciocco G, Martinez FJ, et al. Spectrum of *Aspergillus* infection in lung transplant recipients: case series and review of the literature. Chest 2001;119(1):169–75.

85. Vadnerkar A, Clancy CJ, Celik U, et al. Impact of mold infections in explanted lungs on outcomes of lung transplantation. Transplantation 2010;89(2):253–60.

86. Cahill BC, Hibbs JR, Savik K, et al. *Aspergillus* airway colonization and invasive disease after lung transplantation. Chest 1997;112(5):1160–4.

87. Husain S, Kwak EJ, Obman A, et al. Prospective assessment of Platelia *Aspergillus* galactomannan antigen for the diagnosis of invasive aspergillosis in lung transplant recipients. Am J Transplant 2004;4(5):796–802.

88. Clancy CJ, Jaber RA, Leather HL, et al. Bronchoalveolar lavage galactomannan in diagnosis of invasive pulmonary aspergillosis among solid-organ transplant recipients. J Clin Microbiol 2007;45(6): 1759–65.

89. Husain S, Paterson DL, Studer SM, et al. Aspergillus galactomannan antigen in the bronchoalveolar lavage fluid for the diagnosis of invasive aspergillosis in lung transplant recipients. Transplantation 2007;83(10):1330–6.

90. Wheat LJ. Approach to the diagnosis of invasive aspergillosis and candidiasis. Clin Chest Med 2009;30(2):367–77, viii.

91. Wengenack NL, Binnicker MJ. Fungal molecular diagnostics. Clin Chest Med 2009;30(2):391–408, viii.

92. Hosseini-Moghaddam SM, Husain S. Fungi and molds following lung transplantation. Semin Respir Crit Care Med 2010;31(2):222–33.

93. Husain S, Paterson DL, Studer S, et al. Voriconazole prophylaxis in lung transplant recipients. Am J Transplant 2006;6(12):3008–16.

94. Boussaud V, Daudet N, Billaud EM, et al. Neuromuscular painful disorders: a rare side effect of voriconazole in lung transplant patients under tacrolimus. J Heart Lung Transplant 2008;27(2):229–32.

95. Wang TF, Wang T, Altman R, et al. Periostitis secondary to prolonged voriconazole therapy in lung transplant recipients. Am J Transplant 2009; 9(12):2845–50.

96. Thomas LD, Miller GG. Interactions between antiinfective agents and immunosuppressants. Am J Transplant 2009;9(Suppl 4):S263–6.

97. Singh N, Husain S. Invasive aspergillosis in solid organ transplant recipients. Am J Transplant 2009;9(Suppl 4):S180–91.

98. Walsh TJ, Anaissie EJ, Denning DW, et al. Treatment of aspergillosis: clinical practice guidelines of the Infectious Diseases Society of America. Clin Infect Dis 2008;46(3):327–60.

99. Morales P, Galán G, Sanmartín E, et al. Intrabronchial instillation of amphotericin B lipid complex: a case report. Transplant Proc 2009;41(6):2223–4.

100. Berge M, Guillemain R, Boussaud V, et al. Vorico-nazole pharmacokinetic variability in cystic fibrosis lung transplant patients. Transpl Infect Dis 2009; 11(3):211–9.

101. Howard A, Hoffman J, Sheth A. Clinical application of voriconazole concentrations in the treatment of invasive aspergillosis. Ann Pharmacother 2008; 42(12):1859–64.

102. Armstrong-James D, Teo IA, Shrivastava S, et al. Exogenous interferon-gamma immunotherapy for invasive fungal infections in kidney transplant patients. Am J Transplant 2010;10(8):1796–803.

103. Pappas PG, Silveira FP. *Candida* in solid organ transplant recipients. Am J Transplant 2009; 9(Suppl 4):S173–9.

104. Pappas PG, Kauffman CA, Andes D, et al. Clinical practice guidelines for the management of candidi-asis: 2009 update by the Infectious Diseases Society of America. Clin Infect Dis 2009;48(5): 503–35.

Malignancies Following Lung Transplantation

Hilary Y. Robbins, MD, Selim M. Arcasoy, MD*

KEYWORDS

- Malignancy • Lung transplant • Skin cancer
- Posttransplant lymphoproliferative disorder • Lung cancer

Epidemiologic studies show that recipients of solid organ transplantation (SOT) have an approximately three- to four-fold increased risk of developing cancer compared with the general population.[1–3] Historically, transplant recipients were noted to have a particularly high incidence of skin cancer, lymphoma, Kaposi's sarcoma, cervical cancer, anogenital carcinoma, kidney cancer, and hepatocellular carcinoma.[4–9] Recent data suggest that SOT recipients are also at higher risk for developing common solid organ tumors, such as lung, breast, prostate, and colon cancer.[8] Cancers in transplant recipients tend to occur at an earlier age and, in the case of skin cancers, with multiple lesions.[3,10] Current data from the International Society of Heart and Lung Transplantation Registry indicate that malignancy accounts for 13% of deaths between 5 and 10 years after lung transplantation.[11]

Multiple factors account for the higher incidence of malignancy in transplant patients. Immunosuppressive agents promote cancer partly through a decrease in T-cell mediated immune surveillance. Impaired lymphocyte function seems to be particularly significant in malignancies associated with oncogenic viruses, such as the Epstein-Barr virus (EBV) in post-transplant lymphoproliferative disorder (PTLD) or human herpesvirus 8 in Kaposi's sarcoma. Alternative mechanisms independent of lymphocyte function have also been proposed. Cyclosporine impairs DNA repair mechanisms, induces an invasive cellular phenotype via transforming growth factor ß stimulation, and

promotes angiogenesis through increasing vascular endothelial growth factor concentrations.[12–14] In contrast, mammalian target of rapamycin inhibitors such as sirolimus have antineoplastic properties, including suppression of cell proliferation, tumor growth, angiogenesis, and metastasis.[15] Most clinical trials have shown a lower risk of malignancy with sirolimus-based immunosuppressive regimens.[16–18] Finally, immunosuppressive agents and environmental risk factors for malignancy may be synergistic, as suggested by the finding that ultraviolet A radiation induces higher levels of oxidative DNA damage in an in vitro model of azathioprine therapy.[19]

This article focuses on the two most common malignancies after lung transplantation: skin cancer and PTLD. Bronchogenic carcinoma, which has been considered both an indication for and a complication of lung transplantation, is also addressed.

SKIN CANCER

Epidemiology and Risk Factors

Cutaneous squamous cell carcinoma (SCC) and basal cell carcinoma (BCC) account for most cancers after SOT.[1] The incidence of skin cancer increases over time after transplant, and a reversal of the normal predominance of BCC over SCC occurs. The development of skin cancers is accelerated in transplant recipients compared with immunocompetent hosts, with one series showing an average time from lung transplant to diagnosis of SCC of 19 months.[10,20] In this study the

---

The authors have nothing to disclose.

Lung Transplantation Program, Division of Pulmonary, Allergy, and Critical Care Medicine, Columbia University Medical Center, 622 West 168th Street, PH-14 East Room 104, New York, NY 10032, USA

* Corresponding author.

E-mail address: sa2059@columbia.edu

Clin Chest Med 32 (2011) 343–355

doi:10.1016/j.ccm.2011.02.011

incidence of SCC was 3.1% over a mean follow-up period of 36 months.[20]

A recent population-based cohort study in Denmark showed incidence rates for BCC and SCC of 4 and 6.6 per 1000 person-years, respectively, in the first 4 years after lung transplantation. By 5 to 10 years, the incidence increased to 9.7 per 1000 person-years for BCC and for SCC.[5] Compared with the expected incidence of skin cancers in the Danish population, lung transplant patients had a 26-fold increase in SCC, 4.1-fold increase in BCC, and 2.6-fold increase in malignant melanoma. Incidence rates of skin cancer in the lung transplant population were similar to those in other SOT recipients.

Older age, male gender, high level of sun exposure, and cumulative voriconazole dose have been shown to increase the risk for SCC in lung transplant recipients.[20] Other risk factors for skin cancers in the SOT population include a pretransplant history of nonmelanoma skin cancer, duration and type of immunosuppression, and certain viral infections.[21–23] Several cutaneous malignancies in the immunosuppressed population are associated with viral infection, including SCC, which is linked to human papillomavirus; Kaposi's sarcoma, caused by human herpesvirus 8; and Merkel cell carcinoma, which has been associated with the newly discovered Merkel cell polyomavirus.[24,25] Although both Kaposi's sarcoma and Merkel cell carcinoma are rare tumors in the United States transplant population, their incidence is dramatically increased compared with immunocompetent hosts.

Although the relative contribution of each immunosuppressive agent is difficult to determine, cyclosporine has been associated with a dose-dependent increase in skin cancers.[22,26] Azathioprine seems to increase skin cancer risk through photosensitizing cells to ultraviolet A radiation.[19,27] Mycophenolate mofetil has been shown to reduce the risk of skin cancers in short-term follow-up.[28] Recent studies of sirolimus suggest that it may be protective against the development of nonmelanoma skin cancer.[17]

Risk factors for the de novo development of melanoma in organ transplant recipients are less well defined, but may relate to the presence of atypical nevi, sun exposure, and personal or family history of melanoma.[29] A personal history of melanoma is often considered a contraindication to transplantation, with early literature reporting an approximately 20% recurrence rate.[30] Two recent series have shown no recurrence or metastasis in 17 patients with pretransplant melanoma, although most reported cases were early-stage disease (stage 0-IIC).[31,32]

Presentation

SCC predominantly affects sun-exposed areas, including the back of the hands and the face. BCC also tends to affect sun-exposed areas, with a predominance on the face, upper chest, and back but not the hands.[33] Men may be at greater risk than women for skin cancers on the external ear, scalp, and neck because of hair styles and thickness.[7] The distribution of melanoma is less predictable, with most presenting on the trunk, head, or neck, and less commonly on the upper and lower limbs. Approximately one-third of melanomas develop at the site of a preexisting nevus.[31]

Prevention

Patients should receive education about environmental exposures linked to skin cancer, both before transplant and after. They should be counseled on avoidance of sun exposure particularly between 11 AM and 3 PM, the use of protective clothing and sunscreen effective for ultraviolet A and B radiation with a high sun protection factor, performing self-examination, and obtaining dermatologic screening at least yearly.[34,35]

Treatment

Precancerous lesions, including actinic keratosis and Bowen disease (SCC in situ or disease confined to the epidermis), may be difficult to distinguish from invasive SCC without biopsy. Therefore, the threshold to biopsy should be low in this population. Treatment options for precancerous lesions in SOT include local therapy, such as cryotherapy and electrocautery with curettage, and topical therapy, such as photodynamic therapy or topical 5-fluorouracil, diclofenac, and imiquimod.[36–39]

Treatment guidelines for the management of SCC and other skin cancers in organ transplant patients are largely based on treatment recommendations in the immunocompetent population.[34,35,40–42] For invasive SCC or BCC, excision is recommended using either standard surgical techniques with intraoperative frozen section evaluation or Mohs micrographic surgery.[40] In the general population, surgical margins for excision should be at least 4 to 6 mm, and up to 10 mm in patients with high-risk features; no distinct guidelines exist for SOT recipients.[43] Mohs micrographic surgery is the preferred treatment in high-risk tumors, tumors with positive margins on surgical resection, and recurrent cancers, and for optimal tissue conservation in anatomically sensitive areas.[44] Palpable regional lymphadenopathy should be evaluated with fine needle aspiration or open biopsy. If positive, regional lymph node dissection may be indicated and staging should be performed to exclude the presence of distant metastasis.

Radiation is not recommended for transplant recipients as first-line therapy for SCC or BCC.[34,45] Adjuvant therapy with radiation should be considered in patients who have positive margins when reexcision is not considered feasible or in cases of perineural involvement. Radiation to improve locoregional control should be considered in patients with SCC who have disease metastatic to lymph nodes as adjuvant treatment after lymph node dissection, or in patients considered inoperable.[46]

Few patients with metastatic SCC are treated with chemotherapy, usually as an adjunct to surgery or radiotherapy. Most regimens are extrapolated from data in head and neck cancers, although systemic toxicities must be taken into account when adapting these regimens to lung transplant patients. Common regimens include single-agent or combination regimens with a platinum or taxane, with or without epidermal growth factor receptor (EGFR) inhibition.[47] The anti-EGFR monoclonal antibody cetuximab is approved for use in SCC of the head and neck, but its use was associated with fatal respiratory failure in two lung transplant recipients.[48]

Chemoprophylaxis

Systemic therapy with acitretin, a systemic retinoid, has been shown to significantly reduce the development of new malignant and premalignant lesions in organ transplant recipients.[49–51] Its use may be limited by side effects, including dry skin, alopecia, elevated liver enzymes, and hyperlipidemia. In addition, tumor growth usually continues, or may transiently increase, with cessation of the drug. Conflicting data exist on the efficacy of photodynamic therapy as a preventative option in patients with multiple SCC despite optimal medical and surgical management.[52,53]

Reduction or Change in Immunosuppression

No standard recommendations exist regarding reduction or alteration in immunosuppression in patients with skin cancers. Reduction of immunosuppression (RI) may be considered in patients with multiple skin cancers or rapidly progressive or metastatic disease, and must be weighed against the risk of graft rejection. Tumor regression is well demonstrated in renal transplant recipients with Kaposi sarcoma managed with RI (usually discontinuation of cyclosporine), although with a significant incidence of acute and chronic graft dysfunction.[54] The switch from cyclosporine-based to sirolimus-based immunosuppression has been shown to decrease the time to first skin cancer by approximately 65% in kidney transplant recipients.[17]

Outcomes

In transplant recipients, SCC tends to be more aggressive, with an increase in deep tissue involvement, perineural and lymphatic invasion, and need for radiation or chemotherapy.[55] Recurrence of SCC or BCC is more common in SOT recipients, occurring in 12% to 48% of cases within 3 to 4 years of the initial diagnosis.[2,44,56] The incidence of metastatic skin cancer in SOT recipients is 7%, and occurs at a mean of 1.4 years after the primary diagnosis.[9,57] In one series, 1-year survival after the diagnosis of metastasis was 89% for regional nodal metastasis and 39% for distant metastasis.[57] Poor prognostic features include multiple tumors, a cephalic presentation, older age, metastatic disease, poor histologic differentiation, tumor thickness greater than 5 mm, and deep tissue invasion.[58] Cancer-specific mortality from BCC or SCC in the Israel Penn International Transplant Tumor Registry was 11% and 18%, respectively.[56]

Prognostic features for melanoma in the transplant population are probably similar to those in immunocompetent hosts, and include tumor thickness and nodal status.[59,60] Melanoma with tumor thickness greater than 2 mm has a worse prognosis in SOT recipients than in nontransplanted individuals, with a greater than 11-fold increased risk of death.[31] Melanoma-specific mortality of 13% at a median follow-up of 2.4 years was reported in this study.[31]

POSTTRANSPLANT LYMPHOPROLIFERATIVE DISORDER
Pathology

The term PTLD encompasses a diverse group of lymphoproliferative disorders, separated into four histologic types by the updated 2008 WHO classification.[61] Early lesions include plasmacytic hyperplasia or those resembling infectious mononucleosis, in which a polyclonal plasma cell infiltrate is present but lymph node architecture is preserved. Polymorphic PTLD describes tumors with a polyclonal infiltrate with features of cellular atypia destructive of underlying tissue architecture. Monomorphic PTLD refers to clonal populations of B cells, T cells, and natural killer cells, morphologically similar to non-Hodgkin's lymphomas. Lastly, classical Hodgkin's lymphoma has been reported. Greater than 80% of PTLDs are B-cell tumors; approximately 15% originate from T cells and 1% from natural killer cells. Evidence of EBV infection is present in pathology samples in greater than 80% of cases.[62] Genetic analysis of PTLD tumors suggests that most of these tumors are of recipient origin.[63]

Epidemiology and Risk Factors

The incidence of PTLD in lung transplant recipients has varied widely in the literature, with single-center studies showing a range of 1.8% to 20%.[64–70] A United Network for Organ Sharing analysis from 1988–1999 revealed a PTLD incidence of 3.7% in lung transplant recipients.[71] This study showed that PTLD was more common in thoracic organ recipients than in liver and kidney transplant recipients, with an incidence of 0.9% and 0.6%, respectively. An analysis of the Collaborative Transplant Study database showed a 58.6-fold increase in non-Hodgkin's lymphoma in lung transplant patients compared with a healthy reference population.[6]

Among the most significant risk factors for PTLD after lung transplantation is EBV serostatus, with a 20-fold increased risk for the development of PTLD in EBV-seronegative recipients compared with those who were EBV-seropositive before transplant.[65] EBV infects greater than 90% of the population, resulting in latent B-lymphocyte infection with the viral genome.[72] EBV-specific cytotoxic T-cells are the primary mode of control for EBV infection; therefore, acquired T-cell immunodeficiency after transplantation can result in uncontrolled proliferation of EBV-infected B cells. Most EBV-seronegative SOT recipients develop primary EBV infection within 3 to 6 months after transplant.[73]

Demographic factors that increase PTLD risk in lung transplant recipients include age younger than 18 years, possibly related to EBV-seronegative status in pediatric recipients, and Caucasian race.[71] One report found a higher incidence of PTLD in lung transplant recipients older than 55 years, which may be related to immune senescence.[69] Cytomegalovirus mismatch in combination with EBV-seronegative status has been shown to be synergistic in increasing the risk for PTLD.[66] Finally, more aggressive immunosuppressive therapy is associated with susceptibility to PTLD. The use of lympholytic therapy was associated with a 1.8-fold higher incidence of PTLD in cardiac and renal transplant recipients.[74] Controversy exists regarding the role of calcineurin inhibitors, which in some studies have been shown to increase the risk of PTLD in kidney transplant recipients.[75,76] Neither induction with interleukin 2 (IL-2) receptor antagonists nor the use of azathioprine and mycophenolate mofetil seems to increase PTLD risk after kidney transplantation.[6] Contrary to the antineoplastic profile generally attributed to sirolimus, one study showed a higher incidence of PTLD with its use.[18] The above risk factors do not completely explain the full spectrum of PTLD, such as the development of non–B-cell tumors or B-cell tumors that are EBV-negative.

Presentation and Diagnosis

Greater than 50% of lung transplant recipients who develop PTLD do so within the first year of transplant, and are considered to have early-onset disease.[64–67,69,77,78] Cases have been reported as early as the first posttransplant week.[68,78] The allograft is the most common site of primary disease in early-onset PTLD, which can present as single or multiple pulmonary masses or nodules, or less frequently as airspace consolidation, lymphadenopathy, or pleural effusion (**Fig. 1**A, B).[79,80] Extrapulmonary manifestations can be protean, including intra-abdominal disease, central nervous system disease, or cutaneous lesions (see **Fig. 1**C, D).

Late-onset PTLD, in contrast, is more likely to present in extrathoracic sites, with gastrointestinal involvement the most frequent manifestation.[81] EBV-negative PTLD tends to occur late after transplant. Bakker and colleagues[79] reported a median time to diagnosis of 9 months in EBV-positive PTLD compared with 103 months in EBV-negative disease in kidney and lung transplant recipients.

The diagnosis of PTLD often requires surgical biopsy or excision to ensure adequate sampling of the underlying tissue architecture, although needle aspirate, core biopsy, and transbronchial biopsy may provide sufficient tissue for diagnosis. Pathologic evaluation should include an analysis of morphology, clonality, cellular lineage of origin, flow cytometry, and evaluation for the presence of EBV with EBV-encoded RNA in situ hybridization.[82] Disease staging is typically performed with CT, although positron emission tomography may be useful in detecting unsuspected lesions or in assessing response to treatment.[69]

Surveillance monitoring of EBV in peripheral blood has been assessed as a marker of impending PTLD, with the goal of reducing immunosuppression accordingly to prevent the development of PTLD.[83,84] Studies of EBV viral load in lung transplant recipients have been insufficiently sensitive and specific to predict the future development of PTLD, and this test is not currently recommended by consensus guidelines.[77,82,85,86] A recent report suggests that levels of free plasma EBV may correlate better with the risk of PTLD and response to treatment in patients with PTLD.[87]

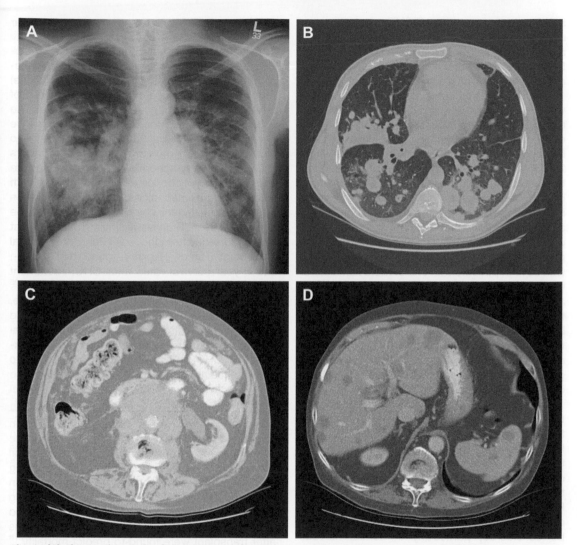

Fig. 1. (*A*) Chest radiograph of a patient with bilateral lung transplantation revealing nodular airspace opacities due to PTLD. (*B*) Axial computed tomography of the same patient, showing multiple bilateral lung nodules with an area of focal consolidation. (*C*) Computed tomography of the abdomen in a second single lung transplant recipient showing a large conglomerate mass of PTLD abutting the vertebral column and encasing the aorta. (*D*) Computed tomography of the abdomen in the same patient as Fig. 1C, demonstrating hepatic and splenic lesions of PTLD.

Prevention

Several retrospective series have shown a reduction in the incidence of PTLD with the use of antiviral therapy compared with historical control groups in whom antiviral prophylaxis was not standard.[88–90] In one study, ganciclovir use protected kidney recipients against PTLD (odds ratio, 0.17; 95% CI, 0.05–056) compared with no prophylaxis. Other longitudinal studies have failed to confirm a reduction in PTLD risk despite the implementation of antiviral prophylaxis.[75] Firm conclusions about prevention are difficult to draw

from these data, given the differences in patient populations, EBV serostatus, and immunosuppression regimens. Antiviral medications such as acyclovir and ganciclovir do not affect episomal replication in latently infected B cells, which uses cellular DNA polymerase, the primary contributor to PTLD. Therefore antiviral medications do not prevent PTLD once EBV infection is established.

Treatment

Treatment recommendations for PTLD in SOT exist, although randomized trials to guide therapy have not been performed.[86,91,92] Initial treatment of PTLD includes RI. Guidelines on RI suggest a reduction in calcineurin inhibitor dose by 25% to 50%, cessation of azathioprine or mycophenolate, and maintenance of prednisone at a dose of 7.5 to 10 mg daily.[91,92] Induction of complete response with RI alone varies widely between studies, ranging from 6% to 80%, likely because of differences in patient and tumor characteristics.[65,93,94] Disease remission with RI typically occurs within 2 to 4 weeks, although case series have reported tumor resolution up to 14 weeks.[95] In one study, independent predictors of RI failure included increased lactate dehydrogenase (LDH), loss of allograft function, and multiorgan disease.[95] A partial or complete response was seen in 89% of patients without any of these risk factors compared with 25% of patients with one or more risk factors. RI carries the risk of acute and chronic rejection, and necessitates close observation of lung function. The optimal duration of RI is unclear, and will be affected by tumor response, clinical status of the patient, and development of rejection. Other mechanisms of immunotherapy are under investigation, including infusion of cytotoxic T lymphocytes and viral gene induction.[96,97]

Localized therapy, such as surgery or radiation therapy, may be an option in a minority of lung transplant patients, usually in conjunction with RI or systemic chemotherapy. Surgical intervention may be useful for tumor debulking or in management of local complications such as gastrointestinal disease with obstruction or bleeding. Radiation therapy has been reported to be a component of multimodality therapy, and should be considered, particularly in central nervous system disease.[98,99]

Rituximab, a monoclonal antibody against the B-cell marker CD20, is the mainstay of therapy in CD20+ B-cell PTLD, and should be considered in all patients with incomplete response to RI or those with aggressive disease. Successful use of rituximab with RI in lung transplant recipients has been reported.[70,100,101] Three uncontrolled phase II clinical trials of rituximab have been performed in SOT recipients with CD20+ B-cell PTLD for whom RI failed, showing complete remission rates of 34% to 42% after the first cycle of therapy.[102,103] Serious adverse events related to rituximab were notable for intestinal perforation in one patient and neutropenia in 2% to 5% of patients. Favorable prognostic factors related to response to rituximab included age younger than 60 years, normal LDH, and Eastern Cooperative Oncology Group performance status of 2 or greater. In patients with all three factors, only one required salvage chemotherapy.[102] Overall

survival in these trials was 73% to 75% at 1 year and 52% to 67% at 2 years.

Multiagent chemotherapy for PTLD in SOT recipients has generally consisted of CHOP (cyclophosphamide, doxorubicin, vincristine, prednisolone) with or without the use of rituximab. Because of the toxicities of multiagent chemotherapy, its use is typically reserved for CD20- or EBV-negative tumors, CD20+ B-cell tumors unresponsive to rituximab, T-cell lymphomas, aggressive tumors such as Burkitt lymphoma–type PTLD, and classical Hodgkin's lymphoma.[91,104] Compared with studies of rituximab alone, complete remission rates with multiagent chemotherapy seem to be higher, but overall survival is similar.[105] The largest published series from the Israel Penn International Transplant Tumor Registry found that 1-, 3-, and 5-year survival rates after CHOP treatment were 58%, 36%, and 24%, respectively.[106] Compared with treatment with rituximab alone, anthracycline-based chemotherapy is associated with higher rates of infection- and treatment-related mortality.[105] However, the addition of rituximab to CHOP (R-CHOP) does not seem to increase the risk of serious adverse events.[107]

Prognosis

Although no prognostic scoring system has been developed for PTLD, the International Prognostic Index (stage, performance status, extranodal disease, LDH, and age) and Ann Arbor staging system for lymphoma have been validated in SOT populations.[108,109] In a series of 104 lung transplant patients with PTLD, disseminated disease and PTLD diagnosis more than 6 months after transplant were found to predict mortality.[78] In a retrospective series of lung and heart–lung transplant recipients from 1988 to 2000, patients with PTLD had reduced survival at 3 and 5 years: 50% and 38%, respectively, compared with 70% and 52% in the cohort as a whole.[81] In other reports, the development of PTLD has not been found to impact posttransplant survival.[77,110]

Retransplantation for bronchiolitis obliterans syndrome in lung transplant recipients after treatment of PTLD has been shown to be a viable option, with no reported recurrence of PTLD.[78,111]

LUNG CANCER
Epidemiology and Risk Factors

The incidence of bronchogenic carcinoma after lung transplantation has been estimated in case series to be 0.25% to 4.0%.[112–119] The epidemiology of bronchogenic carcinoma after lung transplantation has recently been reviewed.[120] The incidence of lung cancer in this series was 0.75

per 100 patient-years, significantly higher than that in the general population. The mean age at recipient diagnosis was 58 years, and approximately half were men. The underlying diagnosis was chronic obstructive pulmonary disease (COPD) in 76% and idiopathic pulmonary fibrosis (IPF) in 19%. Nearly all lung cancers occurred in the native lung of single lung transplant recipients (91%), and most had an extensive smoking history (83%). Histology was documented as non–small cell in 93% of cases.

These demographics reflect known risk factors for bronchogenic carcinoma, including smoking history, older age, and a diagnosis of IPF or COPD.[121–124] In the setting of transplantation, other important factors include procedure type (ie, single vs bilateral transplant), incidental disease noted in the native lung explant, and donor-derived malignancy. In a matched cohort study, a 5.3-fold increase in the risk of lung cancer was shown in patients with a single lung transplant compared with those with a bilateral transplant.[125] Incidental bronchogenic carcinoma noted on explanted lungs is not uncommon, with a pathologic series noting an incidence of 1.4%.[126] Even when the tumor is completely resected at transplant, disease recurrence is common and prognosis is particularly poor in patients with stage II or greater disease.[127] Screening CT of the chest at regular intervals should be considered to exclude malignancy in transplant candidates at high risk for lung cancer. Finally, unusual cases without classic risk factors have been reported, including small cell carcinoma developing in otherwise healthy, nonsmoking young adults with cystic fibrosis. In

one case, genetic analysis suggested that the tumor was of donor origin.[128,129]

Presentation

Most tumors are diagnosed within the first 2 years after transplantation, although lung cancer has been reported as late as 10 years after transplant.[114,120,125] Most patients have nonspecific respiratory symptoms (ie, cough, dyspnea, chest pain), symptoms referable to a site of metastatic disease, or constitutional symptoms. Hemoptysis is a rare presentation.[130] The most common findings on chest imaging are a new lung nodule or mass in 60% of cases, pleural effusion in 12%, and nonresolving infiltrate in 3% (**Fig. 2**); these findings are almost invariably restricted to the native lung of single lung transplant recipients.[120]

Although infection is probably the most common cause of pulmonary nodules in lung transplant patients, neoplastic disease must be considered, especially if occurring in the native lung of a patient with COPD or IPF. Despite frequent chest radiography in this population, tumors may be missed on routine imaging because of existing native lung disease or postoperative changes.

Treatment

Although surgical resection is the preferred modality in early-stage non–small cell lung cancer, fewer than half of reported cases have undergone surgical resection and nearly a third have received palliative treatment alone given the extent of their cancer and comorbid diseases. Immunosuppression is commonly reduced, with unknown benefit,

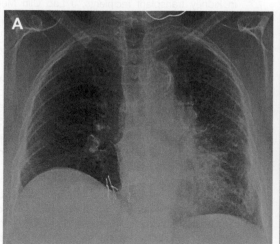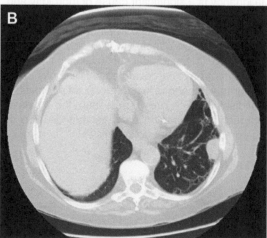

Fig. 2. (*A*) Chest radiograph of a patient with interstitial lung disease following right single lung transplantation. A subtle change in the appearance of the lateral left lower lung zone prompted further imaging. (*B*) Computed tomography of the chest in the same patient shows a pleural-based mass in the left lung base, which was diagnosed as small cell carcinoma metastatic to hilar lymph nodes.

and chemotherapy and radiation are used as otherwise indicated for bronchogenic carcinoma in the nontransplant population.[131] However, medical comorbidities and bone marrow reserve frequently limit aggressive chemotherapy. Prognosis tends to be poor, with a mean survival after cancer diagnosis of less than 1 year and a 5-year survival of 25%. Survival greater than 5 years after resection of stage IA disease has been documented.[125]

Bronchioloalveolar Carcinoma

Bronchioloalveolar carcinoma (BAC) is a rare indication for lung transplantation, constituting 0.1% of all procedures in the United States between 1995 and 2009.[11] The largest case series, compiled via an international survey, includes 26 patients who had a transplant for advanced multifocal BAC and were followed up for up to 10 years (median 21 months).[127] Postoperative mortality was 15%, with all deaths occurring in patients undergoing single lung transplant after prior contralateral pneumonectomy. In the remaining 22 patients, 59% developed recurrent BAC between 5 and 49 months (median, 12 months) after transplant; 3 patients underwent retransplantation for this indication. Of the patients with recurrence, 9 died between 11 and 82 months (median, 22 months) after transplant; 5-year survival for all patients was 39%. Analysis of DNA polymorphisms in resected tissue samples showed that the origin of recurrent BAC was the recipient.[132,133]

SUMMARY

Malignancy is a significant cause of morbidity and mortality after lung transplantation. Preventative efforts should be pursued in all patients, particularly against skin cancer. Malignancy should be considered in the diagnostic evaluation of new symptoms, physical examination findings, and radiographic changes in the transplant population. Multidisciplinary care represents the optimal approach to managing cancers that develop in this complex patient population.

REFERENCES

1. Adami J, Gäbel H, Lindelöf B, et al. Cancer risk following organ transplantation: a nationwide cohort study in Sweden. Br J Cancer 2003;89(7): 1221–7.
2. Lindelöf B, Sigurgeirsson B, Gäbel H, et al. Incidence of skin cancer in 5356 patients following organ transplantation. Br J Dermatol 2000;143(3): 513–9.
3. Webster A, Craig J, Simpson J, et al. Identifying high risk groups and quantifying absolute risk of cancer after kidney transplantation: a cohort study of 15,183 recipients. Am J Transplant 2007;7(9): 2140–51.
4. Penn I. Posttransplant malignancies. Transplant Proc 1999;31(1–2):1260–2.
5. Jensen A, Svaerke C, Farkas D, et al. Skin cancer risk among solid organ recipients: a nationwide cohort study in Denmark. Acta Derm Venereol 2010;90(5):474–9.
6. Opelz G, Döhler B. Lymphomas after solid organ transplantation: a collaborative transplant study report. Am J Transplant 2004;4(2):222–30.
7. Moloney F, Comber H, O'Lorcain P, et al. A population-based study of skin cancer incidence and prevalence in renal transplant recipients. Br J Dermatol 2006;154(3):498–504.
8. Kasiske B, Snyder J, Gilbertson D, et al. Cancer after kidney transplantation in the United States. Am J Transplant 2004;4(6):905–13.
9. Sheil A, Disney A, Mathew T, et al. De novo malignancy emerges as a major cause of morbidity and late failure in renal transplantation. Transplant Proc 1993;25(1 Pt 2):1383–4.
10. Harwood C, Proby C, McGregor J, et al. Clinicopathologic features of skin cancer in organ transplant recipients: a retrospective case-control series. J Am Acad Dermatol 2006;54(2):290–300.
11. Christie J, Edwards L, Kucheryavaya A, et al. The Registry of the International Society for Heart and Lung Transplantation: twenty-seventh official adult lung and heart-lung transplant report–2010. J Heart Lung Transplant 2010;29(10):1104–18.
12. Herman M, Weinstein T, Korzets A, et al. Effect of cyclosporin A on DNA repair and cancer incidence in kidney transplant recipients. J Lab Clin Med 2001;137(1):14–20.
13. Hojo M, Morimoto T, Maluccio M, et al. Cyclosporine induces cancer progression by a cell-autonomous mechanism. Nature 1999;397(6719):530–4.
14. Guba M, von Breitenbuch P, Steinbauer M, et al. Rapamycin inhibits primary and metastatic tumor growth by antiangiogenesis: involvement of vascular endothelial growth factor. Nat Med 2002;8(2):128–35.
15. Baldo P, Cecco S, Giacomin E, et al. mTOR pathway and mTOR inhibitors as agents for cancer therapy. Curr Cancer Drug Targets 2008;8(8):647–65.
16. Kauffman H, Cherikh W, Cheng Y, et al. Maintenance immunosuppression with target-of-rapamycin inhibitors is associated with a reduced incidence of de novo malignancies. Transplantation 2005;80(7): 883–9.
17. Campistol J, Eris J, Oberbauer R, et al. Sirolimus therapy after early cyclosporine withdrawal reduces the risk for cancer in adult renal transplantation. J Am Soc Nephrol 2006;17(2):581–9.

18. Kirk A, Cherikh W, Ring M, et al. Dissociation of depletional induction and posttransplant lymphoproliferative disease in kidney recipients treated with alemtuzumab. Am J Transplant 2007;7(11):2619–25.

19. O'Donovan P, Perrett C, Zhang X, et al. Azathioprine and UVA light generate mutagenic oxidative DNA damage. Science 2005;309(5742):1871–4.

20. Vadnerkar A, Nguyen M, Mitsani D, et al. Voriconazole exposure and geographic location are independent risk factors for squamous cell carcinoma of the skin among lung transplant recipients. J Heart Lung Transplant 2010;29(11):1240–4.

21. Ramsay H, Fryer A, Hawley C, et al. Factors associated with nonmelanoma skin cancer following renal transplantation in Queensland, Australia. J Am Acad Dermatol 2003;49(3):397–406.

22. Jensen P, Hansen S, Møller B, et al. Skin cancer in kidney and heart transplant recipients and different long-term immunosuppressive therapy regimens. J Am Acad Dermatol 1999;40(2 Pt 1):177–86.

23. Caforio A, Fortina A, Piaserico S, et al. Skin cancer in heart transplant recipients: risk factor analysis and relevance of immunosuppressive therapy. Circulation 2000;102(19 Suppl 3):III222–7.

24. Chang Y, Cesarman E, Pessin M, et al. Identification of herpesvirus-like DNA sequences in AIDS-associated Kaposi's sarcoma. Science 1994;266(5192):1865–9.

25. Feng H, Shuda M, Chang Y, et al. Clonal integration of a polyomavirus in human Merkel cell carcinoma. Science 2008;319(5866):1096–100.

26. Dantal J, Hourmant M, Cantarovich D, et al. Effect of long-term immunosuppression in kidney-graft recipients on cancer incidence: randomised comparison of two cyclosporin regimens. Lancet 1998;351(9103):623–8.

27. Terhorst D, Drecoll U, Stockfleth E, et al. Organ transplant recipients and skin cancer: assessment of risk factors with focus on sun exposure. Br J Dermatol 2009;161(Suppl 3):85–9.

28. Crespo-Leiro M, Alonso-Pulpón L, Vázquez de Prada J, et al. Malignancy after heart transplantation: incidence, prognosis and risk factors. Am J Transplant 2008;8(5):1031–9.

29. Zwald F, Christenson L, Billingsley E, et al. Melanoma in solid organ transplant recipients. Am J Transplant 2010;10(5):1297–304.

30. Penn I. Malignant melanoma in organ allograft recipients. Transplantation 1996;61(2):274–8.

31. Matin R, Mesher D, Proby C, et al. Melanoma in organ transplant recipients: clinicopathological features and outcome in 100 cases. Am J Transplant 2008;8(9):1891–900.

32. Dapprich D, Weenig R, Rohlinger A, et al. Outcomes of melanoma in recipients of solid organ transplant. J Am Acad Dermatol 2008;59(3):405–17.

33. Hartevelt M, Bavinck J, Kootte A, et al. Incidence of skin cancer after renal transplantation in The Netherlands. Transplantation 1990;49(3):506–9.

34. Stasko T, Brown M, Carucci J, et al. Guidelines for the management of squamous cell carcinoma in organ transplant recipients. Dermatol Surg 2004;30(4 Pt 2):642–50.

35. Hofbauer G, Anliker M, Arnold A, et al. Swiss clinical practice guidelines for skin cancer in organ transplant recipients. Swiss Med Wkly 2009;139(29–30):407–15.

36. Ulrich C, Bichel J, Euvrard S, et al. Topical immunomodulation under systemic immunosuppression: results of a multicentre, randomized, placebo-controlled safety and efficacy study of imiquimod 5% cream for the treatment of actinic keratoses in kidney, heart, and liver transplant patients. Br J Dermatol 2007;157(Suppl 2):25–31.

37. Ulrich C, Johannsen A, Röwert-Huber J, et al. Results of a randomized, placebo-controlled safety and efficacy study of topical diclofenac 3% gel in organ transplant patients with multiple actinic keratoses. Eur J Dermatol 2010;20(4):482–8.

38. Perrett C, McGregor J, Warwick J, et al. Treatment of post-transplant premalignant skin disease: a randomized intrapatient comparative study of 5-fluorouracil cream and topical photodynamic therapy. Br J Dermatol 2007;156(2):320–8.

39. Wennberg A, Stenquist B, Stockfleth E, et al. Photodynamic therapy with methyl aminolevulinate for prevention of new skin lesions in transplant recipients: a randomized study. Transplantation 2008;86(3):423–9.

40. Miller S. The National Comprehensive Cancer Network (NCCN) guidelines of care for nonmelanoma skin cancers. Dermatol Surg 2000;26(3):289–92.

41. Telfer N, Colver G, Morton C, et al. Guidelines for the management of basal cell carcinoma. Br J Dermatol 2008;159(1):35–48.

42. Dummer R, Hauschild A, Guggenheim M, et al, ESMO Guidelines Working Group. Melanoma: ESMO Clinical Practice Guidelines for diagnosis, treatment and follow-up. Ann Oncol 2010;21(Suppl 5):v194–7.

43. Brodland D, Zitelli J. Surgical margins for excision of primary cutaneous squamous cell carcinoma. J Am Acad Dermatol 1992;27(2 Pt 1):241–8.

44. Rowe D, Carroll R, Day CJ. Prognostic factors for local recurrence, metastasis, and survival rates in squamous cell carcinoma of the skin, ear, and lip. Implications for treatment modality selection. J Am Acad Dermatol 1992;26(6):976–90.

45. Veness M, Harris D. Role of radiotherapy in the management of organ transplant recipients diagnosed with non-melanoma skin cancers. Australas Radiol 2007;51(1):12–20.

46. Veness M, Morgan G, Palme C, et al. Surgery and adjuvant radiotherapy in patients with cutaneous head and neck squamous cell carcinoma metastatic to lymph nodes: combined treatment should be considered best practice. Laryngoscope 2005; 115(5):870–5.

47. Haddad R, Shin D. Recent advances in head and neck cancer. N Engl J Med 2008;359(11):1143–54.

48. Leard L, Cho B, Jones K, et al. Fatal diffuse alveolar damage in two lung transplant patients treated with cetuximab. J Heart Lung Transplant 2007; 26(12):1340–4.

49. Bavinck J, Tieben L, Van der Woude F, et al. Prevention of skin cancer and reduction of keratotic skin lesions during acitretin therapy in renal transplant recipients: a double-blind, placebo-controlled study. J Clin Oncol 1995;13(8):1933–8.

50. George R, Weightman W, Russ G, et al. Acitretin for chemoprevention of non-melanoma skin cancers in renal transplant recipients. Australas J Dermatol 2002;43(4):269–73.

51. Harwood C, Leedham-Green M, Leigh I, et al. Low-dose retinoids in the prevention of cutaneous squamous cell carcinomas in organ transplant recipients: a 16-year retrospective study. Arch Dermatol 2005;141(4):456–64.

52. Willey A, Mehta S, Lee P. Reduction in the incidence of squamous cell carcinoma in solid organ transplant recipients treated with cyclic photodynamic therapy. Dermatol Surg 2010;36(5):652–8.

53. de Graaf Y, Kennedy C, Wolterbeek R, et al. Photodynamic therapy does not prevent cutaneous squamous-cell carcinoma in organ-transplant recipients: results of a randomized-controlled trial. J Invest Dermatol 2006;126(3):569–74.

54. Duman S, Töz H, Aşçi G, et al. Successful treatment of post-transplant Kaposi's sarcoma by reduction of immunosuppression. Nephrol Dial Transplant 2002; 17(5):892–6.

55. Lott D, Manz R, Koch C, et al. Aggressive behavior of nonmelanotic skin cancers in solid organ transplant recipients. Transplantation 2010;90(6): 683–7.

56. Buell J, Hanaway M, Thomas M, et al. Skin cancer following transplantation: the Israel Penn International Transplant Tumor Registry experience. Transplant Proc 2005;37(2):962–3.

57. Martinez J, Otley C, Stasko T, et al. Defining the clinical course of metastatic skin cancer in organ transplant recipients: a multicenter collaborative study. Arch Dermatol 2003;139(3):301–6.

58. Euvrard S, Kanitakis J, Claudy A. Skin cancers after organ transplantation. N Engl J Med 2003; 348(17):1681–91.

59. Balch C, Soong S, Gershenwald J, et al. Prognostic factors analysis of 17,600 melanoma patients: validation of the American Joint Committee on Cancer melanoma staging system. J Clin Oncol 2001; 19(16):3622–34.

60. Debarbieux S, Duru G, Dalle S, et al. Sentinel lymph node biopsy in melanoma: a micromorphometric study relating to prognosis and completion lymph node dissection. Br J Dermatol 2007;157(1): 58–67.

61. Swerdlow S, Webber S, Chadburn A, et al. Post-transplant lymphoproliferative disorders. Lyon (France): International Agency for Research on Cancer (IARC); 2008.

62. Mucha K, Foroncewicz B, Ziarkiewicz-Wróblewska B, et al. Post-transplant lymphoproliferative disorder in view of the new WHO classification: a more rational approach to a protean disease? Nephrol Dial Transplant 2010;25(7):2089–98.

63. Gulley M, Swinnen L, Plaisance KJ, et al. Tumor origin and CD20 expression in posttransplant lymphoproliferative disorder occurring in solid organ transplant recipients: implications for immune-based therapy. Transplantation 2003;76(6):959–64.

64. Levine S, Angel L, Anzueto A, et al. A low incidence of posttransplant lymphoproliferative disorder in 109 lung transplant recipients. Chest 1999;116(5): 1273–7.

65. Aris R, Maia D, Neuringer I, et al. Post-transplantation lymphoproliferative disorder in the Epstein-Barr virus-naïve lung transplant recipient. Am J Respir Crit Care Med 1996;154(6 Pt 1):1712–7.

66. Walker R, Paya C, Marshall W, et al. Pretransplantation seronegative Epstein-Barr virus status is the primary risk factor for posttransplantation lymphoproliferative disorder in adult heart, lung, and other solid organ transplantations. J Heart Lung Transplant 1995;14(2):214–21.

67. Armitage J, Kormos R, Stuart R, et al. Posttransplant lymphoproliferative disease in thoracic organ transplant patients: ten years of cyclosporine-based immunosuppression. J Heart Lung Transplant 1991;10(6):877–86 [discussion: 886–7].

68. Montone K, Litzky L, Wurster A, et al. Analysis of Epstein-Barr virus-associated posttransplantation lymphoproliferative disorder after lung transplantation. Surgery 1996;119(5):544–51.

69. Reams B, McAdams H, Howell D, et al. Posttransplant lymphoproliferative disorder: incidence, presentation, and response to treatment in lung transplant recipients. Chest 2003;124(4):1242–9.

70. Knoop C, Kentos A, Remmelink M, et al. Post-transplant lymphoproliferative disorders after lung transplantation: first-line treatment with rituximab may induce complete remission. Clin Transplant 2006; 20(2):179–87.

71. Dharnidharka V, Tejani A, Ho P, et al. Post-transplant lymphoproliferative disorder in the United States: young Caucasian males are at highest risk. Am J Transplant 2002;2(10):993–8.

72. Cohen J. Epstein-Barr virus infection. N Engl J Med 2000;343(7):481–92.
73. Savoie A, Perpête C, Carpentier L, et al. Direct correlation between the load of Epstein-Barr virus-infected lymphocytes in the peripheral blood of pediatric transplant patients and risk of lymphoproliferative disease. Blood 1994;83(9):2715–22.
74. Opelz G, Henderson R. Incidence of non-Hodgkin lymphoma in kidney and heart transplant recipients. Lancet 1993;342(8886–8887):1514–6.
75. Gao S, Chaparro S, Perlroth M, et al. Post-transplantation lymphoproliferative disease in heart and heart-lung transplant recipients: 30-year experience at Stanford University. J Heart Lung Transplant 2003;22(5):505–14.
76. Pirsch J. Cytomegalovirus infection and posttransplant lymphoproliferative disease in renal transplant recipients: results of the U.S. multicenter FK506 Kidney Transplant Study Group. Transplantation 1999;68(8):1203–5.
77. Wheless S, Gulley M, Raab-Traub N, et al. Post-transplantation lymphoproliferative disease: Epstein-Barr virus DNA levels, HLA-A3, and survival. Am J Respir Crit Care Med 2008;178(10):1060–5.
78. Raj R, Frost A. Lung retransplantation after posttransplantation lymphoproliferative disorder (PTLD): a single-center experience and review of literature of PTLD in lung transplant recipients. J Heart Lung Transplant 2005;24(6):671–9.
79. Bakker N, van Imhoff G, Verschuuren E, et al. Early onset post-transplant lymphoproliferative disease is associated with allograft localization. Clin Transplant 2005;19(3):327–34.
80. Pickhardt P, Siegel M, Anderson D, et al. Chest radiography as a predictor of outcome in posttransplantation lymphoproliferative disorder in lung allograft recipients. AJR Am J Roentgenol 1998;171(2):375–82.
81. Paranjothi S, Yusen R, Kraus M, et al. Lymphoproliferative disease after lung transplantation: comparison of presentation and outcome of early and late cases. J Heart Lung Transplant 2001; 20(10):1054–63.
82. Parker A, Bowles K, Bradley J, et al. Diagnosis of post-transplant lymphoproliferative disorder in solid organ transplant recipients - BCSH and BTS Guidelines. Br J Haematol 2010;149(5):675–92.
83. Lee T, Savoldo B, Rooney C, et al. Quantitative EBV viral loads and immunosuppression alterations can decrease PTLD incidence in pediatric liver transplant recipients. Am J Transplant 2005;5(9): 2222–8.
84. Smets F, Latinne D, Bazin H, et al. Ratio between Epstein-Barr viral load and anti-Epstein-Barr virus specific T-cell response as a predictive marker of posttransplant lymphoproliferative disease. Transplantation 2002;73(10):1603–10.
85. Benden C, Aurora P, Burch M, et al. Monitoring of Epstein-Barr viral load in pediatric heart and lung transplant recipients by real-time polymerase chain reaction. J Heart Lung Transplant 2005;24(12): 2103–8.
86. Epstein-Barr virus and lymphoproliferative disorders after transplantation. Am J Transplant 2004; 4(Suppl 10):59–65.
87. Tsai D, Douglas L, Andreadis C, et al. EBV PCR in the diagnosis and monitoring of posttransplant lymphoproliferative disorder: results of a two-arm prospective trial. Am J Transplant 2008;8(5):1016–24.
88. Malouf M, Chhajed P, Hopkins P, et al. Anti-viral prophylaxis reduces the incidence of lymphoproliferative disease in lung transplant recipients. J Heart Lung Transplant 2002;21(5):547–54.
89. Darenkov I, Marcarelli M, Basadonna G, et al. Reduced incidence of Epstein-Barr virus-associated posttransplant lymphoproliferative disorder using preemptive antiviral therapy. Transplantation 1997;64(6):848–52.
90. Funch D, Walker A, Schneider G, et al. Ganciclovir and acyclovir reduce the risk of post-transplant lymphoproliferative disorder in renal transplant recipients. Am J Transplant 2005;5(12):2894–900.
91. Parker A, Bowles K, Bradley J, et al. Management of post-transplant lymphoproliferative disorder in adult solid organ transplant recipients - BCSH and BTS Guidelines. Br J Haematol 2010;149(5):693–705.
92. Paya C, Fung J, Nalesnik M, et al. Epstein-Barr virus-induced posttransplant lymphoproliferative disorders. ASTS/ASTP EBV-PTLD Task Force and The Mayo Clinic Organized International Consensus Development Meeting. Transplantation 1999;68(10):1517–25.
93. Knight J, Tsodikov A, Cibrik D, et al. Lymphoma after solid organ transplantation: risk, response to therapy, and survival at a transplantation center. J Clin Oncol 2009;27(20):3354–62.
94. Ghobrial I, Habermann T, Maurer M, et al. Prognostic analysis for survival in adult solid organ transplant recipients with post-transplantation lymphoproliferative disorders. J Clin Oncol 2005; 23(30):7574–82.
95. Tsai D, Hardy C, Tomaszewski J, et al. Reduction in immunosuppression as initial therapy for posttransplant lymphoproliferative disorder: analysis of prognostic variables and long-term follow-up of 42 adult patients. Transplantation 2001;71(8):1076–88.
96. Merlo A, Turrini R, Dolcetti R, et al. The interplay between Epstein-Barr virus and the immune system: a rationale for adoptive cell therapy of EBV-related disorders. Haematologica 2010;95(10):1769–77.
97. Mentzer S, Perrine S, Faller D. Epstein–Barr virus post-transplant lymphoproliferative disease and virus-specific therapy: pharmacological re-activation of viral target genes with arginine butyrate. Transpl Infect Dis 2001;3(3):177–85.

98. Buell J, Gross T, Hanaway M, et al. Posttransplant lymphoproliferative disorder: significance of central nervous system involvement. Transplant Proc 2005; 37(2):954–5.

99. Cavaliere R, Petroni G, Lopes M, et al, Group IPCNSLC. Primary central nervous system post-transplantation lymphoproliferative disorder: an International Primary Central Nervous System Lymphoma Collaborative Group Report. Cancer 2010;116(4):863–70.

100. Cook R, Connors J, Gascoyne R, et al. Treatment of post-transplant lymphoproliferative disease with rituximab monoclonal antibody after lung transplantation. Lancet 1999;354(9191):1698–9.

101. Reynaud-Gaubert M, Stoppa A, Gaubert J, et al. Anti-CD20 monoclonal antibody therapy in Epstein-Barr Virus-associated B cell lymphoma following lung transplantation. J Heart Lung Transplant 2000; 19(5):492–5.

102. Choquet S, Leblond V, Herbrecht R, et al. Efficacy and safety of rituximab in B-cell post-transplantation lymphoproliferative disorders: results of a prospective multicenter phase 2 study. Blood 2006;107(8): 3053–7.

103. González-Barca E, Domingo-Domenech E, Capote F, et al. Prospective phase II trial of extended treatment with rituximab in patients with B-cell post-transplant lymphoproliferative disease. Haematologica 2007;92(11):1489–94.

104. Frey NV, Tsai DE. The management of posttransplant lymphoproliferative disorder. Med Oncol 2007;24(2):125–36.

105. Elstrom R, Andreadis C, Aqui N, et al. Treatment of PTLD with rituximab or chemotherapy. Am J Transplant 2006;6(3):569–76.

106. Buell J, Gross T, Hanaway M, et al. Chemotherapy for posttransplant lymphoproliferative disorder: the Israel Penn International Transplant Tumor Registry experience. Transplant Proc 2005;37(2):956–7.

107. Evens A, David K, Helenowski I, et al. Multicenter analysis of 80 solid organ transplantation recipients with post-transplantation lymphoproliferative disease: outcomes and prognostic factors in the modern era. J Clin Oncol 2010;28(6):1038–46.

108. Carbone P, Kaplan H, Musshoff K, et al. Report of the Committee on Hodgkin's Disease Staging Classification. Cancer Res 1971;31(11):1860–1.

109. A predictive model for aggressive non-Hodgkin's lymphoma. The International Non-Hodgkin's Lymphoma Prognostic Factors Project. N Engl J Med 1993;329(14):987–94.

110. Metcalfe M, Kutsogiannis D, Jackson K, et al. Risk factors and outcomes for the development of malignancy in lung and heart-lung transplant recipients. Can Respir J 2010;17(1):e7–13.

111. Johnson S, Cherikh W, Kauffman H, et al. Retransplantation after post-transplant lymphoproliferative disorders: an OPTN/UNOS database analysis. Am J Transplant 2006;6(11):2743–9.

112. de Perrot M, Wigle D, Pierre A, et al. Bronchogenic carcinoma after solid organ transplantation. Ann Thorac Surg 2003;75(2):367–71.

113. Spiekerkoetter E, Krug N, Hoeper M, et al. Prevalence of malignancies after lung transplantation. Transplant Proc 1998;30(4):1523–4.

114. Arcasoy S, Hersh C, Christie J, et al. Bronchogenic carcinoma complicating lung transplantation. J Heart Lung Transplant 2001;20(10):1044–53.

115. Choi Y, Leung A, Miro S, et al. Primary bronchogenic carcinoma after heart or lung transplantation: radiologic and clinical findings. J Thorac Imaging 2000;15(1):36–40.

116. McAdams H, Erasmus J, Palmer S. Complications (excluding hyperinflation) involving the native lung after single-lung transplantation: incidence, radiologic features, and clinical importance. Radiology 2001;218(1):233–41.

117. Schulman L, Htun T, Staniloae C, et al. Pulmonary nodules and masses after lung and heart-lung transplantation. J Thorac Imaging 2000;15(3):173–9.

118. Stagner L, Allenspach L, Hogan K, et al. Bronchogenic carcinoma in lung transplant recipients. J Heart Lung Transplant 2001;20(8):908–11.

119. Collins J, Kazerooni E, Lacomis J, et al. Bronchogenic carcinoma after lung transplantation: frequency, clinical characteristics, and imaging findings. Radiology 2002;224(1):131–8.

120. Minai O, Shah S, Mazzone P, et al. Bronchogenic carcinoma after lung transplantation: characteristics and outcomes. J Thorac Oncol 2008;3(12):1404–9.

121. Sasco A, Secretan M, Straif K. Tobacco smoking and cancer: a brief review of recent epidemiological evidence. Lung Cancer 2004;45(Suppl 2):S3–9.

122. Woloshin S, Schwartz L, Welch H. The risk of death by age, sex, and smoking status in the United States: putting health risks in context. J Natl Cancer Inst 2008;100(12):845–53.

123. Hubbard R, Venn A, Lewis S, et al. Lung cancer and cryptogenic fibrosing alveolitis. A population-based cohort study. Am J Respir Crit Care Med 2000;161(1):5–8.

124. Turner M, Chen Y, Krewski D, et al. Chronic obstructive pulmonary disease is associated with lung cancer mortality in a prospective study of never smokers. Am J Respir Crit Care Med 2007; 176(3):285–90.

125. Dickson R, Davis R, Rea J, et al. High frequency of bronchogenic carcinoma after single-lung transplantation. J Heart Lung Transplant 2006;25(11): 1297–301.

126. Abrahams N, Meziane M, Ramalingam P, et al. Incidence of primary neoplasms in explanted lungs: long-term follow-up from 214 lung transplant patients. Transplant Proc 2004;36(9):2808–11.

127. de Perrot M, Chernenko S, Waddell T, et al. Role of lung transplantation in the treatment of bronchogenic carcinomas for patients with end-stage pulmonary disease. J Clin Oncol 2004;22(21):4351–6.

128. Picard C, Grenet D, Copie-Bergman C, et al. Small-cell lung carcinoma of recipient origin after bilateral lung transplantation for cystic fibrosis. J Heart Lung Transplant 2006;25(8):981–4.

129. De Soyza A, Dark J, Parums D, et al. Donor-acquired small cell lung cancer following pulmonary transplantation. Chest 2001;120(3):1030–1.

130. Speziali G, McDougall J, Midthun D, et al. Native lung complications after single lung transplantation for emphysema. Transpl Int 1997; 10(2):113–5.

131. Ettinger D, Akerley W, Bepler G, et al. Non-small cell lung cancer. J Natl Compr Canc Netw 2010; 8(7):740–801.

132. Garver RJ, Zorn G, Wu X, et al. Recurrence of bronchioloalveolar carcinoma in transplanted lungs. N Engl J Med 1999;340(14):1071–4.

133. Gómez-Román J, Del Valle C, Zarrabeitia M, et al. Recurrence of bronchioloalveolar carcinoma in donor lung after lung transplantation: microsatellite analysis demonstrates a recipient origin. Pathol Int 2005;55(9):580–4.

Airway Complications Following Lung Transplantation

Jonathan Puchalski, MD, MEd[a], Hans J. Lee, MD[b],
Daniel H. Sterman, MD[c],*

KEYWORDS

- Stenosis • Stent • Bronchoscopy • Lung transplant
- Anastomosis

The most common indications for lung transplantation include emphysema, idiopathic pulmonary fibrosis (IPF), cystic fibrosis (CF), and idiopathic pulmonary arterial hypertension. The 5-year overall posttransplant survival rate is 52%.[1] One of the major issues that affect the outcome of lung transplantation is the development of complications at or near the anastomosis between the donor and recipient bronchus. The incidence of airway complications from lung transplantation reported in the medical literature varies, but ranges from 7% to 18%; with mortality related to these complications approximating 2% to 5%.[2,3] There are 6 major types of airway complications: necrosis and dehiscence, infection, granulation tissue formation, malacia, fistulae, and stenosis (**Table 1**).[2] This article reviews the risk factors for developing airway complications after lung transplantation, the clinical features of the complications, and treatment options for these problems.

GENERAL RISK FACTORS FOR AIRWAY COMPLICATIONS AFTER TRANSPLANTATION

Airway complications following lung transplantation are believed to be related to several factors including ischemia of the donor bronchus, immunosuppression, rejection, inadequate organ preservation, surgical techniques, and infections.[4] Donor lung quality is an important factor contributing to early success of lung allografts, and may also affect the incidence of airway complications. Ideal lung donors are typically no more than 50 years old, have less than a 20-pack-year smoking history, and have a po_2 greater than 300 mm Hg with a 100% fraction of inspired oxygen (Fio_2) challenge.[2]

It is suggested that segmental, nonanastomotic, large airway stenosis after transplantation may have a different cause than anastomotic complications. Acute cellular rejection is more common in patients with nonanastomotic complications, especially when airway inflammation is present. The endothelial injury may promote vasospasm and decreased blood flow to the proximal airways. Infection caused by loss of neural connections, decreased microbial clearance, and constant exposure to microorganisms in the setting of immunosuppression is also hypothesized to contribute to the development of postanastomotic complications.[4]

The extent of airway injury ranges from no injury and complete circumferential mucosal healing to airway wall healing without mucosal healing, to extensive necrosis of the mucosa and airway wall.[5] Although grading systems have been

The authors have nothing to disclose.
[a] Yale Pulmonary & Critical Care Medicine, Winchester Building, 25 York Street, 2nd Floor, New Haven, CT 06510, USA
[b] MCV Campus, Pulmonary/Critical Care Division, PO Box 980050, Richmond, VA 23298, USA
[c] Pulmonary, Allergy, & Critical Care Division, University of Pennsylvania Medical Center, 833 West Gates Building, 3400 Spruce Street, Philadelphia, PA 19104, USA
* Corresponding author.
E-mail address: daniel.sterman@uphs.upenn.edu

Clin Chest Med 32 (2011) 357–366
doi:10.1016/j.ccm.2011.03.001
0272-5231/11/$ – see front matter © 2011 Elsevier Inc. All rights reserved.

Table 1
Airway complications following lung transplant

Complications	Time	Endoscopic Management
Stenosis	Late (2–9 mo)	Balloon bronchoplasty Stent placement (silicone) Antiinflammatory injections
Excessive granulation tissue	Late	Forceps debulkment Ablation techniques Antiinflammatory injections
Necrosis and dehiscence	Early (<1 mo)	Stent placement (silicone/SEMS)
Bronchomalacia	Early (<4 mo)	Stent placement (silicone)
Fistulae	Early/late	Fibrin glue/blood patch Unidirectional valve Stent placement (SEMS)
Infections	Early/late	Removal of granulation/necrotic tissue

Abbreviation: SEMS, self-expanding metallic stent.

proposed, there is no universally accepted method for grading airway injury.[3]

Ischemia

Lung transplantation is unique among solid organ transplantation because systemic arterial blood supply is not routinely restored during implantation. Because the bronchial arterial circulation is typically not re anastomosed, perfusion is dependent on blood supply from the pulmonary arterial circulation. Pulmonary arterial blood flow may be insufficient in the perioperative period, particularly in the setting of intraoperative and postoperative hypotension and vasopressor administration, and may result in ischemic injury to the anastomosis and/or postanastomotic bronchus. This ischemic injury plays an important role in the cause of anastomotic complications. Pretransplantation cold ischemia of the donor bronchus may also contribute to the development of posttransplant anastomotic complications. Ideally, allograft cold ischemic times should be limited to a maximum of 6 hours to minimize the risk of injury.[1]

Following heart-lung transplantation, the donor's tracheobronchial circulation is maintained and tracheal anastomoses are perfused with coronary collaterals. In contrast, it may take up to 4 weeks for revascularization of the donor organ by the recipient's bronchial arteries following isolated lung transplantation. Factors such as hypotension, dehydration, and low cardiac output may worsen ischemic insult. Bronchial artery revascularization (BAR) may significantly restore bronchial blood flow, but the technical complexity and resultant prolonged graft ischemic time and need for cardiopulmonary bypass have precluded general acceptance of this procedure.[2] Efforts to maintain vascularized peribronchial soft tissue undisturbed during transplantation to maintain collateral microvasculature are advocated as a less complicated means of maximizing perfusion and decreasing risk of anastomotic complication. The use of heparin and prostaglandins to increase microcirculatory flow and retrograde perfusion of the donor bronchus has been advocated by some investigators, but is not widely used.[3]

Rejection and Immunosuppression

Acute cellular rejection has been identified as an independent risk factor for bronchial complications.[3] Acute inflammation of the bronchial mucosa as seen in acute rejection may cause submucosal edema and increased vascular resistance to collateral flow, leading to reduction in graft perfusion.[2] The use of more effective immunosuppression regimens and more aggressive rejection surveillance has been associated with decreased rates of airway complications, although it is unclear whether there is a causal relationship.[6] Although contrary to earlier opinion, most transplant centers believe that corticosteroids are not detrimental to proper healing of the anastomosis. Corticosteroids may decrease the formation of anastomotic granulation tissue and concomitantly decrease the incidence of allograft rejection.[2] However, some immunosuppressive agents may worsen the risk of anastomotic injury. For example, severe impairment in postoperative wound healing, including anastomotic dehiscence, has been seen in association with sirolimus, prompting a warning to avoid sirolimus until bronchial anastomotic healing is complete.[7]

Surgical Techniques

Surgical techniques have changed since the first successful lung transplantation almost 30 years ago. The early technique of using an omental wrap to improve anastomotic perfusion has been abandoned. The telescoping bronchus technique that succeeded this approach has, in turn, been replaced by an end-to-end anastomosis in many institutions because of lower anastomotic complications with this surgical method.[3,8] A simple interrupted suture or figure-of-eight suture to accomplish the end-to-end anastomosis is preferred to a mattress suture because the latter has been associated with more complications.[6] Avoiding stretch on the anastomosis and using minimal telescoping for size-discrepant bronchi may be beneficial in decreasing incidence of anastomotic injury.[8] Using a short donor bronchus, within 1 to 2 cartilaginous rings of the upper lobe take-off, in conjunction with a longer native bronchus, may theoretically improve blood supply.[2,8]

Infections

An association between the presence of *Aspergillus* in the airways following transplantation and subsequent occurrence of airway complications has been shown. The incidence of these complications is higher in the presence of *Aspergillus* and necrosis than in the presence of necrosis alone, suggesting an independent and/or synergistic role for *Aspergillus* infection.[9] Additional risks for airway complications include infections with *Pseudomonas* and *Actinomyces*. It is hypothesized that infection with these organisms can cause inflammation, scarring, and compromised blood supply.[10]

Miscellaneous

Factors such as age, weight, height, gender, diagnosis leading to transplantation, cytomegalovirus status, preoperative corticosteroid use, induction therapy, operation time, ischemia time, and prolonged postoperative mechanical ventilation have not consistently been shown to be risk factors for airway complications.[2] However, prolonged donor mechanical ventilation time is suggested to play a role.[11] A larger recipient height may be a risk factor related to a larger bronchial circumference, resulting in donor/recipient bronchial mismatch and possible need for telescoping.[2,12] Additional factors, such as postoperative pneumonia, severe primary graft failure, and the requirement for postoperative hemodialysis, may also be risks for airway complications.[13]

CLASSIFICATION OF AIRWAY HEALING AND COMPLICATIONS

There have been several proposals for classification of airway healing.[14] However, none of these classification systems have been adopted universally. The Couraud grading system (**Box 1**) has been shown to be predictive of subsequent anastomotic complications.[15] This grading system relies on bronchoscopic inspection on the 15th postoperative day and ranges from complete mucosal healing (grade 1) to limited focal necrosis/extensive necrosis (grade 3A/B).

Airway complications may be categorized by their time of occurrence after transplantation: early (<3 months) or late (>3 months). When multiple, complications can occur concomitantly or in a continuum.[2] For example, an initial ischemic injury can cause concurrent necrosis and dehiscence, and subsequent infection or stenosis. The risk of airway complications increases after being treated for a prior complication; up to 35% of patients with an initial complication will experience a second, and 70% of those with 2 episodes will subsequently experience a third or more.[2,8]

There are 6 categories of airway complications (**Fig. 1**; see **Table 1**), which are described in detail later.

Anastomotic Necrosis and Dehiscence

Bronchial necrosis/dehiscence is an ischemic complication that occurs within several weeks of

---

Box 1
Couraud grading system

Grade 1

    Complete circumferential primary mucosal healing

Grade 2A

    Complete circumferential primary healing of the airway wall without necrosis and with partial primary mucosal healing

Grade 2B

    Complete circumferential primary healing of the airway wall without necrosis but with no primary mucosal healing

Grade 3A

    Limited focal necrosis (extending less than 0.5 cm from the anastomotic line)

Grade 3B

    Extensive necrosis

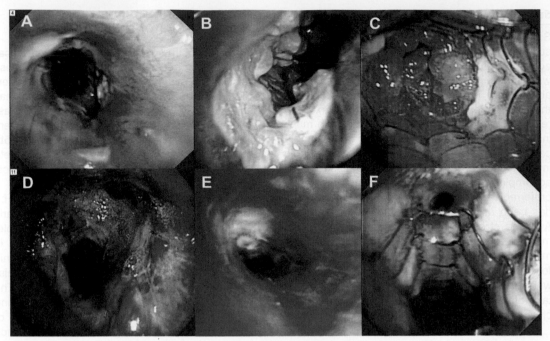

Fig. 1. Types of airway complication. (*A*) Ischemia with scarring, (*B*) necrosis, (*C*) granulation tissue, (*D*) anastomotic stenosis/necrosis, (*E*) nonanastomotic stenosis, (*F*) fistulae.

transplantation. The severity may range from mild focal necrotic sloughing (commonly at the anastomosis site) to perforation of the bronchial wall from extensive necrosis (**Box 2**). Severe complications (grade III and IV) have a high mortality,[9,16,17]

Box 2
Bronchial necrosis/dehiscence grading

Grade I

No slough or necrosis reported. Anastomosis healing well

Monitoring or conservative treatment

Grade II

Any necrotic mucosal slough reported, but no bronchial wall necrosis

Conservative treatment

Grade III

Bronchial wall necrosis within 2 cm of anastomosis

Bronchoscopic treatment

Grade IV

Extensive bronchial wall necrosis extending >2 cm from anastomosis

Bronchoscopic or surgical treatment

---

whereas grade I findings are commonly seen at the anastomosis site and can be managed with conservative management and surveillance bronchoscopy.

Bronchial necrosis or dehiscence may be seen on surveillance bronchoscopy or clinically manifest by dyspnea, failure to wean, or sepsis. Additional clinical features of dehiscence include subcutaneous emphysema, pneumomediastinum, pneumothorax, or persistent air leaks. The chest radiograph (CXR) is often unreliable but computed tomography (CT) can detect bronchial wall defects, bronchial narrowing, irregularities of the airway wall, or extraluminal air around the anastomosis. Several studies have suggested that chest CT has a high sensitivity and specificity for detecting dehiscence but bronchoscopy remains the gold standard.[2]

Bronchial necrosis/dehiscence is associated with the subsequent development of other airway complications. Bronchial stenosis is commonly seen as a late sequela.[18] The necrotic tissue may also create a nidus for subsequent fungal infection with *Aspergillus* or *Candida*. Mechanical debulking of necrotic areas and sloughed mucosa may be needed to treat or prevent infections in severe cases. Fistula formation with the mediastinum, pleura, and vascular structures is another grave complication related to bronchial necrosis. Insertion of thoracostomy tubes may be needed to manage pneumothoraces associated with bronchial dehiscence.

The use of covered metallic stents was unsuccessful in managing dehiscence.[19] More recently, placement of uncovered metallic stent to provoke granulation tissue formation has been successfully used as a means of facilitating healing.[20] After placement of a bare metal stent for a prescribed period of time, the stent should be removed before becoming embedded within the airway by exuberant granulation tissue. Serious airway injuries, including perforation, may occur with delayed removal. Adhesive agents such as fibrin glue and α-cyanoacrylate glue have also been described, but are typically limited in efficacy by the size of the dehiscence.[19,21]

Bronchial Fistulae

Bronchopleural fistula following transplantation is usually encountered in the setting of a bronchial anastomotic dehiscence as described earlier. It may also occur with rupture of a peripheral cavitary pneumonia or abscess. Conservative management with nutrition and chest tube placement may be the initial management strategy while waiting for the fistula to heal and close spontaneously. Bronchoscopic management with fibrin glue or placement of a blood patch may suffice in some cases. The US Food and Drug Administration (FDA) has also approved an endobronchial valve (IBV Valve, Spiration/Olympus Inc, Redmond, WA, USA) as a humanitarian use device in certain postoperative situations, but not yet in the posttransplant setting. This unidirectional valve is placed bronchoscopically and allows air to escape from, but not enter, the airway, providing time for the injury to heal.[22] If conservative management fails, surgical management may be required.

Bronchomediastinal fistulas may present with bacteremia, abscess formation, or cavitation and are often lethal. The inciting cause is often an infection and treatment may therefore include antibiotics. If a single fistula is present, it may be closed bronchoscopically with a stent or adhesive; for more complex fistulae, surgical closure may be necessary.

Bronchovascular fistula development is a rare and often fatal complication with descriptions in case reports and small case series. Hemoptysis is the most common early symptom; air embolism and sepsis have also been reported. Fungal infection of the bronchial anastomosis, with erosion into an adjacent pulmonary artery, is the most common mechanism.[23] Surgical intervention is often required, although this carries a high risk of morbidity and mortality.[24] Surgical treatment of bronchovascular fistulae may involve pneumonectomy in the setting of bilateral lung transplantation, or resection of the fistula with reconstruction of the pulmonary artery and bronchial anastomosis.[25]

Bronchial Stenosis

The most common posttransplant airway complication is bronchial stenosis, which may occur at the bronchial anastomosis or more distally (segmental nonanastomotic bronchial stenosis). A common nonanastomotic site is the bronchus intermedius, which may lead to complete obliteration of the airway, referred to as the vanishing bronchus intermedius syndrome.[2]

Bronchial stenosis is usually identified between 2 and 9 months following transplantation. It may be discovered incidentally during surveillance bronchoscopy or detected when the patient experiences dyspnea, wheezing, cough, or recurrent pneumonia. Detection may be facilitated by monitoring spirometry, with demonstration of suboptimal values typically in an obstructive pattern. Flattening of the expiratory limb of the flow volume is another important clue to the presence of large airway obstruction. Although the CXR may reveal segmental or lobar atelectasis, more sophisticated imaging with spiral, three-dimensional, and multiplanar reconstruction CT is typically more helpful.[2]

Transplant-related bronchial stenosis is usually managed bronchoscopically, with techniques that include balloon bronchoplasty and stenting. Rarely, surgical interventions such as lobectomy, sleeve resection, and retransplantation are used.

Excessive Endoluminal Granulation Tissue

Excessive granulation tissue in the transplanted airway occurs from ischemic injury, infection, or as the result of trauma from treatment of airway complications with balloon dilation, stents, or lasers. Similar to other complications, patients who develop granulation tissue may present with a cough, dyspnea, hypoxemia, or postobstructive pneumonia. Decreasing spirometry may be an early clinical finding. Diagnostic strategies include bronchoscopy and CT scanning.[2]

Bronchomalacia

In contrast with bronchial stenosis and excessive granulation tissue, which cause fixed airway narrowing, bronchomalacia leads to dynamic airway collapse. It is usually seen within 4 months of transplantation and presents with signs and symptoms similar to those of other airway complications, including cough, dyspnea, wheezing, or recurrent infections. Clinically significant malacia is defined as greater than or equal to 50% narrowing of the airway lumen on expiration. The exact mechanism for bronchial malacia is not well understood but it is suspected that the airway wall becomes weakened from an ischemic injury, infection, or the immunosuppression regimen.[18] Malacia may occur at the anastomosis site alone or it may occur beyond the anastomosis and even affect the entire airway. The forced expiratory volume in 1 second (FEV_1), forced expiratory flow (FEF) of 25% to 75%, and peak expiratory flow rates are diminished. Expiratory or dynamic inspiratory-expiratory CT scans are suggestive, whereas bronchoscopy is confirmatory.[2]

INTERVENTIONS FOR AIRWAY COMPLICATIONS
Balloon Bronchoplasty

Bronchoplasty using a high-pressure balloon is often the initial management for a stenotic airway, and can be easily performed under moderate sedation and in an outpatient setting. It is one of the least technically involved procedures with the lowest morbidity and least potential for causing other airway complications. Potential problems include transient hypoxemia from obstructing the transplanted airway, mucosal bleeding, and airway rupture or tearing.[26,27] There have been no deaths reported directly related to balloon bronchoplasty in published series of lung transplant recipients.

There have been mixed reports on the effectiveness of balloon bronchoplasty alone in the management of transplant-related stenosis. This variation in outcome stems from the inherent differences in the extent and severity of the stenotic airway. Mildly stenotic airways are more likely to respond to single or repeat balloon dilation, whereas repeat procedures may be unrealistic for severe stenosis. Stenoses that are focal, circumferential, fibrotic, or webbed have the best outcome from balloon dilation. Other adjunct modalities, such as electrocautery and laser radial incisions, may augment the success of balloon bronchoplasty.[26]

Antiinflammatory and antiproliferative agents such as corticosteroids and mitomycin have been injected locally at the stenosis site.[28] The injections have been performed either alone or before balloon bronchoplasty to control the underlying inflammation and prevent recurrent granulation tissue formation. The data on this technique are minimal and limited to case reports or small case series, with mixed causes for the bronchial stenosis.

Airway Stenting

There are 3 main categories of airway stents, based on the material from which they are made:

silicone, metallic, and hybrid (**Fig. 2**). All 3 have been used for anastomotic stenosis. They splint open the airway mechanically to restore patency, and can offer immediate clinical benefits, including improvement in symptoms and in spirometry.

Silicone stents are the preferred prosthesis in all nonmalignant airway stenoses, including posttransplant anastomotic stenosis. This is largely because silicone stents are easily removed even after a prolonged insertion period. The disadvantages of silicone stents include the need for nebulization therapy for airway clearance and the requirement for placement via rigid bronchoscopy. The largest series of silicone stents for stenosis in a mixed patient population (not limited to lung transplant recipients) reported migration (9.5%), obstruction by secretions (3.6%), and granulation (7.9%) as the most common serious complications.[29] The issue of migration has improved with newer stent designs that include using external studs, hourglass shapes, and Y-configuration to maintain stability. However, mucus plugging is particularly problematic with silicone stents because they have a lower internal/external diameter ratio than metal stents. Nebulizer treatments with hypertonic saline and n-acetyl cysteine (Mucomyst) are commonly prescribed to loosen secretions and facilitate expectoration.[29]

The popularity of metallic stents stems from their ease of placement by flexible bronchoscopy. However, the complications of metallic stents are considerable, including the formation of excessive granulation tissue leading to airway obstruction, erosion of airways, fracture, and excessive mucus production. The excess mucus leads to colonization of the airways with bacteria and fungi. Early exchange of metallic stents before complications occur has been advocated by some investigators with limited success.[30,31] Another major disadvantage of the metallic stents is the difficulty of removal after a prolonged time, especially beyond 3 to 4 weeks.[32] In 2005, the FDA issued a black box warning discouraging the use of metallic airway stents in benign diseases of the airways.

Hybrid stents are typically made of Nitinol and fully covered with polyurethane. Like metallic stents, hybrid stents are easily placed via flexible bronchoscopy. Like silicone stents, hybrid stents are easily removed, even after prolonged periods of implantation. However, one study of 49 stent placements in a non–transplant focused population described complications such as granulation tissue formation (20%) or migration (18%).[30] There have also been reports of hybrid stent fracture, particularly when placed in the tracheal position.

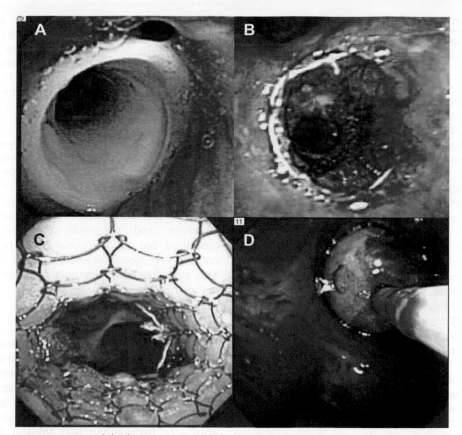

Fig. 2. Airway interventions. (*A*) Silicone stent, (*B*) hybrid stent, (*C*) metallic stent, (*D*) balloon dilation.

Permanent stent placement may not be necessary in many cases of posttransplant anastomotic stenosis. In one series of 22 stents placed for this indication, 18 were successfully removed in approximately 12 months (mean duration 362.3 days, range 185–567 days).[31] The investigators described difficulties with stent removal in diffuse bronchial stenosis, possibly because of a more advanced stage of the disease. The mechanism of resolution of the stenosis is not clear, but is believed to be related to resolution of the initial inflammation and fibrotic stricture in nonmalacic airways. Some stenotic complications have been reported to resolve in as little as 6 months.[3] There is no consensus on when a trial of stent removal should be undertaken. Such a decision should take into account the severity and complexity of the airway stenosis, the technical challenges involved in reinserting a stent should removal prove unsuccessful, and the difficulties (if any) encountered by the patient in maintaining the stent in place.

When malacia involves a focal area like the anastomosis site, airway stenting to maintain patency is often an effective treatment. The preferred stent in patients receiving transplants remains the silicone stent, which allows for removal if stenting does not result in improved pulmonary function and airway clearance and/or if serious complications develop from the stent. The constant dynamic airway movement and irritation around the stent may increase the risk of stent-related complication, including granulation tissue formation and stent migration.[33] There are reports of using metallic stents for malacia in patients receiving lung transplants; however, the use of metallic stents should only be considered after all other therapies have failed, because of their increased risk of complications.[31,32] When there is distal or diffuse malacia, airway stenting may not be feasible because the choke point migrates distally after stent placement.[34] In these cases, continuous positive airway pressure (CPAP) may be an alternative, and acts by creating a pneumatic stent. Surgical resection of the involved airway and retransplantation are additional options that may be considered for severe cases.[35]

Bronchoscopic Ablation of Granulation Tissue

The severity of obstruction by endoluminal granulation tissue formation often dictates the initial treatment. Limited granulation tissue may be easily debulked bronchoscopically with forceps. More severe obstructions may be managed with laser ablation, argon plasma coagulation, electrocautery, cryotherapy, endobronchial brachytherapy, and photodynamic therapy.[36] Airway stents may be placed to maintain patency of the airway; however, stents inherently cause granulation tissue. Granulation tissue recurs following interventions in 10% to 50% of cases.[36] Endobronchial injection of antifibrotic and inflammatory agents has been used to reduce the recurrence rate. There are scant data for the usefulness of these agents; however, there have seldom been complications from such attempts. Mitomycin-C, an antineoplastic agent, at low doses (<1 mg/mL) prevents fibroblast proliferation in vitro and in vivo.[28,37] Topical steroids such as triamcinolone, effective in the treatment of keloids, may also prevent recurrent granulation tissue in the airway.[38,39] The optimal doses for local injections have not been established. Doses of triamcinolone greater than or equal to 20 mg have been shown to decrease serum cortisol levels and should be used sparingly.[40]

In refractory cases of excessive granulation tissue, high-dose brachytherapy may be a consideration.[41–43] Intense intraluminal radiation therapy can be delivered via bronchoscopically placed catheters. Radiation emitted from the catheter (photons released from the ^{192}Ir source) has a limited (1–2 cm) range beyond the bronchus because of the initial energy level. The short-term recurrence rate (<6 months) is low, and long-term response may be optimized by performing a debulking procedure 24 hours before brachytherapy.[42,43]

Management of Airway Infections

Approximately 5% of lung transplant recipients develop fungal infections of the airways, typically following an initial ischemic injury. These infections may be localized to the devitalized bronchial anastomosis or may more diffusely present as bronchitis with pseudomembranes. *Aspergillus* species predominate but *Candida* species may occasionally be responsible. Occurring within the first 6 months after transplantation, these airway infections are usually asymptomatic and detected only by surveillance bronchoscopy. Oral azoles and nebulized amphotericin are usually effective in treating these infections. Rarely, these infections may lead to anastomotic dehiscence or to bronchovascular fistulas and massive hemoptysis.

An increased risk of bronchial stenosis and bronchomalacia has been reported following resolution of these airway infections. To decrease the likelihood of developing fungal superinfection, antifungal prophylaxis is often initiated in patients with significant ischemic damage to the anastomosis or bronchial mucosa.

Surgical Management

Most patients with posttransplant airway complications can be managed bronchoscopically; however, in severe cases, surgical intervention may be necessary. Complex surgical interventions such as bronchial anastomosis repair, sleeve resection, and retransplantation have been described, but are often challenging because of ongoing immunosuppression, medical comorbidities, poor functional status, and adhesions from prior surgery.

SUMMARY

Lung transplantation has improved the survival and quality of life of many patients with advanced lung disease. However, airway complications still present many challenges in the posttransplant period. The treatment of these complications requires expertise and a multidisciplinary approach. Recognizing and treating the posttransplant airway complications can minimize morbidity and maximize the benefits of the transplantation.

REFERENCES

1. Denlinger CE, Meyers BF. Update on lung transplantation for emphysema. Thorac Surg Clin 2009;19: 275–83.
2. Santacruz JF, Mehta AC. Airway complications and management after lung transplantation: ischemia, dehiscence, and stenosis. Proc Am Thorac Soc 2009;6:79–93.
3. Weder W, Inci I, Koram S, et al. Airway complications after lung transplantation: risk factors, prevention and outcome. Eur J Cardiothorac Surg 2009;35: 293–8.
4. Hasegawa T, Iacono AT, Orons PD, et al. Segmental nonanastomotic bronchial stenosis after lung transplantation. Ann Thorac Surg 2000;69:1020–4.
5. Couraud L, Nashef S, Nicolini P, et al. Classification of airway anastomotic healing. Eur J Cardiothorac Surg 1992;6:496–7.
6. Date H, Trulock EP, Arcidi JM, et al. Improved airway healing after lung transplantation. J Thorac Cardiovasc Surg 1995;110:1424–33.
7. Groetzner J, Kur F, Spelsberg F, et al. Airway anastomosis complications in de novo lung

transplantation in sirolimus-based immunosuppression. J Heart Lung Transplant 2004;23(5): 632–8.

8. Murthy SC, Blackstone EH, Gildea TR, et al. Impact of anastomotic complications after lung transplantation. Ann Thorac Surg 2007;84:401–9.

9. Herrera JM, McNeil KD, Higgins RS, et al. Airway complications after lung transplantation: treatment and long-term outcome. Ann Thorac Surg 2001;71: 989–94.

10. Thistlethwaite PA, Yung G, Kemp A, et al. Airway stenosis after lung transplantation: incidence, management and outcome. J Thorac Cardiovasc Surg 2008;136:1569–75.

11. Mordant P, Bonnette P, Puyo P, et al. Advances in lung transplantation for cystic fibrosis that may improve outcome. Eur J Cardiothorac Surg 2010; 38(5):637–43.

12. Van De Wauwer C, Van Raemdonck D, Verleden GM, et al. Risk factors for airway complications within the first year after lung transplantation. Eur J Cardiothorac Surg 2007;31:703–10.

13. Fadel E, de Perrot M, Pierre A. Factors affecting airway complications after lung transplantation: a single-center experience of 460 patients. J Heart Lung Transplant 2008;27(2):S106–7.

14. Chhajed PN, Tamm M, Glanville AR. Role of flexible bronchoscopy in lung transplantation. Semin Respir Crit Care Med 2004;25:413–23.

15. Couraud L, Nashef S, Jougon J. Classification of airway anastomotic healing. Eur J Cardiothorac Surg 1992;6:496–7.

16. Kshettry V, Kroshus T, Hertz M, et al. Early and late airway complications after lung transplantation: incidence and management. Ann Thorac Surg 1997;63: 1576–83.

17. Kirk AJ, Conacher ID, Corris PA, et al. Successful surgical management of bronchial dehiscence after single-lung transplantation. Ann Thorac Surg 1990; 49:147–9.

18. Schafers H, Haydock DA, Cooper J. The prevalence and management of bronchial anastomotic complications in lung transplantation. J Thorac Cardiovasc Surg 1991;101:1044–52.

19. Chhajed P, Malouf M, Tamm M, et al. Interventional bronchoscopy for the management of airway complications following lung transplantation. Chest 2001;120:1894–9.

20. Mughal MM, Gildea TR, Murthy S, et al. Short-term deployment of self-expanding metallic stents facilitates healing of bronchial dehiscence. Am J Respir Crit Care Med 2005;172:768–71.

21. Maloney J, Weigel T, Love R. Endoscopic repair of bronchial dehiscence after lung transplantation. Ann Thorac Surg 2001;72:2109–11.

22. Gillespie CT, Sterman DH, Cerfolio RJ, et al. Endobronchial valve treatment for prolonged air leaks of

the lung: a case series. Ann Thorac Surg 2011; 91(1):270–3.

23. Knight J, Elwing JM, Milstone A. Bronchovascular fistula formation: a rare airway complication after lung transplantation. J Heart Lung Transplant 2008; 27:1179–85.

24. Guth S, Mayer E, Fischer B, et al. Bilobectomy for massive hemoptysis after bilateral lung transplantation. J Thorac Cardiovasc Surg 2001;121: 1194–5.

25. Samano M, Saka J, Caramori M, et al. Fatal bronchovascular fistula after a single lung transplantation: a case report. Clinics 2009;64:1031–3.

26. McArdle J, Gildea T, Mehta A. Balloon bronchoplasty: its indications, benefits, and complications. J Bronchol 2005;12:123–7.

27. Redel-Montero J, Cosano-Povedano A, Munoz-Cabrea L, et al. Endoscopic treatment of main airway disruption. J Bronchol 2005;12:25–7.

28. Erard A, Monnier P, Spiliopoulos A, et al. Mitomycin C for control of recurrent bronchial stenosis: a case report. Chest 2001;120:2103–5.

29. Dumon J, Cavaliere S, Diaz-Jimenez P, et al. Seven year experience with the Dumon prosthesis. J Bronchol 1996;3:6–10.

30. Fernandex-Bussy S, Akindipe O, Kulkarni V, et al. Clinical experience with a removable tracheobronchial stent in the management of airway complications after lung transplantation. J Heart Lung Transplant 2009;28:683–8.

31. Alazemi S, Lunn W, Majid A, et al. Outcomes, healthcare resources use, and cost of endoscopic removal of metallic airway stents. Chest 2010;138:350–6.

32. Noppen M, Stratakos G, D'Haese J, et al. Removal of covered self-expandable metallic airway stents in benign disorders: indications, technique, and outcomes. Chest 2005;127:482–7.

33. Murgu S, Colt H. Complications of silicone stent insertion in patients with expiratory central airway collapse. Ann Thorac Surg 2007;84:1870–7.

34. Miyazawa T, Miyazu Y, Iwamoto Y, et al. Stenting at the flow-limiting segment in tracheobronchial stenosis due to lung cancer. Am J Respir Crit Care Med 2004;169(10):1096–102.

35. Osaki S, Maloney J, Meyer K, et al. Redo lung transplantation for acute and chronic lung allograft failure: long term follow-up in a single center. Eur J Cardiothorac Surg 2008;34:1191–7.

36. Sonett JR, Keenan RJ, Ferson PF, et al. Endobronchial management of benign, malignant, and lung transplantation airway stenoses. Ann Thorac Surg 1995;59:1417–22.

37. Penafiel A, Lee P, Hsu A, et al. Topical mitomycin-C for obstructing endobronchial granuloma. Ann Thorac Surg 2006;82:e22–3.

38. Niwa T, Nakamura A, Kato T, et al. Bronchoscopic intralesional injection of triamcinolone acetonide

treated against bronchial obstruction caused by peanut aspiration. Respir Med 2005;99:645–7.

39. Yotaro I, Yuta M, Ryoichi K, et al. Three cases of airway stenosis caused by granulation successfully treated by bronchoscopic intralesional injection of triamcinolone acetonide. J Jpn Soc Bronch 1999; 21:358–64.

40. Aoyama H, Izawa Y. Effect of intrakeloidal injection of triamcinolone acetonide on serum cortisol level. J Jpn Orthop Assoc 1982;2:847–51.

41. Kennedy A, Sonett J, Orens J, et al. High dose rate brachytherapy to prevent recurrent benign hyperplasia in lung transplant bronchi: theoretical and clinical considerations. J Heart Lung Transplant 2000;19:155–9.

42. Tendulkar R, Fleming P, Reddy C, et al. High-dose-rate endobronchial brachytherapy for recurrent airway obstruction from hyperplastic granulation tissue. Int J Radiat Oncol Biol Phys 2008;70:701–6.

43. Madu C, Machuzak M, Sterman D, et al. High-dose-rate (HDR) brachytherapy for the treatment of benign obstructive endobronchial granulation tissue. Med Img Anal 2006;66:1450–6.

Lung Retransplantation

Steven M. Kawut, MD, MS

KEYWORDS

• Lung transplantation • Retransplantation • Ethics

Lung transplantation is a therapeutic option for patients with advanced lung disease. Early or late graft failure or airway compromise may lead to significant morbidity and mortality after lung transplantation. Although there are no curative medical or surgical interventions for many of these complications, lung retransplantation is one potential therapy. Retransplantation raises many of the same considerations faced in initial transplantation in terms of indications, selection of candidates, surgical approach, and outcomes, but is complicated by short-term or long-term intensive immunosuppression, infection, and technical issues attributable to the previous transplant. Perhaps the most important (and controversial) aspect of retransplantation is whether allocating a second (or third)[1] lung allograft to one patient while potentially depriving another patient of an initial transplant is ethically justifiable.

Until recently, the issues surrounding lung retransplantation were more theoretical than real because so few were performed. However, changes in the method of lung allocation in the United States have increased the frequency of retransplantation and brought many of these controversies to bear on lung transplant allocation committees and transplant centers. Unfortunately, there is no consensus regarding the medically and ethically appropriate retransplant candidate.

FREQUENCY OF LUNG RETRANSPLANTATION

Four hundred and sixty-six (2.4%) of the 19,524 transplants performed from 2000 to 2008 and reported to the International Society for Heart and Lung Transplantation (ISHLT) Registry were retransplants.[2] There has been a statistically significant increase in the number and percentage of lung transplants that were retransplants performed over the years 2000 to 2008 (both $P \le .003$) (**Fig. 1**). During the years 2000 to 2004, 40 or fewer retransplants were performed yearly, whereas 60 to 110 were performed yearly between 2005 and 2008. Similarly, less than 2% of all lung transplants in the ISHLT Registry were retransplants between 2000 and 2004, whereas 2% to 4% of transplants were retransplants between 2005 and 2008. Both the mean yearly number of retransplants (77 vs 32) and the mean yearly proportion of lung transplants that were retransplants (2.9% vs 1.7%) were significantly greater for the years 2005 to 2008 than for the years 2000 to 2004 (both $P = .01$).

Lung retransplantation has become more common particularly in the United States.[3] The number of new retransplant candidates and the proportion of new transplant candidates who were retransplant candidates added to the waiting list each year were unchanged over the years 2000 to 2009 (both $P = .10$; **Fig. 2**A). There were no differences in the mean yearly number of patients listed for retransplantation between 2005 and 2009 compared with those listed between 2000 and 2004 (78 vs 69, respectively; $P = .46$). However, there may have been a slight increase in the mean yearly proportion of newly listed patients who were retransplant candidates in 2005 to 2009 compared with 2000 to 2004, but this was not statistically significant (4.1% vs 3.6%, respectively; $P = .08$). Despite the stability in the rates of listing for retransplantation, both the absolute number of retransplants performed and the percentage of transplants that were retransplants significantly increased between 2000

Pulmonary, Allergy, and Critical Care Division, Department of Medicine, and the Center for Clinical Epidemiology and Biostatistics, University of Pennsylvania School of Medicine, 711 Blockley Hall, 423 Guardian Drive, Philadelphia, PA 19104, USA
E-mail address: kawut@upenn.edu

Clin Chest Med 32 (2011) 367–377
doi:10.1016/j.ccm.2011.02.013

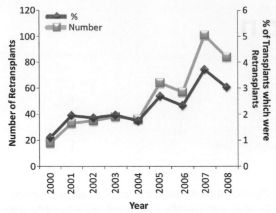

Fig. 1. Adult lung retransplants performed (number and percent of transplants) by year from 2000 to 2008 in the ISHLT Registry ($P = .001$ and $P = .003$ for associations between number and percent with time). (*Data from* Christie JD, Edwards LB, Kucheryavaya AY, et al. The Registry of the International Society for Heart and Lung Transplantation: twenty-seventh official adult lung and heart-lung transplant report–2010. J Heart Lung Transplant 2010;29(10): 1104–18.)

and 2009 (both $P \leq .003$; see **Fig. 2B**). The mean yearly number of retransplants (62 vs 27) and the mean yearly proportion of lung transplants that were retransplants (4.2% vs 2.6%) were significantly greater for the years 2005 to 2008 than for the years 2000 to 2004 (both $P = .01$).

These changes in the frequency of lung retransplantation coincided with (and were likely caused by) the introduction of the Lung Allocation Score (LAS) priority system for lung allocation in May 2005 in the United States (see the article by Eberlein and colleagues elsewhere in this issue for further exploration of this topic). Before the LAS system, lung allografts were allocated by time accrued on the list, in addition to geography, body size, and blood type. The LAS system prioritizes patients based on calculations of estimated 1-year survival with and without lung transplantation, favoring those patients with a combination of high net survival benefit (ie, the difference between survival with and without transplantation) and high medical urgency (ie, low estimated survival without transplantation). Because retransplant candidates, specifically with bronchiolitis obliterans syndrome (BOS), had 1-year wait list survival similar to that of idiopathic pulmonary fibrosis, they were included in group D (restrictive lung diseases) in the LAS calculation and are thereby afforded high priority (see the article by Eberlein and colleagues elsewhere in this issue for further exploration of this topic).[4] Retransplant candidates who would not have remained suitable candidates (or alive) long enough with the previous allocation system can now receive a lung offer in a timely fashion under the LAS system. Indeed, the median wait time for retransplantation was much shorter for patients listed under the LAS system than for those listed before May 2005 (25 days [interquartile range (IQR), 3–66 days] vs 180 days [IQR, 32–569 days] respectively; $P<.001$).[5] Patients listed for retransplantation had median LAS scores within the upper quintile for patients on the active waiting list from 2006 to 2008,

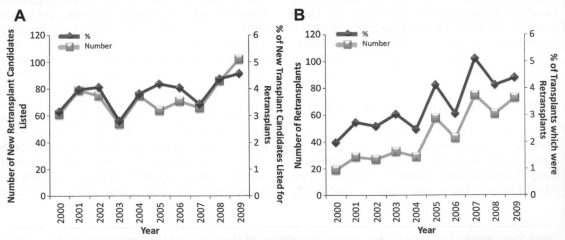

Fig. 2. (*A*) Adult lung retransplantation candidates newly listed (number and percent of candidates) ($P = .10$ for associations between number and percent with time) and (*B*) adult lung retransplants performed (number and percent of total transplants) by year from 2000 to 2009 in the United States ($P<.001$ and $P = .003$ for associations between number and percent with time). (*Data from* OPTN as of December 3, 2010. Available at: http://optn. transplant.hrsa.gov.)

explaining the shortened wait times and increase in retransplantation in the United States.[6]

SELECTION OF CANDIDATES

Lung retransplantation may be indicated for lung transplant recipients with severe lung allograft dysfunction which is not amenable to medical or other surgical therapies. The selection criteria for lung retransplantation are similar to those for initial lung transplantation.[7] Absolute contraindications include recent nondermatologic malignancy; untreatable advanced disease of another main organ system; noncurable chronic extrapulmonary infection, including chronic active viral hepatitis B, hepatitis C, and human immunodeficiency virus; significant chest wall/spinal deformity; documented medical nonadherence; untreatable psychiatric condition associated with the inability to cooperate or comply with medical therapy; lack of a consistent or reliable social support system; and active or recent substance addiction. Relative contraindications include older age; unstable clinical status; severely limited functional status; colonization with highly resistant or highly virulent bacteria, fungi, or mycobacteria; obesity; severe or symptomatic osteoporosis; mechanical ventilation; and inadequately treated other medical conditions. Although there are no defined criteria for when lung transplant recipients should be considered for retransplantation, most patients retransplanted in recent years were 1 or more years out from their initial transplant (median 3.1 years; IQR, 1.0–6.5).[5] Key factors that affect outcomes after retransplantation include the indication (in terms of type and timing of allograft failure) and the requirement for mechanical ventilation (see later discussion), so that these factors must figure into the decision to evaluate or list someone for retransplantation. The most common indication for both listing and performance of lung retransplantation in the United States during the past decade was BOS (**Table 1**). A total of 20% of retransplants were performed for primary graft dysfunction (PGD) or acute rejection.

TYPE OF PROCEDURE

There are several operative approaches to the retransplant candidate. Patients who have undergone initial bilateral lung transplant may receive either a single or bilateral lung retransplant.[5] Patients who have undergone initial single lung transplantation may undergo ipsilateral or contralateral single lung retransplantation or a bilateral lung retransplantation.

The decision regarding which type of retransplantation to perform is based on a variety of

Table 1
Indications for listing and transplanting lung retransplant candidates in the United States between 2000 and 2009

	New Lung Retransplant Candidates Listed (N = 733)		Lung Retransplant Recipients (N = 447)	
BOS	462	63%	292	65%
Primary graft dysfunction	110	15%	77	17%
Acute rejection	28	4%	14	3%
Other	133	18%	64	14%

Data from OPTN as of December 3, 2010. Available at: http://optn.transplant.hrsa.gov/.

factors. The presence of suppurative infection in the initial allograft (or remaining native lung) warrants explantation and replacement to prevent early infectious complications in the new allograft. Even if not infected, it may still be advantageous to explant the failed allograft that could be a source of ongoing immune stimulation,[8] although most recent retransplantation procedures in the United States leave the allograft behind while having better outcomes than historical retransplant procedures.[5] Technical issues relating to the choice of single lung transplantation for the initial transplant (contralateral chest wall deformity or pleural disease) might dictate the need for ipsilateral single lung retransplantation. Over time, single-single (ipsilateral) retransplant procedures have become less common and bilateral-single retransplant procedures have become more common, likely reflecting the increasing frequency of initial bilateral lung transplantation.[5] Although unadjusted analyses suggest that ipsilateral single lung retransplantation may be associated with a higher risk of death (and contralateral single lung retransplantation associated with a lower risk of death), these findings were not significant predictors of outcome after adjustment for other covariates and were likely confounded by factors, such as indication and timing of retransplantation.[5]

OUTCOMES

The risk of death on the waiting list for patients listed for lung retransplantation in the United States is double or triple that of patients listed for initial lung transplantation.[6] The mean annual death rate on the list for lung retransplant candidates was 295.6 per 1000 person-years for 2005 to 2008, whereas it was 118.2 per 1000 person-years for all lung transplant candidates.

Only a handful of small studies of the risk factors and outcomes in lung retransplantation have been published. A prospective multicenter registry enrolled 230 retransplant recipients from 47 centers between 1985 and 1996.[9–14] Twenty-six centers were located in North America, 20 in Europe, and 1 in Australia. The final publication from this study showed a 1-year survival of 47% and 3-year survival of 33%.[14] A total of 63% of patients were retransplanted for BOS. Patients who were either nonambulatory or dependent on mechanical ventilation had a significantly increased risk of death. Retransplantation performed before 1992 was also associated with a higher mortality compared with retransplant performed after that date. Patients without these risk factors had outcomes similar to those of patients undergoing initial lung transplantation. Although rates of BOS after retransplantation overall were similar to those reported after initial transplantation, those retransplanted less than 2 years after their initial transplant had a significantly higher risk of BOS at 2 years, and those retransplanted for BOS demonstrated a more rapid postretransplant decline in forced expiratory volume in 1 second than those retransplanted for other indications. The identification of retransplant patients with outcomes similar to those of initial transplant recipients was suggested to justify retransplantation as a viable and ethical option for certain lung transplant recipients with failing allografts. The limitations in this study are its voluntary registry design and the historical nature of the data.

Brugiere and colleagues[15] presented 15 patients who underwent lung retransplantation for BOS at their center between 1988 and 2002. The 1-year and 5-year survival was 60% and 45%, respectively, outcomes similar to those of initial single lung transplantation at the investigators' center. The median time between initial transplantation and retransplantation was 31 months (range, 12–39 months). All were clinically stable at the time of retransplantation, although 6 required tracheostomy and mechanical ventilation and 6 were not ambulatory. All patients underwent single lung retransplantation (4 ipsilateral, 9 contralateral, and 2 after initial bilateral lung transplantation). The retained allograft was the source of fatal infection in 4 of the recipients. Such infections related to the allograft always occurred in the presence of suppuration, even though bronchiectasis was minimal or absent at relisting for transplant, leading the investigators to propose explantation of the initial allograft whenever possible during retransplantation.

Schafers and colleagues[16] published a cohort of 14 patients who underwent lung retransplantation at their center from 1987 to 1994. One-year and 2-year survival was 77% and 64%, respectively, which was somewhat lower than initial transplantation at this center. These investigators found that preoperative mechanical ventilation was associated with significantly more days in the intensive care unit (61 days vs 13 days; $P<.05$) as was early retransplantation (<90 days from initial transplant) (72 days vs 16 days; $P<.05$). These factors may also have been associated with higher early mortality. The risk of BOS with retransplantation was also higher than that with initial transplant.

Osaki and colleagues[17] published a cohort of 17 patients who underwent lung retransplantation (2 of whom underwent retransplantation twice). One-year and 5-year survival was 59% and 42%, respectively, outcomes that were significantly worse than those with initial transplant at their center. The 1-year and 5-year survival rates for the patients retransplanted for BOS (N = 12) were 67% and 44%, respectively. The need for mechanical ventilation (or extracorporeal life support) appeared to be associated with an increased risk of death ($P = .09$); however, the presence of a retained allograft was not ($P = .31$).

Investigators from the Hannover Thoracic Transplant Program recently published a cohort of 54 consecutive patients who underwent lung retransplantation before January 1, 2004.[18] A total of 37 patients were retransplanted for BOS, 10 for PGD, and 7 for airway complications (5 with severe dehiscence and 2 with airway scarring). Survival in those patients retransplanted for BOS mirrored that of patients undergoing initial transplantation from this center (**Fig. 3**). However, the patients with PGD and airway complications had

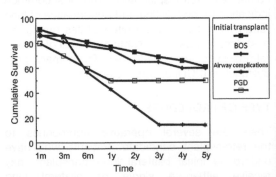

Fig. 3. Survival of lung retransplant recipients (by indication) and initial lung transplant recipients before January 2004 ($P = .001$ for PGD and airway complications vs BOS and initial transplant). (*Adapted from* Strueber M, Fischer S, Gottlieb J, et al. Long-term outcome after pulmonary retransplantation. J Thorac Cardiovasc Surg 2006;132(2):407–12; with permission.)

a significantly worse survival, leading the investigators to avoid retransplantation for these indications in the latter portion of the study period and, potentially, to confounding by time.

Aigner and colleagues[19] published data from 46 patients who underwent lung retransplantation between 1995 and 2006 in Vienna. They found that patients retransplanted for BOS (N = 19) had 1-year and 5-year survival of 72.5% and 61.3%, respectively, which was significantly better than the survival of patients retransplanted for PGD (N = 23; **Fig. 4**). These estimates did not account for 3 patients who required re-retransplantation. There appeared to be improvement in outcomes over time with retransplant recipients from 2002 to 2006 having better survival than recipients from 1995 to 2001.

The largest retrospective cohort study of lung retransplantation compared modern lung retransplantation to both modern initial lung transplantation and to historical retransplantation in 79 centers in the United States.[5] Patients in the modern retransplant cohort received a first lung retransplantation between January 2001 and May 2006 (N = 205; **Table 2**). Patients who underwent initial lung transplant during this time period were included in the modern initial transplant cohort (N = 5657). Patients who underwent a first lung retransplant between January 1990 and

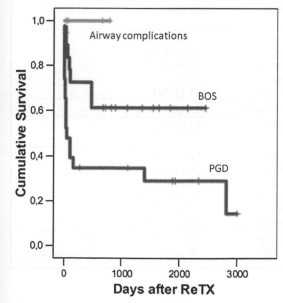

Fig. 4. Survival after lung retransplantation between 1995 and 2006 (*P* = .02 for PGD vs BOS, other differences were not significant). (*Adapted from* Aigner C, Jaksch P, Taghavi S, et al. Pulmonary retransplantation: is it worth the effort? A long-term analysis of 46 cases. J Heart Lung Transplant 2008;27(1):60–5; with permission.)

December 2000 comprised the historical retransplant cohort (N = 184). The modern retransplant cohort was significantly older than the historical retransplant cohort but younger than the modern initial transplant cohort (see **Table 2**). Most of the patients in the 3 cohorts had either chronic obstructive pulmonary disease or diffuse parenchymal lung disease as the indication for initial lung transplantation. These diagnoses were less frequent in the modern retransplant patients than in the initial transplant patients, and pulmonary arterial hypertension and cystic fibrosis/bronchiectasis were more frequent. Hypertension, renal failure, and corticosteroid use were significantly more common in the modern retransplant cohort than in the modern initial transplant cohort, and diabetes mellitus was more common in the modern retransplant cohort than both of the other cohorts.

Modern and historical retransplant patients were more likely to require mechanical ventilation at the time of transplant than were initial transplant recipients, and more than half of the modern and historical retransplant procedures were performed for BOS. Half of the modern retransplant patients received initial bilateral lung or heart-lung transplantation, and most of these patients went on to receive bilateral lung retransplantation. Modern retransplant patients more often underwent single lung retransplantation after initial bilateral lung transplant than did historical retransplant patients and less frequently underwent ipsilateral single lung retransplantation.

Survival estimates at 1 and 5 years after modern lung retransplantation were 62% and 45%, respectively (**Fig. 5**). Patients undergoing modern lung retransplantation had a significantly lower risk of death after the procedure than that of the historical retransplant cohort, independent of recipient and donor variables, pulmonary diagnosis, and mechanical ventilation at the time of transplant (**Fig. 6**, **Table 3**). On the other hand, patients undergoing modern lung retransplantation still had a 30% higher risk than that of patients undergoing modern initial transplantation (bivariate model, see **Table 3**). Adjustment for recipient and surgical factors attenuated the effect estimates, indicating that differences in these factors explained some, but not all, of the increased risk associated with retransplantation (multivariate models 1 and 2, see **Table 3**). Further adjustment for the presence of renal failure reduced the hazard ratio even further, showing that kidney disease accounted for much of the increased risk of death seen in the retransplantation recipients when compared with initial transplant patients (multivariate model 3, see **Table 3**). Retransplant

Table 2
Recipient and procedure characteristics of modern retransplant recipients (2001–2006), historical retransplant recipients (1990–2000), and modern initial transplant recipients (2001–2006) in the United States

Characteristic	Modern Retransplant (N = 205)	Historical Retransplant (N = 184)	Modern Initial Transplant (N = 5657)
Age, y	43 ± 16	39 ± 17[a]	50 ± 14[b]
Gender, female	109 (53%)	103 (56%)	2721 (48%)
Race/ethnicity			
Non-Hispanic white	182 (89%)	169 (92%)	4935 (87%)
Black	13 (6%)	12 (6%)	414 (7%)
Other	10 (5%)	3 (2%)	308 (5%)
Body mass index, kg/m^2	22 ± 5 (N = 202)	22 ± 6 (N = 172)	24 ± 5[b] (N = 5456)
Initial diagnosis			
Chronic obstructive pulmonary disease	66 (32%)	70 (38%)	2505 (44%)
Diffuse parenchymal lung disease	52 (25%)	32 (17%)	1690 (30%)
Pulmonary arterial hypertension	24 (12%)	28 (15%) [b]	240 (4%) [a]
Cystic fibrosis/bronchiectasis	53 (26%)	33 (18%)	977 (17%)
Other	10 (5%)	21 (11%)	245 (4%)
Diabetes mellitus	74 (36%)	22 (17%)[b] (N = 128)	608 (11%)[b] (N = 5595)
Hypertension	80 (40%) (N = 199)	45 (36%) (N = 125)	993 (18%)[b] (N = 5540)
Renal failure	72 (36%) (N = 200)	56 (30%) (N = 133)	486 (9%)[b] (N = 5583)
Corticosteroid use	151 (79%) (N = 191)	106 (82%) (N = 129)	1881 (35%)[b] (N = 5425)
Mechanical ventilation at time of transplant procedure	40 (20%)	45 (25%)	145 (3%)[b]
Indication for retransplantation			
Bronchiolitis obliterans syndrome	107 (52%)	103 (56%)	—
Primary graft dysfunction	32 (16%)	16 (9%)	—
Acute rejection	7 (3%)	4 (2%)	—
Other or unknown	59 (27%)	61 (33%)	—
Median time from initial transplant, y	3.1 (1.0–6.5)	1.9 (0.5–3.1)[a]	—
Early retransplant (<30 d from initial transplant)	22 (11%)	31 (17%)	—
Procedure type (initial-retransplant)	(N = 201)	(N = 173)	—
Bilateral-bilateral (en bloc included)	67 (33%)	56 (32%)	—
Bilateral-single	41 (20%)	13 (8%) [a]	—
Single-bilateral	31 (15%)	30 (17%)	—
Single-single (ipsilateral)	9 (4%)	33 (19%)	—
Single-single (contralateral)	53 (26%)	41 (24%)	—
Ischemic time, h	5.2 ± 1.9 (N = 182)	5.0 ± 1.8 (N = 157)	4.8 ± 1.7[c] (N = 4934)

Abbreviation: SD, standard deviation.
Data are mean +/− SD, median (interquartile range), or N (%).
[a] $P<.001$ versus modern retransplant.
[b] $P<.01$ versus modern retransplant.
[c] $P<.05$ versus modern retransplant.
Data from Kawut SM, Lederer DJ, Keshavjee S, et al. Outcomes after lung retransplantation in the modern era. Am J Respir Crit Care Med 2008;177(1):114–20; with permission.

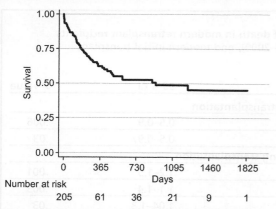

Fig. 5. Kaplan-Meier survival estimate of lung retransplant recipients in the United States from 2001 to 2006. (*From* Kawut SM, Lederer DJ, Keshavjee S, et al. Outcomes after lung retransplantation in the modern era. Am J Respir Crit Care Med 2008;177(1):114–20, Official Journal of the American Thoracic Society, Diane Gern, Publisher; with permission.)

patients had twice the risk of BOS as initial transplant patients (95% confidence interval [CI] 1.4–3.0; *P*<.001).

Although mechanical ventilation at the time of retransplantation and early retransplantation (<30 days from the initial transplant) were both significantly associated with an increased risk of death in unadjusted analyses in the modern retransplant cohort (**Table 4**), only early retransplantation and

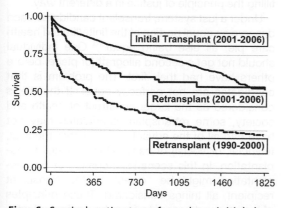

Fig. 6. Survival estimates of modern initial lung transplantation (2001–2006), modern lung retransplantation (2001–2006), and historical lung retransplantation (1990–2000) recipients after adjustment for age (55 years), sex (female), race/ethnicity (non-Hispanic white), procedure type (bilateral), mechanical ventilation (none), and pulmonary diagnosis (chronic obstructive pulmonary disease) (*P*<.05 for all comparisons). (*From* Kawut SM, Lederer DJ, Keshavjee S, et al. Outcomes after lung retransplantation in the modern era. Am J Respir Crit Care Med 2008;177(1):114–20, Official Journal of the American Thoracic Society, Diane Gern, Publisher; with permission.)

male donor gender were independently associated with an increased risk of death. The 1-year survival for the 22 patients who underwent early retransplantation was only 31%, whereas it was 66% for the others.

This study showed that outcomes after lung retransplantation in the United States have improved over time; however, survival after lung retransplantation was still not as good as that after initial lung transplantation. Based on the multivariate analyses, these differences seemed attributable to a higher prevalence of renal failure and other recipient characteristics. The presence of renal failure in retransplant recipients is likely attributable to long-standing use of calcineurin inhibitors and has been associated with poor outcomes in nonrenal solid-organ transplant recipients.[20] Renal failure is associated with a variety of medical comorbidities that could shorten survival. Alternatively, the presence of renal failure may just serve as a surrogate marker for either the duration and intensity of calcineurin inhibitor-based immunosuppression or the degree of disease of the microcirculation in other organs leading to higher risk after retransplantation.

Early retransplantation independently conferred a high risk for a poor outcome in the modern retransplant cohort. Mechanical ventilation was also associated with an increased risk of death. After adjusting for timing of retransplantation, however, mechanical ventilation was no longer associated with mortality. Therefore, mechanical ventilation may not be a risk factor for patients who are farther out from the initial transplant (eg, with BOS).

In summary, the 1-year and 5-year survival estimates for retransplantation in the modern era are approximately 60% to 80% and 45% to 65%, respectively. Retransplantation for BOS leads to survival estimates in the upper portions of these ranges. Early retransplantation (eg, for PGD) results in poor outcomes, whereas selected patients receiving mechanical ventilation farther out from initial transplant may do well. There is an increased risk of BOS after retransplantation, which may explain the worse outcomes compared with initial transplant, but recipient characteristics and specifically renal failure may also contribute to poor outcomes.

IS RETRANSPLANTATION ETHICALLY JUSTIFIED?

Although the indications, selection criteria, and outcomes for retransplantation are reasonably straightforward, the ethical justification for retransplantation is less so in the setting of scarce organs.

Table 3
Proportional hazards models comparing the risks of death in modern retransplant recipients (2001–2006), historical retransplant recipients (1990–2000), and modern initial transplant recipients (2001–2006) in the United States

	Hazard Ratio	95% CI	*P* value
Modern lung retransplantation vs historical lung retransplantation			
Bivariate	0.7	0.5–0.9	.006
Multivariate[a]	0.7	0.5–0.97	.03
Modern lung retransplantation vs modern initial lung transplantation			
Bivariate	1.3	1.2–1.5	.001
Multivariate model 1[b]	1.2	1.1–1.4	.003
Multivariate model 2[c]	1.2	1.04–1.3	.03
Multivariate model 3[d]	1.1	1.0–1.3	.11

Abbreviation: CI, confidence interval.
  [a] Adjusted for recipient age, gender, race/ethnicity, initial diagnosis, single/bilateral retransplantation, indication for retransplantation, ischemic time, mechanical ventilation, donor age, race, and mode of death, early retransplantation, diabetes mellitus, and renal failure.
  [b] Adjusted for recipient age, gender, race/ethnicity, body mass index, initial diagnosis, single/bilateral transplantation, ischemic time, and mechanical ventilation.
  [c] Model 1 + adjustment for hypertension, diabetes mellitus, corticosteroid use.
  [d] Model 2 + adjustment for renal failure.
  Data from Kawut SM, Lederer DJ, Keshavjee S, et al. Outcomes after lung retransplantation in the modern era. Am J Respir Crit Care Med 2008;177:114–20.

Because organ donation comes from the deceased and their families and "donated organs belong to the community,"[21,22] the populace views regarding retransplantation are therefore important to consider. A recent systematic review summarized 15 studies eliciting community preferences for organ allocation.[23] Sixty percent or more of respondents preferred allocating organs to initial transplant candidates rather than to retransplant candidates. However, some thought that those who had already received a transplant that failed for medical reasons might have proved themselves able to care for the transplant, warranting priority for another allograft. The vast majority of respondents preferred allocating organs to those with the best chance at survival and improved quality of life with transplant, making these guiding principles for retransplantation.

Several investigators have directly addressed the ethics of solid-organ retransplantation.[24–27] The principle of justice mandates there be equity in distribution of benefits and harms among transplant candidates; however, a rational planner could either discount or favor retransplantation under this principle. For example, it would be rational for an individual (unaware of the future) to prefer a system where the maximal number of people get the opportunity for initial transplantation, rather than one where some undergo retransplantation before others get an initial transplant. In a different scenario, allocating a second organ to a particular patient who has already proven themselves capable of adhering to the complicated medical regimen might increase the chance of success of that transplant and provide greater overall benefit to the population of transplant candidates, still fulfilling the principle of justice in a different way.

Under a just system, transplant candidates each deserve an equal portion of the finite/limited health care pie, all else being equal.[26] One individual should not get a second allograft (or piece) before others have had their first. The problem is that candidates are not perfectly equal. If the pie is considered as the larger construct of health and society, some retransplant candidates may not have had all of the advantages (whether medical, financial, or social) of candidates for initial transplantation. In this scenario, a chance at retransplantation might be "owed" to the transplant recipient, all things considered. These principles of justice would seem to favor lung retransplantation in certain instances, but by themselves are not sufficient to justify retransplant.

Maximizing efficacy (or utilitarianism) refers to the goal of increasing total benefits to transplant candidates overall by targeted organ allocation to those most likely to benefit. Utilitarianism would mandate that initial transplantation be prioritized over retransplantation, because retransplant recipients generally demonstrate a worse survival.[28] Even with initial transplantation, patients with some diagnoses (eg, pulmonary hypertension or

Table 4
Association of recipient and donor characteristics with the risk of death in modern lung retransplant recipients (2001–2006) in the United States

Variable	Hazard Ratio	95% CI	*P* value
Bivariate models			
Recipient			
Age (per 10-y increment)	0.9	0.8–1.1	.45
Male gender	1.4	0.8–2.2	.23
Race/ethnicity: others vs non-Hispanic white	1.6	0.8–3.2	.21
Body mass index (per 5-unit increment)	1.0	0.9–1.0	.92
Initial diagnosis (vs chronic obstructive pulmonary disease)			
Diffuse parenchymal lung disease	1.5	0.7–2.8	.27
Cystic fibrosis/Bronchiectasis	1.3	0.7–2.5	.43
Pulmonary arterial hypertension	1.2	0.6–2.5	.67
Renal failure	1.3	0.8–2.2	.30
Mechanical ventilation at the time of retransplantation	2.0	1.1–3.4	.02
Indication for retransplantation (vs BOS)			
Primary graft dysfunction	1.1	0.6–2.1	.72
Acute rejection	1.2	0.4–3.8	.81
Other or unknown	0.9	0.5–1.7	.80
Donor			
Age (per 10-y increment)	1.1	0.9–1.3	.26
Male gender	1.7	1.0–3.0	.04
Procedure			
Early retransplant (<30 d from initial transplant)	2.6	1.4–4.9	.003
Procedure type (initial-retransplant) (vs bilateral-bilateral)			
Bilateral-single	0.9	0.4–1.7	.71
Single-bilateral	1.1	0.6–2.2	.74
Single-single (ipsilateral)	2.3	0.9–6.1	.09
Single-single (contralateral)	0.5	0.2–1.0	.05
Ischemic time (per 1-h increment)	1.1	0.9–1.2	.44
Multivariate model			
Early retransplant (<30 d from initial transplant)	2.8	1.5–5.4	.001
Donor male gender	1.9	1.1–3.2	.02

Data from Kawut SM, Lederer DJ, Keshavjee S, et al. Outcomes after lung retransplantation in the modern era. Am J Respir Crit Care Med 2008;177:114–20.

sarcoid) have poorer outcomes than patients with other diagnoses (eg, cystic fibrosis and chronic obstructive pulmonary disease). Full pursuit of a utilitarian approach could dictate that all lung allografts be used for those with the best post-transplant survival (or the maximal net benefit), potentially eliminating patients with certain lung disease diagnoses (or requiring retransplant) from candidacy. This approach of course would appear inequitable and unpalatable for initial transplant, and the lung transplant community has already factored efficacy differences into the allocation system to balance utilitarianism with justice and urgency (eg, the appeal process for severely ill

patients with pulmonary hypertension), suggesting that neither the community nor policymakers are fully at ease with a utilitarian priority system that sacrifices egalitarianism.[26] Because retransplantation has similar or better outcomes than initial transplant in certain cases, a utilitarian approach seemingly justifies the allocation of allografts for lung retransplantation in such instances.

Prioritarianism favors the worst off[28,29] and directs the allocation of organs to the sickest first, no matter what the outcomes. This approach is not justifiable for either initial transplant or retransplantation in the setting of scarce allograft resources, as efficacy would be significantly compromised and it only considers the sickest at the current time and neglects others who may progress. Similarly, transplant physicians and surgeons may understandably feel bound to prioritize for retransplantation patients whom they have transplanted and cared for (often for years), appropriately regarding the interests of their own patients as paramount.[30,31] However, it is not only acceptable to prioritize the needs of other patients over ones own patients when considering retransplantation (just as with initial transplantation or other scenarios requiring triage or rescue), but the exceptions are also frequent enough that some have suggested professional guidelines for such situations.[30]

A youngest-first strategy (where organs for retransplantation of a significantly younger individual could be prioritized over the initial transplant of an older individual) might be justifiable, beyond the impact of age on urgency or benefit. Public preference strongly supports the allocation of scarce life-saving interventions to younger individuals.[23,28,32] "Because [all people] age, treating people of different ages differently does not mean that we are treating persons unequally."[28,33] Although possibly viewed as ageism, all 66 year olds were once 25 years old and had they needed a lung retransplantation would have had an advantage extended to them under such a system, therefore providing equal opportunity.

In the United States, urgency and efficacy (in terms of net survival benefit at 1 year) determine priority of lung offers within the constraints of geography, compatible blood type, and body size. The policy of the United Network for Organ Sharing is to enhance the overall availability of allografts, balance medical utility (net benefit to all transplant patients as a group) and justice (equity in distribution of benefits and burdens among transplant patients), provide organ offers within comparable time periods for patients depending on their circumstances, and respect the autonomy of persons.[21] Accordingly, retransplantation would (and should) be prioritized lower than many, but not all, initial transplants, but appears ethically justifiable by the same principles that guide all organ allocation.

A key element to the fair allocation of organs for retransplantation lies in the accuracy of the metric of net benefit used to distribute organs. The LAS system is based on survival at 1 year; whether this is the best measure of benefit is controversial. Also, the LAS system did not derive a prediction model specifically for retransplant candidates because of the small population. Therefore, the LAS scores assigned to retransplant candidates are derived from models based on patients with idiopathic pulmonary fibrosis.[4] If the efficacy of lung retransplantation is overestimated by the model, the recent increase in retransplantation procedures under the LAS could be unjustified and jeopardize the ethical stance of lung allocation for retransplantation. For example, 10% of recent LAS scores for retransplant candidates overestimated posttransplant survival by greater than or equal to 231 days and 10% underestimated survival greater than or equal to 83 days, demonstrating somewhat greater variability than for transplant candidates overall.[6] To maintain the appropriate and ethical prioritization of organs for retransplantation in the United States, there should be focused efforts on refining the net benefit calculus for this group, lest misclassification or a spuriously high or low calculated priority threaten just allocation of lung allografts.

In summary, there is a growing number of lung allografts used for retransplantation and a greater percentage of lung transplants that are retransplantations, even though the absolute numbers remain small. The criteria for retransplantation are similar to those for initial transplant, but the optimal technical approach is not clear. Survival after lung retransplantation has improved over time, although it is still worse than after initial transplant. Retransplantation early after initial transplant continues to pose a prohibitive risk and should be avoided. Retransplant is ethically justified; however, prioritization of lung allografts for both initial transplant and retransplantation needs to be guided by the principles of justice and efficacy and must be based on accurate estimates of net benefit. Future efforts should focus on understanding the mechanisms of the increased risk of BOS and higher mortality after retransplantation, honing the selection of optimal candidates and technical approach, and refining the ethical allocation of organs for this procedure.

ACKNOWLEDGMENTS

The author thanks Scott D. Halpern, MD, PhD, MBE for his insightful comments after review of this manuscript. This work was supported in part by Health Resources and Services Administration contract 234-2005-37011C. The content is the responsibility of the author alone and does not necessarily reflect the views or policies of the Department of Health and Human Services, nor does mention of trade names, commercial products, or organizations imply endorsement by the US Government.

REFERENCES

1. Vakil N, Mason DP, Yun JJ, et al. Third-time lung transplantation in a patient with cystic fibrosis. J Thorac Cardiovasc Surg 2011;141(1):e3–5.

2. Christie JD, Edwards LB, Kucheryavaya AY, et al. The Registry of the International Society for Heart and Lung Transplantation: twenty-seventh official adult lung and heart-lung transplant report–2010. J Heart Lung Transplant 2010;29(10): 1104–18.

3. Data from OPTN as of December 3, 2010. Available at: http://optn.transplant.hrsa.gov. Accessed December 3, 2010.

4. Egan TM, Murray S, Bustami RT, et al. Development of the new lung allocation system in the United States. Am J Transplant 2006;6(5 Pt 2):1212–27.

5. Kawut SM, Lederer DJ, Keshavjee S, et al. Outcomes after lung retransplantation in the modern era. Am J Respir Crit Care Med 2008;177(1):114–20.

6. 2009 Annual Report of the U.S. Organ Procurement and Transplantation Network and the Scientific Registry of Transplant Recipients: transplant data 1999–2008. Rockville (MD): U.S. Department of Health and Human Services, Health Resources and Services Administration, Healthcare Systems Bureau, Division of Transplantation; 2009.

7. Orens JB, Estenne M, Arcasoy S, et al. International guidelines for the selection of lung transplant candidates: 2006 update–a consensus report from the Pulmonary Scientific Council of the International Society for Heart and Lung Transplantation. J Heart Lung Transplant 2006;25(7):745–55.

8. Keshavjee S. Retransplantation of the lung comes of age. J Thorac Cardiovasc Surg 2006;132(2):226–8.

9. Novick RJ, Andreassian B, Schafers HJ, et al. Pulmonary retransplantation for obliterative bronchiolitis. Intermediate-term results of a North American-European series. J Thorac Cardiovasc Surg 1994;107(3):755–63.

10. Novick RJ, Kaye MP, Patterson GA, et al. Redo lung transplantation: a North American-European experience. J Heart Lung Transplant 1993;12(1 Pt 1):5–15 [discussion: 15–6].

11. Novick RJ, Schafers HJ, Stitt L, et al. Recurrence of obliterative bronchiolitis and determinants of outcome in 139 pulmonary retransplant recipients. J Thorac Cardiovasc Surg 1995;110(5):1402–13 [discussion: 1413–4].

12. Novick RJ, Schafers HJ, Stitt L, et al. Seventy-two pulmonary retransplantations for obliterative bronchiolitis: predictors of survival. Ann Thorac Surg 1995;60(1):111–6.

13. Novick RJ, Stitt L, Schafers HJ, et al. Pulmonary retransplantation: does the indication for operation influence postoperative lung function? J Thorac Cardiovasc Surg 1996;112(6):1504–13 [discussion: 1513–4].

14. Novick RJ, Stitt LW, Al-Kattan K, et al. Pulmonary retransplantation: predictors of graft function and survival in 230 patients. Pulmonary Retransplant Registry. Ann Thorac Surg 1998;65(1):227–34.

15. Brugiere O, Thabut G, Castier Y, et al. Lung retransplantation for bronchiolitis obliterans syndrome: long-term follow-up in a series of 15 recipients. Chest 2003;123(6):1832–7.

16. Schafers HJ, Hausen B, Wahlers T, et al. Retransplantation of the lung. A single center experience. Eur J Cardiothorac Surg 1995;9(6):291–5 [discussion: 296].

17. Osaki S, Maloney JD, Meyer KC, et al. Redo lung transplantation for acute and chronic lung allograft failure: long-term follow-up in a single center. Eur J Cardiothorac Surg 2008;34(6):1191–7.

18. Strueber M, Fischer S, Gottlieb J, et al. Long-term outcome after pulmonary retransplantation. J Thorac Cardiovasc Surg 2006;132(2):407–12.

19. Aigner C, Jaksch P, Taghavi S, et al. Pulmonary retransplantation: is it worth the effort? A long-term analysis of 46 cases. J Heart Lung Transplant 2008;27(1):60–5.

20. Ojo AO, Held PJ, Port FK, et al. Chronic renal failure after transplantation of a nonrenal organ. N Engl J Med 2003;349(10):931–40.

21. Egan TM. Ethical issues in thoracic organ distribution for transplant. Am J Transplant 2003;3(4):366–72.

22. Childress JF. The gift of life: ethical issues in organ transplantation. Bull Am Coll Surg 1996;81(3):8–22.

23. Tong A, Howard K, Jan S, et al. Community preferences for the allocation of solid organs for transplantation: a systematic review. Transplantation 2010; 89(7):796–805.

24. Mentzer SJ, Reilly JJ Jr, Caplan AL, et al. Ethical considerations in lung retransplantation. J Heart Lung Transplant 1994;13(1 Pt 1):56–8.

25. Novick RJ. Heart and lung retransplantation: should it be done? J Heart Lung Transplant 1998;17(6):635–42.

26. Ubel PA, Arnold RM, Caplan AL. Rationing failure. The ethical lessons of the retransplantation of scarce vital organs. JAMA 1993;270(20):2469–74.

27. Kotloff RM. Lung retransplantation: all for one or one for all? Chest 2003;123(6):1781–2.

28. Persad G, Wertheimer A, Emanuel EJ. Principles for allocation of scarce medical interventions. Lancet 2009;373(9661):423–31.

29. Parfit D. Equality and priority. Ratio 1997;10:202–21.

30. Wendler D. Are physicians obligated always to act in the patient's best interests? J Med Ethics 2010; 36(2):66–70.

31. AMA. Principles of medical ethics. Available at: http://www.ama-assn.org/ama/pub/physician-resources/medical-ethics/code-medical-ethics/principles-medical-ethics.shtml. Accessed December 1, 2010.

32. Tsuchiya A, Dolan P, Shaw R. Measuring people's preferences regarding ageism in health: some methodological issues and some fresh evidence. Soc Sci Med 2003;57(4):687–96.

33. Daniels N. Am I my parents' keeper? An essay on justice between the young and the old. Oxford, 1988.

Alternatives to Lung Transplantation: Lung Volume Reduction for COPD

Gerard J. Criner, MD

KEYWORDS

- Lung volume reduction surgery
- National Emphysema Treatment Trial • COPD
- Bronchoscopic lung volume reduction

Emphysema is a progressive and debilitating disease that is recalcitrant to medical interventions. Hyperinflation is the sentinel complication of emphysema that decreases exercise performance and quality of life, impairs respiratory muscle and chest wall mechanics, increases breathlessness, prolongs respiratory failure requiring mechanical ventilation, and increases mortality[1–4] Recent evidence suggests that hyperinflation has implications that go far beyond the respiratory system and may also exert its negative effects on exercise performance and mortality by reducing cardiac chamber size and impairing right and left ventricular function.[5–7] It may also heighten systemic inflammation.[8]

Lung volume reduction surgery (LVRS) was devised with the intent of mitigating the degree and impact of hyperinflation. Before the National Emphysema Treatment Trial (NETT), data regarding LVRS consisted mainly of uncontrolled, single-center studies that were characterized by small patient numbers, substantial variability in patient selection criteria and surgical approach, duration of follow-up, and definitions of complications and outcomes.[9–17] NETT was a randomized, controlled, prospective, multicenter, long-term trial designed to provide definitive answers regarding the independent effects of LVRS in comparison with medical therapy on survival as well as exercise performance, lung function, patient symptoms, and quality of life.[18] NETT demonstrated a 5.2% 90-day postoperative mortality compared with 1.5% with optimal medical therapy. This risk is acceptable to many severely impaired patients with emphysema, but other patients remain apprehensive and forego LVRS and await less invasive therapeutic options.[19,20] In May 2003, soon after the publication of NETT results, interest grew in nonsurgical bronchoscopic approaches to lung volume reduction (BLVR).[21–29]

Herein I review the effects of LVRS in comparison with medical therapy, characterize the optimum candidate for LVRS, and provide an up-to-date review of the various experimental bronchoscopic lung reduction techniques that are currently undergoing investigation.

LUNG VOLUME REDUCTION SURGERY

In 2003, the results of the NETT were published, detailing the effects of LVRS on survival and maximum exercise capacity in 1218 patients with emphysema who were randomized to LVRS or medical treatment between January 1998 and July 2002 and followed for a mean of 2.4 years.[30] NETT also reported the effects of LVRS on pulmonary function, oxygen requirement, 6-minute walk distance (6MWD), quality of life, respiratory

Division of Pulmonary and Critical Care Medicine and Temple Lung Center, Temple University School of Medicine, 745 Parkinson Pavilion, 3401 North Broad Street, Philadelphia, PA 19140, USA
E-mail address: crinerg@tuhs.temple.edu

Clin Chest Med 32 (2011) 379–397
doi:10.1016/j.ccm.2011.02.014
0272-5231/11/$ – see front matter © 2011 Elsevier Inc. All rights reserved.

symptoms, and health care use. In 2006, the NETT Research Group published updated analyses of survival and functional measures data with a median follow-up of 4.3 years.[31] These analyses included 40% more patients with functional measures at 2 years after randomization compared with the original 2003 outcomes report. Subsequent NETT publications reported on the prevalence and duration of air leaks,[32] optimum surgical approach to perform LVRS,[33] and cost effectiveness of the procedure.[34,35] The major findings of these reports are summarized as follows.

Major Outcomes in NETT: All Patients

Between January 1998 and July 2002, 3777 patients were screened for NETT and 1218 underwent randomization: 608 to LVRS and 610 to medical treatment. Baseline characteristics (**Table 1**) were similar between groups. Of 608 patients assigned to LVRS, 580 (95.4%) underwent LVRS (406 [70%] by median sternotomy, 174 [30%] by video-assisted thoracoscopic surgery), 21 (3.5%) declined LVRS, and 7 (1.2%) were considered unsuitable by the surgeon for LVRS.

Ninety-day mortality rate was 7.9% (95% confidence interval [CI], 5.9%–10.3%) in the LVRS group compared with 1.3% in the medical group (95% CI, 0.6%–2.6%, $P<.001$). At a mean follow-up of 29.2 months after randomization, 160 patients assigned to medical treatment died compared with 157 patients assigned to LVRS. There was no difference in mortality rates at this time point between groups, although a higher initial mortality rate was identified in the LVRS group soon after the operation (**Fig. 1**A).

Exercise capacity improved 10 W or more in 28%, 22%, and 15% of LVRS patients after 6, 12, and 24 months, respectively compared with 4%, 5%, and 3% of medical control patients ($P<.001$ at each time point, **Fig. 2**, **Table 2**). Additionally, patients who underwent LVRS were more likely to demonstrate improvements in 6MWD, % predicted forced expiratory volume in 1 second (FEV_1), severity of dyspnea, and general as well as disease-specific quality of life assessments compared with the control group (see **Fig. 2**; **Table 2**).

Identifying a Patient Subgroup at High Risk of Death Following LVRS

Before NETT commenced, a 30-day surgical mortality greater than 8% in either treatment group was defined as a stopping end point. In May 2001,

a subgroup defined by FEV_1 of less than or equal to 20% predicted and either a diffusing capacity for carbon monoxide (DL_{CO}) of less than or equal to 20% predicted or homogeneous emphysema met the prespecified stopping criteria because of excessive mortality with LVRS.[36] The 30-day mortality in those who received LVRS was 16% (95% CI, 8.2%–26.7%, $P<.001$) compared with no deaths in the medical group. For those "high-risk profile" LVRS-treated patients who survived 6 months after randomization, there was little or no difference in functional and quality-of-life outcomes compared with the medically treated group: exercise capacity increased by 4.5 ± 13.0 W versus a decrease of 4.4 ± 14.8 W ($P = .06$), 6MWD increased by 14.9 ± 63.7 m versus a decrease of 21.6 ± 56.7 m ($P = .03$), and FEV_1 increased by 5.5% ± 6.9% predicted versus a decrease of 0.4% ± 1.9% predicted ($P<.001$). At 6 months, the Quality of Well-Being score showed a similar decrease (0.01 units) for both groups.

As described by the previous data, patients with severe emphysema characterized by an FEV_1 of less than or equal to 20% predicted and either a homogeneous pattern of emphysema on chest CT or a DL_{CO} of less than or equal to 20% predicted have high postoperative LVRS mortality and little chance of clinically meaningful improvements in lung function, exercise tolerance, or quality of life. As a result, these types of patients are not approved for LVRS by the Centers for Medicare and Medicaid Services (CMS) or by the Joint Commission for the Accreditation of Healthcare Organization (JCAHO) guidelines.

Results of NETT: Outcomes in Non–High-Risk Patients

Among 1078 NETT patients who were not high risk, the 30-day mortality after LVRS was 2.2% and 0.2% after medical treatment ($P<.001$). Ninety-day mortality rate was 5.2% with LVRS and 1.5% with medical therapy ($P = .001$; **Table 3**). At a mean 29.2 months follow-up after randomization into NETT, LVRS provided no survival benefit over medical treatment, even with exclusion of the high risk for death subgroup. Patients who underwent LVRS more likely had improvements in 6MWD, maximum exercise capacity, FEV_1% predicted, and quality of life (disease specific and general) compared with continued medical treatment ($P<.001$ for each comparison; see **Fig. 2**).

Preoperative Predictors of LVRS Outcomes in Non–High-Risk NETT Patients

The baseline factors associated with differences in mortality, functional outcomes, and quality-of-life

Table 1
Characteristics of all 1218 patients at baseline[a]

Characteristic	Surgery Group (n = 608)	Medical-Therapy Group (n = 610)
Age at randomization, y	66.5 ± 6.3	66.7 ± 5.9
Race or ethnic group, n (%)		
Non-Hispanic white	581 (96)	575 (94)
Non-Hispanic black	19 (3)	23 (4)
Other	8 (1)	12 (2)
Sex, n (%)[b]		
Female	253 (42)	219 (36)
Male	355 (58)	391 (64)
Distribution of emphysema on CT, n (%)[c]		
Predominantly upper lobe	385 (63)	405 (67)
Predominantly non–upper lobe	223 (37)	204 (33)
Heterogeneous	330 (54)	336 (55)
Homogeneous	278 (46)	274 (45)
Perfusion ratios[d]	0.30 ± 0.21	0.28 ± 0.23
Maximal workload, W	38.7 ± 21.1	39.4 ± 22.2
Distance walked in 6 min, ft[e]	1216.5 ± 312.6	1219.0 ± 316.0
FEV_1 after bronchodilator use, % of predicted value	26.8 ± 7.4	26.7 ± 7.0
Total lung capacity after bronchodilator use, % of predicted value	128.0 ± 15.3	128.5 ± 15.0
Residual volume after bronchodilator use, % of predicted value	220.5 ± 49.9	223.4 ± 48.9
Carbon monoxide diffusing capacity, % of predicted value	28.3 ± 9.7	28.4 ± 9.7
PaO_2, mm Hg	64.5 ± 10.5	64.2 ± 10.1
$PaCO_2$, mm Hg	43.3 ± 5.9	43.0 ± 5.8
Total score on St George's Respiratory Questionnaire[f]	52.5 ± 12.6	53.6 ± 12.7
Average daily Quality of Well-Being score[g]	0.58 ± 0.12	0.56 ± 0.11
Total UCSD Shortness of Breath score[h]	61.6 ± 18.1	63.4 ± 18.6

Abbreviations: CT, computed tomography; FEV_1, forced expiratory volume in one second; PaO_2, partial pressure on arterial oxygen; $PaCO_2$, partial pressure of arterial carbon dioxide.

[a] P Baseline measurements were obtained after rehabilitation but before randomization, except for the carbon monoxide–diffusing capacity, which was measured before rehabilitation. Plus-minus values are means ± SD.

[b] P for homogeneity = .04.

[c] Upper lobe predominance of emphysema was judged subjectively by each center's radiologist, who described the distribution of disease as predominantly upper lobe, predominantly lower lobe, diffuse, or predominantly affecting superior segments of the lower lobes. The latter 3 choices were grouped as predominantly non–upper lobe. The classification of the emphysema as heterogeneous or homogeneous was based on subjective scores assigned by each center's radiologist to each of 3 zones in each lung. Data on upper lobe versus non–upper lobe distribution were missing for 1 patient.

[d] The perfusion ratio is derived from the radionuclide perfusion scan. Each lung is divided into 3 zones, and a percentage of total perfusion is assigned to each zone. The ratio is calculated as the sum of the percentages assigned to the 2 upper zones divided by the sum of the percentages assigned to the 4 middle and lower zones.

[e] To convert values from feet to meters, divide by 3.28.

[f] The St George's Respiratory Questionnaire is a 51-item questionnaire on the health-related quality of life with regard to respiratory symptoms that is completed by the patient; the total score ranges from 0 to 100, with lower scores indicating better health-related quality of life.

[g] The Quality of Well-Being scale is a 77-item quality-of-life questionnaire completed by the patient. The average daily score ranges from 0 to 1, with higher scores indicating better quality of life.

[h] The University of California, San Diego (UCSD), Shortness of Breath Questionnaire is a 24-item questionnaire about dyspnea that is completed by the patient; the total score ranges from 0 to 120, with lower scores indicating less shortness of breath.

Data from Fishman A, Martinez F, Naunheim K, et al. A randomized trial comparing lung-volume-reduction surgery with medical therapy for severe emphysema. N Engl J Med 2003;348:2059–73.

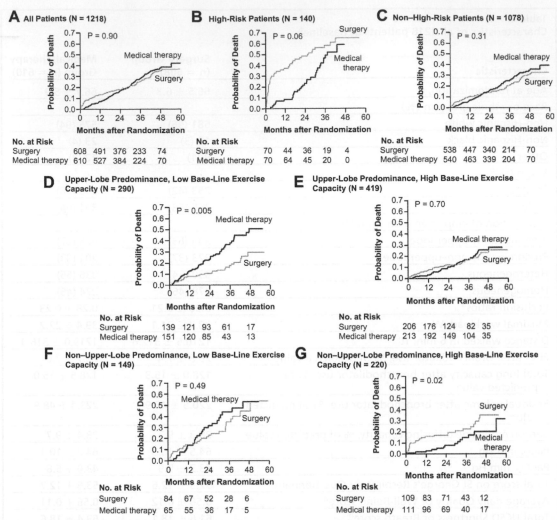

Fig. 1. Probability of death as a function of the number of months after randomization (Kaplan-Meier estimates). High-risk patients were defined as FEV_1 ≤20% predicted and either homogeneous emphysema or DL_{CO} ≤20% predicted. Low baseline exercise capacity was defined as a maximal workload at or below the sex-specific 40th percentile (25 W for women and 40 W for men); high exercise capacity was defined as a workload above this threshold. P values were derived by Fisher's exact test for e comparison between groups over a mean follow-up period of 29.2 months. (*From* Fishman A, Martinez F, Naunheim K, et al. A randomized trial comparing lung-volume-reduction surgery with medical therapy for severe emphysema. N Engl J Med 2003;348(21):2059–73; with permission.)

outcomes between the treatment groups were the craniocaudal distribution of emphysema on chest CT (presence or absence of upper lobe predominant emphysema, P for interaction = .02) and post-rehabilitation exercise test maximum wattage (low or high exercise, P for interaction = .01).

Based on combinations of high and low exercise maximum wattage with upper lobe or non–upper lobe predominant emphysema by chest CT analyses, patients were divided into 4 subgroups. In the 290 patients with upper lobe predominant emphysema and low exercise capacity, LVRS had a lower risk of death than medical therapy

(relative risk (RR) 0.47, P = .005, see **Fig. 1**D; see **Table 3**). This LVRS subgroup more likely achieved greater than or equal to 10 W improvement in maximum exercise wattage at 24 months (30% vs 0%; P<.001, see **Table 2**) and a greater than or equal to 8-point improvement in St George's Respiratory Questionnaire (SGRQ) score at 24 months (48% vs 10%, P<.001, see **Table 2**). In 419 patients with upper lobe predominant emphysema and high exercise wattage, LVRS had no impact on survival (RR 0.98; P = .70). However, LVRS patients were more likely to have greater than or equal to10-W improvement in

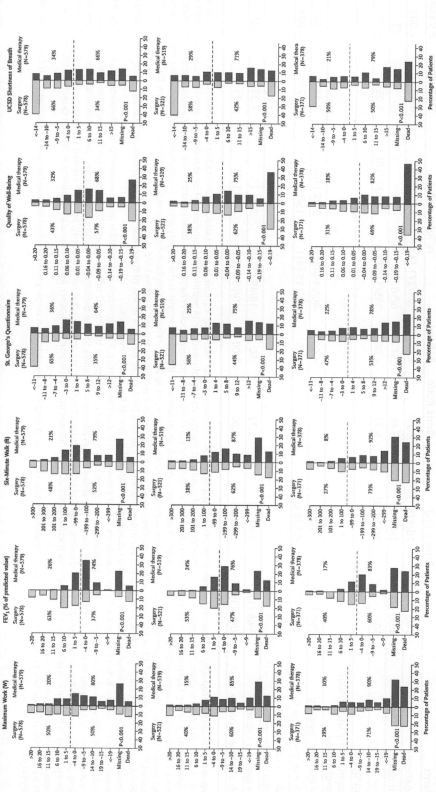

Fig. 2. Changes from post-rehabilitation baseline in exercise capacity (maximal workload), percentage of predicted FEV₁, 6-minute walk distance, health-related quality of life (St George's Respiratory Questionnaire), quality of life (Quality of Well-Being Scale), and dyspnea (UCSD Shortness of Breath Questionnaire) after 6, 12, and 24 months of follow-up for all patients shown in the first, second, and third rows of data, respectively. The category Missing includes patients too ill to complete the procedure or who declined to complete the procedure but did not explain why. For the Quality of Well-Being Scale, patients who died were assigned a score of 0 for the visit, and patients who did not complete the questionnaire were assigned a score equal to half the lowest score observed for the visit. The degree to which the bars are shifted to the upper left of the chart indicates the degree of relative benefit of LVRS over medical treatment. The percentage shown in each quadrant is the percentage of patients in the specified treatment group with a change in the outcome falling in that quadrant. *P* values were determined by the Wilcoxon rank-sum test. (*From* Fishman A, Martinez F, Naunheim K, et al. A randomized trial comparing lung-volume-reduction surgery with medical therapy for severe emphysema. N Engl J Med 2003;348(21):2059–73; with permission.)

Table 2
Improvement in exercise capacity and health-related quality of life at 24 months[a]

Patients	Improvement in Exercise Capacity				Improvement in Health-Related Quality of Life			
	Surgery Group n/Total n (%)	Medical Therapy Group n/Total n (%)	Odds Ratio	P Value	Surgery Group n/Total n (%)	Medical Therapy Group n/Total n (%)	Odds Ratio	P Value
All patients	54/371 (15)	10/378 (3)	6.27	<.001	121/371 (33)	34/378 (9)	4.90	<.001
High risk[b]	4/58 (7)	1/48 (2)	3.48	.37	6/58 (10)	0/48	—	.03
Other	50/313 (16)	9/330 (3)	6.78	<.001	115/313 (37)	34/330 (10)	5.06	<.001
Subgroups[c]								
Predominantly upper-lobe emphysema	—	—	—	—	—	—	—	—
Low exercise capacity	25/84 (30)	0/92	—	<.001	40/84 (48)	9/92 (10)	8.38	<.001
High exercise capacity	17/115 (15)	4/138 (3)	5.81	.001	47/115 (41)	15/138 (11)	5.67	<.001
Predominantly non–upper-lobe emphysema	—	—	—	—	—	—	—	—
Low exercise capacity	6/49 (12)	3/41 (7)	1.77	.50	18/49 (37)	3/41 (7)	7.35	.001
High exercise capacity	2/65 (3)	2/59 (3)	0.90	1.00	10/65 (15)	7/59 (12)	1.35	.61

[a] Improvement in exercise capacity in patients followed for 24 months after randomization was defined as an increase in the maximal workload of more than 10 W from the patient's post-rehabilitation baseline value. Improvement in the health-related quality of life in patients followed for 24 months after randomization was defined as a decrease in the score on the St George's Respiratory Questionnaire of more than 8 points (on a 100-point scale) from the patient's post-rehabilitation baseline score. For both analyses, patients who died or who missed the 24-month assessment were considered not to have improvement. Odds ratios are for improvement in the surgery group as compared with the medical therapy group. P values were calculated by Fisher's exact test. A low baseline exercise capacity was defined as a post-rehabilitation base-line maximal workload at or below the sex-specific 40th percentile (25 W for women and 40 W for men); a high exercise capacity was defined as a workload above this threshold.

[b] High-risk patients were defined as those with a forced expiratory volume in 1 second (FEV_1) that was 20% or less of the predicted value and either homogeneous emphysema on computed tomography or a carbon monoxide diffusing capacity that was 20% or less of the predicted value.

[c] High-risk patients were excluded from the subgroup analyses. For improvement in exercise capacity, P for interaction = .005; for improvement in health-related quality of life, P for interaction = .03. These P values were derived from binary logistic-regression models with terms for treatment, subgroup, and the interaction between the 2, with the use of an exact-score test with 3 degrees of freedom. Other factors that were considered as potential variables for the definition of subgroups included the baseline FEV_1, carbon monoxide diffusing capacity, partial pressure of arterial carbon dioxide, residual volume, ratio of residual volume to total lung capacity, ratio of expired ventilation in 1 minute to carbon dioxide excretion in 1 minute, distribution of emphysema (heterogeneous vs. homogeneous), perfusion ratio, score for health-related quality of life and Quality of Well-Being score; age; race or ethnic group; and sex.

Data from Fishman A, Martinez F, Naunheim K, et al. A randomized trial comparing lung-volume-reduction surgery with medical therapy for severe emphysema. N Engl J Med 2003; 348:2059–73.

Table 3
Mortality among all patients and in subgroups[a]

Patients	90-Day Mortality			Total Mortality				
	Surgery Group	Medical-Therapy Group		Surgery Group		Medical-Therapy Group		Risk Ratio	P Value
	No. of Deaths/Total no. (% [95% CI])	No. of Deaths/Total no. (% [95% CI])	P Value	No. of Deaths/Total no.	No. of Deaths/Person-yr	No. of Deaths/Total no.	No. of Deaths/Person-yr	Risk Ratio	P Value
All patients	48/608 (7.9 [5.9–10.3])	8/610 (1.3 [0.6–2.6])	<.001	157/608	0.11	160/610	0.11	1.01	.90
High risk[b]	20/70 (28.6 [18.4–40.6])	0/70 (0 [0–5.1])	<.001	42/70	0.33	30/70	0.18	1.82	.06
Other	28/538 (5.2 [3.5–7.4])	8/540 (1.5 [0.6–2.9])	.001	115/538	0.09	130/540	0.10	0.89	.31
Subgroups[c]									
Patients with predominantly upper lobe emphysema									
Low exercise capacity	4/139 (2.9 [0.8–7.2])	5/151 (3.3 [1.1–7.6])	1.00	26/139	0.07	51/151	0.15	0.47	.005
High exercise capacity	6/206 (2.9 [1.1–6.2])	2/213 (0.9 [0.1–3.4])	.17	34/206	0.07	39/213	0.07	0.98	.70
Patients with predominantly non-upper lobe emphysema									
Low exercise capacity	7/84 (8.3 [3.4–16.4])	0/65 (0 [0–5.5])	.02	28/84	0.15	26/65	0.18	0.81	.49
High exercise capacity	11/109 (10.1 [5.1–17.3])	1/111 (0.9 [0.02–4.9])	.003	27/109	0.10	14/111	0.05	2.06	.02

[a] Mortality was measured from the date of randomization in both treatment groups. Total mortality rates are based on a mean follow-up of 29.2 months. P values were calculated by Fisher's exact test. Risk ratios are for the risk in the surgery group as compared with the risk in the medical-therapy group. A low baseline exercise capacity was defined as a post-rehabilitation baseline maximal workload at or below the sex-specific 40th percentile (25 W for women and 40 W for men); a high exercise capacity was defined as a workload above this threshold. CI denotes confidence interval.

[b] High-risk patients were defined as those with a forced expiratory volume in 1 second (FEV_1) that was 20% or less of the predicted value and either homogeneous emphysema on computed tomography or a carbon monoxide diffusing capacity that was 20% or less of the predicted value.

[c] High-risk patients were excluded from the subgroup analyses. For total mortality, P for interaction = .004; this P value was derived from binary logistic-regression models with terms for treatment, subgroup, and the interaction between the 2, with the use of an exact-score test with 3 degrees of freedom. Other factors that were considered as potential variables for the definition of subgroups included the baseline FEV_1, carbon monoxide diffusing capacity, partial pressure of arterial carbon dioxide, residual volume, ratio of residual volume to total lung capacity, ratio of expired ventilation in 1 minute to carbon dioxide excretion in 1 minute, distribution of emphysema (heterogeneous vs. homogeneous), perfusion ratio, score for health-related quality of life, and Quality of Well-Being score; age; race or ethnic group; and sex.

Data from Fishman A, Martinez F, Naunheim K, et al. A randomized trial comparing lung-volume-reduction surgery with medical therapy for severe emphysema. N Engl J Med 2003; 348:2059–73.

maximum exercise wattage at 24 months (15% vs 3%, $P = .001$, see **Table 2**) and a greater than or equal to 8-point improvement in SGRQ (41% vs 11%, $P<.001$, see **Table 2**) compared with medical therapy. In 149 patients with non–upper lobe predominant disease and low exercise capacity, LVRS had no impact on risk of death (RR 0.81; $P = .49$) or maximum exercise capacity at 24 months (12% vs 7%, $P = .50$). However, LVRS was more likely to improve SGRQ at 24 months (37% vs 7%, $P = .001$, see **Table 2**). In 220 patients with non–upper lobe predominant emphysema and high exercise at baseline, LVRS increased the risk for death (RR 2.06, $P = .02$) and had no effect on maximum exercise capacity at 24 months (3% both groups, $P = 1.0$) or SGRQ (15% vs 12%, $P = .61$; see **Table 2**).

NETT: Long-term Follow-up

At the time of the initial NETT publication, mean follow-up was only 2.4 years. An assessment of follow-up at a later time point was proposed by the NETT Steering Committee to establish the durability of benefits from LVRS on functional and physiologic performance, and also to assess the effect of LVRS on long-term survival. Enrolled patients continued to have regularly scheduled follow-up tests, telephone interviews, clinic visits, and completed quality of life questionnaires. Long-term survival was updated by clinical center reports and review of the Social Security Master Death file. **Fig. 3**A shows probability of death as a function of years after LVRS or medical treatment in all 1218 patients, with a median follow-up of 4.3 years.[31] Total mortality rate was 0.11 deaths per person-year with LVRS and 0.13 with medical therapy, respectively (RR 0.85, $P = .02$). Survival was improved with LVRS compared with medical treatment despite the expected higher earlier postoperative mortality following LVRS.

Exercise capacity improved by greater than or equal to 10 W in 23%, 15%, and 9% of LVRS patients compared with 5%, 3%, and 1% of the medical patients at follow-up of 1, 2, and 3 years ($P<.001$ at each time point). After LVRS, SGRQ decreased more than 8 units in 40%, 32%, 20%, 10%, and 13% compared with 9%, 8%, 8%, 4%, and 7% following medical care at 1 to 5 years of follow-up ($P<.001$, years 1–3; $P = .005$, year 4; $P = .12$, year 5).

Effect of LVRS Subgroup Classification on Long-term Survival and Functional Outcome Following LVRS

The updated analyses provided additional support for assessing the differential risks and benefits of LVRS by classifying patients using the pattern of emphysema on chest CT and maximum wattage attained on post–pulmonary rehabilitation exercise testing. In 290 patients with upper lobe predominant emphysema and low exercise capacity, LVRS provided a substantial survival advantage compared with medical treatment (RR 0.57, $P = .01$, see **Fig. 3**C). Those patients who underwent LVRS also had significantly improved exercise capacity and quality of life (**Fig. 4**C and **Fig. 5**C, respectively).

Operative Mortality and Cardiopulmonary Morbidity following LVRS

A secondary goal of NETT was to develop predictors of LVRS mortality and morbidity.[37] A number of predictors of mortality and morbidity were analyzed in 511 non–high-risk patients who underwent LVRS. These factors included demographic characteristics, pulmonary function, the extent and pattern of emphysema on chest CT, maximum wattage attained during exercise testing, dyspnea, and quality of life. Major pulmonary morbidity was defined as tracheostomy, failure to wean from mechanical ventilation, pneumonia, re-intubation, or mechanical ventilation for more than 3 days within 30 days of surgery. Major cardiovascular morbidity was defined as myocardial infarction, pulmonary embolus, or cardiac arrhythmia requiring treatment within 30 days of LVRS.

Within 90 days of LVRS, the incidence of operative mortality was 5.5%; major pulmonary and cardiovascular morbidity occurred in 29.8% and 20.0% of patients, respectively. Intraoperatively, 91.0% of patients had no complications, 2.2% had transient hypoxemia, and 1.2% had an arrhythmia; 58.7% of patients had at least 1 postoperative complication within 30 days of LVRS. Arrhythmia was the most common complication and occurred in 23.5% of patients. Pneumonia developed in 18.2% of patients, 21.8% required at least 1 re-intubation, 11.7% were readmitted to the ICU, 8.2% underwent tracheostomy, and 5.1% of patients failed weaning from mechanical ventilation within 3 days after LVRS.

The presence of non–upper lobe predominant emphysema was the sole predictor of operative mortality (relative odds 2.99, $P = .009$). Pulmonary morbidity was greater in older patients (relative odds 1.05, $P = .02$), and those with lower FEV_1 (relative odds 0.97, $P = .05$) or DL_{CO} (relative odds 0.97, $P = .01$). Cardiovascular morbidity was higher in older patients (relative odds 1.07, $P = .004$), those who used oral steroids (relative odds 1.72, $P = .04$), or those with non–upper

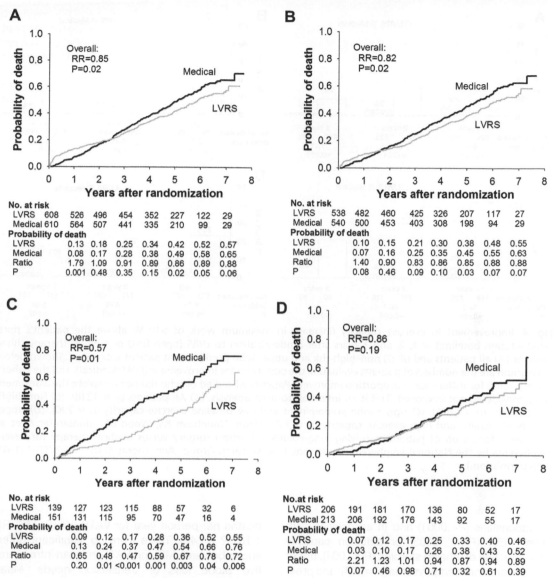

Fig. 3. Kaplan-Meier estimates of the cumulative probability of death as a function of years after randomization to LVRS (*gray line*) or medical therapy (*black line*) for (A) all patients and (B–D) non–high-risk and upper lobe predominant subgroups of patients. The P value is from the Fisher's exact test for difference in the proportions of patients who died during the 4.3 years (median) of follow-up. Shown below each graph are the numbers of patients at risk, the Kaplan-Meier probabilities, the ratio of the probabilities (LVRS:Medical), and P value for the difference in these probabilities. This is an intention-to-treat analysis. (A) All patients (n = 1218). (B) Non–high-risk patients (n = 1078). (C) Upper lobe predominant and low baseline exercise capacity (n = 290). (D) Upper lobe predominant and high exercise capacity (n = 419). RR, relative risk. (*From* Naunheim KS, Wood DE, Mohsenifar Z, et al. Long-term follow-up of patients receiving lung-volume-reduction surgery versus medical therapy for severe emphysema by the National Emphysema Treatment Trial Research Group. Ann Thorac Surg 2006;82(2):431–43; with permission.)

lobe predominant emphysema (relative odds 2.67, P<.001).

LVRS and Air Leaks

Air leaks are common after LVRS and may be prolonged. NETT investigated the effects of a variety

of buttressing products and techniques on preventing postoperative air leaks.[32] Following LVRS, 496 (89.8%) of the 552 patients had air leaks at some point within 30 days of surgery. The median duration of air leaks was 7 days, but 66 patients (11.9%) had air leaks for 30 days or more postoperatively. Air leak duration was longer

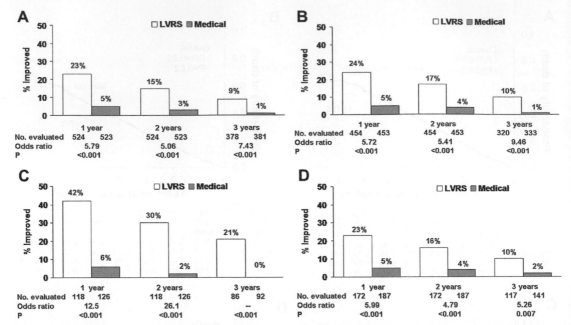

Fig. 4. Improvement in exercise capacity (increase in maximum work of >10 W above the patient's post-rehabilitation baseline) at 1, 2, and 3 years after randomization to LVRS (open box) or medical therapy (filled box) for (A) all patients and (B–D) non–high-risk and upper lobe predominant patient subgroups. Shown below each graph are the numbers of patients evaluated, the odds ratio for improvement (LVRS:Medical), and the Fisher's exact P value for difference in proportion improved. Patients who died or who did not complete the assessment were considered not improved. This is an intention-to-treat analysis. (A) All patients (n = 1218). (B) Non–high-risk patients (n = 1078). (C) Upper lobe predominant and low baseline exercise capacity (n = 290). (D) Upper lobe predominant and high exercise capacity (n = 419). (From Naunheim KS, Wood DE, Mohsenifar Z, et al. Long-term follow-up of patients receiving lung-volume-reduction surgery versus medical therapy for severe emphysema by the National Emphysema Treatment Trial Research Group. Ann Thorac Surg 2006;82(2):431–43; with permission.)

in Caucasians ($P<.0001$) and in association with lower FEV_1 ($P = .0003$) or diffusion capacity ($P = .06$), use of inhaled steroids ($P = .004$), upper lobe predominant emphysema ($P = .04$), and presence of pleural adhesions ($P = .007$). Surgical approach (median sternotomy [MS] vs video-assisted thorascopic surgery [VATS]) and the use of buttressing materials and stapler brand did not influence air leak duration. Postoperative complications were greater in patients with air leaks (57% vs 30%, $P = .0004$) and postoperative stay was longer (11.8 ± 6.5 days vs 7.6 ± 4.4 days, $P = .0005$).

Surgical Approach and LVRS Outcomes

NETT also compared the effects of LVRS surgical approaches via MS or VATS on patient mortality, morbidity, and functional outcomes.[33] Ninety-day mortality was similar for the 2 groups: 5.9% for MS and 4.6% for VATS ($P = .67$). Overall mortality was 0.08 deaths per person-year for MS and 0.10 deaths per person-year for VATS (VATS: MS; RR 1.18, $P = .42$). There were no significant differences between MS and VATS in mean intraoperative blood loss or transfusion needs. Mean operating time was 21.7 minutes shorter for MS than VATS ($P<.001$), hypoxemia was less frequent with MS than VATS (0.8% vs 5.3%, $P = .004$), and intraoperative complications were less with MS compared with VATS (93% vs 86.2% no intraoperative complications, $P = .02$).

Median hospital length of stay was longer for MS than VATS but the difference was not statistically significant (10 vs 9 days; $P = .1$). At 30 days following LVRS, 70.5% of MS patients were living independently compared with 80.9% of VATS patients ($P = .02$). Functional outcomes were similar between groups at 12 and 24 months of follow-up. Costs related to LVRS and associated hospitalization were less for VATS compared with MS ($P = .03$), as were total costs (medical and nonmedical) during the 6 months after LVRS ($P = .005$).

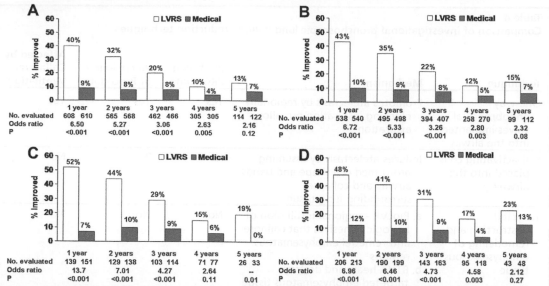

Fig. 5. Improvement in health-related quality of life (decrease in St George's Respiratory Questionnaire total score of >8 units below the patient's post-rehabilitation baseline) at 1, 2, 3, 4, and 5 years after randomization to LVRS (*open box*) or medical therapy (*filled box*) for (*A*) all patients and (*B–D*) non–high-risk and upper lobe predominant subgroups of patients. Shown below each graph are the numbers of patients evaluated, the odds ratio for improvement (LVRS:Medical), and the Fisher's exact *P* value for difference in proportion improved. Patients who died or who did not complete the assessment were considered not improved. This is an intention-to-treat analysis. (*A*) All patients (n = 1218). (*B*) Non–high-risk patients (n = 1078). (*C*) Upper-lobe predominant and low baseline exercise capacity (n = 290). (*D*) Upper lobe predominant and high exercise capacity (n = 419). (*From* Naunheim KS, Wood DE, Mohsenifar Z, et al. Long-term follow-up of patients receiving lung-volume-reduction surgery versus medical therapy for severe emphysema by the National Emphysema Treatment Trial Research Group. Ann Thorac Surg 2006;82(2):431–43; with permission.)

LUNG VOLUME REDUCTION: INVESTIGATIONAL APPROACHES

Despite the many benefits that may result from LVRS, many patients find the operative risks to be unacceptable and forego surgery. In 2004, only 254 Medicare beneficiaries underwent LVRS at 42 approved centers; in 2005 and 2006 only 120 and 105 Medicare beneficiaries underwent LVRS, respectively. Soon after the initial NETT results were published in 2003, scientific and commercial interest grew in nonsurgical approaches to lung volume reduction (LVR) in an attempt to achieve similar physiologic and functional benefits to LVRS but with less morbidity and mortality.[21–29]

Investigative approaches to LVR can be broken down into 5 main categories: (1) one-way endobronchial valves implanted into the airway, (2) self-activating coils placed into the airway, (3) targeted destruction and remodeling of emphysematous tissue, (4) bypass tract airway stenting, and (5) transpleural ventilation (**Table 4**). One-way endobronchial valves work by promoting atelectasis by regionally blocking inspiration but permitting expiration. Self-activating coils that are placed

into the airway induce atelectasis and volume reduction by assuming their preformed coil shape and bending the airway and collapsing the surrounding lung tissue. Targeted destruction and remodeling of emphysematous tissue has been accomplished by biologic lung volume reduction (BioLVR), which is the regional instillation of biologic adhesives that collapse and remodel emphysematous regions; and by Bronchoscopic Thermal Vapor Ablation (BTVA), which heats and destroys targeted emphysematous lung tissue. During airway bypass tract stenting, stents are placed endobronchially into emphysematous lung tissue to enhance the emptying of damaged lung tissue with prolonged expiratory time constants. The same rationale is used with transpleural ventilation techniques in which modified chest tubes are placed transthoracically into emphysematous lung tissue to empty damaged lung externally outside the chest cavity.

The previously mentioned techniques all attempt to achieve sustained reductions in end-expiratory lung volume, but all differ in the approach, the effect of collateral ventilation, or nonintact pleural fissures on success in achieving lung reduction and also the reversibility or

Table 4
Comparison of investigational bronchoscopic lung volume reduction techniques

Technique	Mechanism	Published PRCT Data	Reversibility of Procedure	Affected by Collateral Ventilation
One-way endobronchial valves implanted into the airway	Promotes atelectasis by regionally blocking inspiration but allows expiration	Yes	Yes	Yes
Self-activating coils placed into the airway	Induces atelectasis by assuming preformed coil shape and bends airway and collapses surrounding lung tissue	No	?	No
Targeted destruction and remodeling of emphysematous tissue	a. BioLVR - regional instillation of biologic adhesives that collapse and remodel emphysematous regions b. BTVA heats and destroys targeted emphysematous tissue	No	No	No
Bypass tract airway stenting	Stents placed endobronchially into emphysematous tissue to enhance emptying of damaged lung tissue	Pending	Yes	No
Transpleural ventilation	Modified chest tubes are placed transthoracically into emphysematous tissue to empty damaged lung externally	No	Yes	No

Abbreviations: BioLVR, biologic lung volume reduction; bTVA, bronchoscopic thermal vapor ablation.

irreversibility of the treatment intervention. Each of the previously mentioned techniques is discussed in detail as follows. **Table 4** compares the major features of each of the approaches.

Endobronchial 1-Way Valves

Endobronchial valve systems are deployed into segmental or subsegmental bronchi through a flexible or rigid bronchoscope using a catheter or guide wire. Their design prevents regional inspiration but facilitates expiration and secretion drainage. Regionalized lung volume reduction may occur through progressive deflation and absorption atelectasis.

The 2 most studied valve systems have similar characteristics. The valves expand to fill the airway lumen and are available in multiple diameters designed to occlude airways ranging from approximately 4.0 to 8.5 mm in diameter. Expiratory gas and secretions escape around the outside edges of the flexible Spiration valve (Spiration Incorporated, Redmond, WA, USA) and through the valve lumen of the Zephyr valve (Emphasys Medical, Redwood City, CA, USA; Pulmonx Inc, Redwood City, CA, USA). The Spiration Intrabronchial Valve system has an "umbrella design" in which an occlusive cover is stretched over a titanium wire frame. The Emphasys EBV is a biocompatible cylindrical device with a "duck bill" one-way valve seated in a nitinol wire cage. Both are easily removable if the need arises.

Analysis of the first 98 patients who underwent BLVR with Emphasys endobronchial valves at 9 international centers reported small but significant improvements in FEV_1, forced vital capacity (FVC), residual volume (RV), and 6MWD.[38] In the first 90 days, 8 patients had serious complications including 1 nonprocedural death in a patient with prior lobectomy secondary to lung cancer, 3 pneumothoraces requiring surgical intervention, and 4 air leaks lasting longer than 7 days. Minor complications included chronic obstructive pulmonary disease (COPD) exacerbations in 17 patients. Physiologic improvement was most pronounced in the subset (n = 70) that achieved complete lobar exclusion. Change from baseline to 90-day assessment in FEV_1 and 6MWD were significantly greater after treatment in those who achieved complete lobar exclusion versus those who did not: 14.0% ± 29.3% versus 3.2% ± 15.7% change in FEV_1 ($P = .02$) and 13.9 ± 45.5-m versus 26.7 ± 58.8-m change in 6 MWD ($P = .001$).

The Spiration system Intrabronchial Valve (IBV) phase II trial assessed safety in a multicenter pilot study that treated 91 patients with severe obstruction, hyperinflation, and predominantly upper lobe emphysema with 609 valves placed bilaterally in upper lobe segmental or subsegmental bronchi (mean 6.7 valves, median of 6.0 valves per patient).[29] Valves were placed in the desired airways with 99.7% technical success and no evidence of migration or airway wall erosion. There were no reported procedural deaths and 30-day morbidity and mortality was 5.5% and 1.1%, respectively. Significant improvements in SGRQ quality of life at 6 months after implantation were reported (-8.2 ± 16.2, $P = .001$). Improvements in quality of life correlated with a decrease in lung volume (-294 ± 427 mL, $P = .007$) in treated lobes without visible atelectasis. FEV_1, 6MWD and lower extremity ergometry testing did not significantly change post-IBV implantation. A quantitative CT analysis of lung volume changes in 57 subjects before and after IBV endobronchial valve implantation of the treated and nontreated lobes was reported.[39] Treated upper lobes had a decrease in volume (335 ± 444 mL) in 88% of the cohort, whereas untreated lobes had a simultaneous 11.6% increase in volume. The regional changes in lung volume were associated with clinically important improvements in quality of life (SGRQ, -8.95 ± 16.22) but not clinically important changes in lung function tests. The mechanisms for improvements in quality of life with the redistribution in ventilation following IBV treatment are unexplained at present and require further study.

Phase III Endobronchial 1-Way Valve Trials

The VENT (Endobronchial Valve for Emphysema Palliation Trial) is the first prospective randomized multicenter trial to evaluate BLVR using the Zephyr endobronchial valve (Emphasys Medical Inc) compared with medical care in patients with severe heterogeneous emphysema.[28]

VENT randomized 321 patients (aged 40–75) to implantation with endobronchial valves (n = 220) or to medical management (n = 101) as defined by the GOLD 2001 guidelines. The primary efficacy end points were percent changes in FEV_1 and 6MWD at 6 months compared with baseline for each group analyzed by intention to treat. Secondary end points included mean changes in quality of life as assessed by SGRQ, incremental cycle exercise capacity, dyspnea measured by a modified Medical Research Council score (mMRC), the amount of target lobe volume reduction measured by quantitative HRCT, and daily oxygen usage. The primary safety end point was

a difference between the 2 groups in a Major Complication Composite (MCC) rate at 180 days after randomization. The MCC included death, massive hemoptysis, empyema, pneumonia distal to valves, and ventilator dependency for greater than or equal to 24 hours. Before randomization, all patients underwent 6 to 8 weeks of outpatient pulmonary rehabilitation and optimization of their medical management at the discretion of the treating physician per GOLD guidelines. High-resolution chest CT (HRCT) was performed at baseline and 180 days after randomization. HRCT images were analyzed at a core laboratory to provide quantitative and visual indices of lobar emphysema severity and fissure integrity to determine patient eligibility and lung structural characterization. HRCT scans were used to target treatment; the lobe with the highest percentage of emphysema and greatest degree of heterogeneity (difference in % emphysema between ipsilateral lung lobes) was selected for EBV treatment.

Conscious sedation (71.5% patients) or general anesthesia (28.5% patients) were used to place the valves in a single lobe using flexible bronchoscopy alone (98.6%) or in combination with rigid bronchoscopy. The mean number of valves placed in the targeted lobe was 3.8 per subject (range 1–9). Mean procedure time was 33.8 ± 20.5 minutes. The lobes targeted for EBV included right upper lobe (52.3%), right lower lobe (9.3), left upper lobe (24.3%), and left lower lobe (14.0%).

At 6 months after randomization, the FEV_1 increased 4.3% in the EBV group while it decreased 2.5% in the control group; thus FEV_1 was a mean of 6.8% greater after treatment following EBV compared with the control group ($P = .005$). At 6 months, 6MWD increased 2.6% in the EBV group and decreased 3.2% in the medical group; thus, there was a mean increase of 5.8% for 6MWD following EBV compared with medical therapy ($P = .04$). The secondary outcomes also showed modest improvements at 6 months following EBV therapy in comparison with medical treatment. In this regard, supplemental oxygen use was slightly less in the EBV group ($P = .005$), and SGRQ differed by a mean of -3.4 ($P = .04$), mMRC by -0.3 ($P = .04$), and cycle ergometry peak workload by 3.8 W ($P = .05$), all favoring EBV over medical therapy alone.

At 6 months, medically treated patients had an MCC rate of 1.2% compared with a rate of 6.1% in EBV subjects. Included in the MCC at 6 months was a 2.8% mortality rate in the EBV group versus no deaths in the controls ($P = .19$). Pneumonia developed distal to the EBV valve in 4.2% of EBV subjects; all pneumonias resolved with antibiotic therapy. Hemoptysis occurred in 5.6% of EBV subjects over 6 months after implantation and in no controls ($P = .02$). Hemoptysis was most likely caused by oozing from granulation tissue at the implantation site. COPD exacerbations requiring hospitalization occurred more commonly following EBV (7.9%) versus controls (1.2%) ($P<.03$). In 12 months of follow-up, 31 patients had valves removed; reasons for this included retrieval of migrated valve (n = 8), patient's request (n = 7), pneumonia distal to valve (n = 3), placement in the incorrect lobe (n = 3), recurring COPD exacerbations (n = 2), and hemoptysis (n = 1).

Heterogeneity (difference in the % of emphysema between lobes in the treated lung) and fissure integrity proved to be predictive in determining the magnitude of improvements in FEV_1 and 6MWD. The enhancing effect of heterogeneity on changes in FEV_1 and 6MWD was significant within any quartile of emphysema % and overall was greater with increasing degrees of heterogeneity (**Fig. 6**). At a 15% median cutoff, the high heterogeneity subgroup had relatively greater improvements in FEV_1 and 6MWD at 6 months follow-up. EBV subjects with intact fissures had incremental improvements in FEV_1 at 6 months of 16.2% ($P<.001$) and 17.9% at 12 months ($P<.001$) in comparison with those with incomplete fissures who had insignificant changes of 2.0% and 2.8% at 6 and 12 months, respectively.

EBV subjects also had a greater reduction in quantitative treated lobe volume, as assessed by HRCT, at 6 months compared with medically treated controls (−378.4 vs −16.3 mL, $P<.002$), an effect that was further enhanced in the setting of complete fissures (−712.5 vs +2.2 mL, $P<.001$). Targeted lobe volume reduction measured by HRCT correlated inversely with the change in FEV_1 (r = −0.53, $P<.001$).

Emphasys received expedited review by the Food and Drug Administration (FDA) for the "Zephyr" endobronchial valve and their application was denied FDA approval in December 2008. The panel commented that the mean changes in FEV_1 and 6MWD were not clinically meaningful and that additional data regarding long-term safety of the device were needed. Emphasys dissolved as a company 8 weeks later and the Zephyr valve was purchased by Pulmonx Inc (Redwood City, CA, USA). Plans for future investigation using the Zephyr valve are being developed but hopefully will use the patient characteristics that were identified by VENT (eg, high heterogeneity, intact fissures, and complete lobar exclusion) to be associated with clinically meaningful improvements.

The Spiration Intrabronchial Valve (IBV) system is currently enrolling patients in a pivotal phase III study.

Lung Volume Reduction via Biologic Remodeling of Emphysematous Tissue

Biologic lung volume reduction is a process in which a biodegradable sclerosant gel (BioLVR, Aeris Therapeutics Inc, Woburn, MA, USA) is used to polymerize the small airways and alveolar airspace.[25,26] The fibrin-based hydrogel contains fibroblast growth factor-1 complexed with condroitin sulfate. Focal lung volume loss occurs as collapse, remodeling, and scaring take place over a period of weeks. A theoretical advantage of this method of lung reduction is that it induces its effects distally at the small airway and alveolar level and may work even in the presence of collateral ventilation.

In an open-labeled, multicenter phase 2 dose-ranging study, BioLVR Hydrogel was administered to 8 subsegmental sites (4 pulmonary subsegments in each upper lobe) involving (1) low-dose treatments (n = 28) with 10 mL per site (LD); and (2) high-dose treatments (n = 22) with 20 mL per site (HD).[40] Safety was assessed by the incidence of serious medical complications that followed treatment. Efficacy was assessed by changes from baseline in lung function, dyspnea score, 6MWD, and quality of life. There were no deaths and the 4 serious treatment-related complications all resolved with medical treatment. A reduction in RV/total lung capacity (TLC) at 12 weeks (primary efficacy outcome) was reported with both LD (−6.4% ± 9.3%, $P = .002$) and HD (−5.5% ± 9.4%, $P = .028$) treatments. Improvements in lung function at 6 months were greater with HD (FEV_1 + 15.6% [$P = .002$], FVC + 9.1% [$P = .034$]) than with LD (FEV_1 + 6.7% [$P = .021$], FVC + 5.1% [$P = .139$]). LD-treated and HD-treated groups both demonstrated improved symptom scores and health-related quality of life (HRQOL). Overall, the improvement was larger, and responses more durable with 20 mL/site dosing than 10 mL/site dosing.

BioLVR was also administered to 25 patients with homogeneous emphysema in an open-label phase II study; 8 subjects received low-dose (LD) treatment with 10 mL per site at 8 subsegments and 17 received high-dose (HD) treatment with 20 mL per site at 8 subsegments.[41] There were no deaths or serious medical complications from study treatment. A statistically significant reduction in air trapping was seen at 3-month follow-up in HD patients but not LD patients. At 6 months, changes from baseline in FEV_1, FVC, RV/TLC, dyspnea scores, and SGRQ were better with HD than LD treatment, but only attained statistical significance in HD for FEV_1 (+13.8 ± 20.2, $P = .007$), dyspnea (−0.8 ± 0.7 mMRC score, $P = .001$) and SGRQ total score (−12.2 ± 12.3, $P = .0001$).

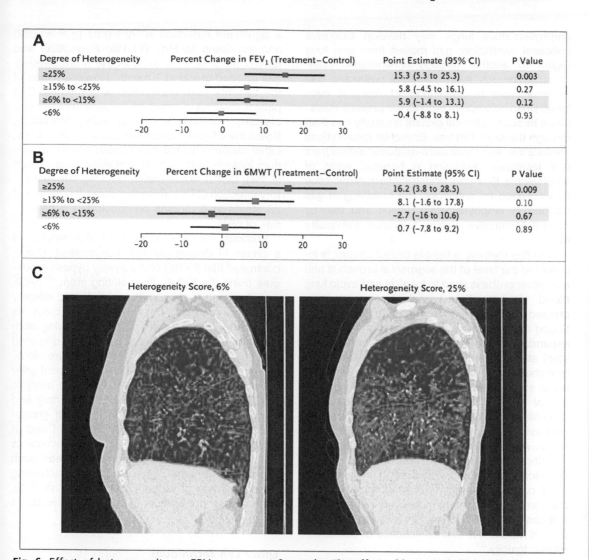

A

Degree of Heterogeneity	Percent Change in FEV₁ (Treatment−Control)	Point Estimate (95% CI)	P Value
≥25%		15.3 (5.3 to 25.3)	0.003
≥15% to <25%		5.8 (−4.5 to 16.1)	0.27
≥6% to <15%		5.9 (−1.4 to 13.1)	0.12
<6%		−0.4 (−8.8 to 8.1)	0.93

B

Degree of Heterogeneity	Percent Change in 6MWT (Treatment−Control)	Point Estimate (95% CI)	P Value
≥25%		16.2 (3.8 to 28.5)	0.009
≥15% to <25%		8.1 (−1.6 to 17.8)	0.10
≥6% to <15%		−2.7 (−16 to 10.6)	0.67
<6%		0.7 (−7.8 to 9.2)	0.89

C

Heterogeneity Score, 6%   Heterogeneity Score, 25%

Fig. 6. Effect of heterogeneity on EBV response at 6 months. The effect of heterogeneity on change in FEV₁ (*Panel A*) and 6MWD (*Panel B*) at 6 months after EBV implantation. % heterogeneity was the difference in quantitative emphysema score (the proportion of pixels of less than −910 Hounsfield units) between EBV-treated and ipsilateral non-treated lobes. In Panel C, sagittal HRCT views with density mask views show low (6%, left subpanel) and high heterogeneity (25%, right subpanel). Darker areas represent pixels < −910 Hounsfield units, consistent with emphysema. (*From* Sciurba FC, Ernst A, Herth FJ, et al. A randomized study of endobronchial valves for advanced emphysema. N Engl J Med 2010;363(13):1233–44; with permission.)

Aeris Therapeutics notified participating clinical investigative sites in November 2008 that planning of a phase III trial of BioLVR was being halted and the company moved toward development of a new polymeric sealant named AeriSeal.[42] AeriSeal is currently undergoing active investigation in Europe. Preliminary data presented in 15 patients with upper lobe predominant emphysema treated in 2 to 4 subsegments showed a reduction in CT measured lung volume in treated lobes and an increase in ipsilateral volume in nontreated lobes. The reductions in lobar volume correlated with a reduction in gas trapping (RV/TLC, r = 0.59,

$P = .02$), increased FEV₁ ($r = -0.65$, $P = .009$) and 6MWD ($r = 0.48$, $P = .07$). Future prospective randomized controlled phase III trials with AeriSeal are planned.

Airway Bypass Tract

Airway bypass transbronchial fenestration is a bronchoscopic technique using a needle-tipped catheter designed to create extra-anatomic bronchial fenestrations that are maintained open with drug-eluting stents (Broncus Technologies, Mountain View, CA, USA). Compared with normal lungs, emphysematous lungs may develop extensive collateral ventilation; gas moves from one lung region to another through nonanatomic pathways.[43] Through these collateral pathways, gas communicates between lung lobules and even lobes when incomplete fissures are present. Resistance through collateral circuits is usually less than through the bronchial tree. Bronchial fenestrations create a low resistance extra-anatomic airflow tract that facilitates ventilation in targeted areas of emphysema. Bronchial fenestrations may decrease hyperinflation by enhancing the emptying of gas trapped in emphysematous tissue and thereby potentially improve exercise tolerance and quality of life.

With this method, a flexible bronchoscope is inserted to the level of the segmental bronchus and a Doppler probe is used to localize and avoid lung blood vessels. Transbronchial openings are created with a 25-gauge transbronchial needle-tipped catheter and a 2.5-mm balloon dilator. An expandable silicone-coated, 3 × 3-mm stainless steel stent is inserted and anchored within the bronchial wall.[44,45] Early efficacy data are based on an ex-vivo trial on explanted human lungs and animal studies.[46] In early animal trials, stent stenosis limited stent function, a problem partially overcome by adding antiproliferative drugs to the stents. A randomized trial demonstrated the superior efficacy of weekly bronchoscopic applications of topical mitomycin C versus saline in maintaining stent patency in dogs.[44] A randomized trial of paclitaxel-eluting versus non–drug-eluting stents in a canine model showed 12-week patency rates of 65% versus 0% and an absence of paclitaxel-related toxicity.[47]

The safety and clinical results of a multicenter evaluation of airway bypass with paclitaxel-eluting stents for 35 patients with severe bilateral emphysema have been published.[45] All had post-bronchodilator residual volume (RV) greater than or equal to 220% of predicted, total lung capacity (TLC) greater than or equal to 133% of predicted and FEV_1 less than 40% of predicted, and all but 2 patients had homogeneously distributed emphysema. A median of 8 stents (range 2–12) were inserted bilaterally in each upper and lower lobe. Standard pulmonary function parameters, 6MWD, dyspnea as measured by mMRC scale, and SGRQ scores were assessed in follow-up. At 6 months, there were statistically significant reductions from post-rehabilitation baseline in RV (5.34 ± 1.13 L to 4.98 ± 1.25 L [$P = .04$]) and dyspnea (−0.5; $P = .025$) but no changes in TLC, FVC, FEV_1, 6MWD, or SGRQ. A subgroup analysis of patients above and below the RV/TLC median of 0.67 demonstrated a significant reduction in RV (−0.87 L; $P = .022$) and increases in FVC (11.1%; $P = .026$) and 6MWD (28.6 m, $P = .021$) in the more severely gas trapped group at 1 month. However, none of the benefits were maintained at 6 months. One patient died as a result of intraoperative airway bleeding, resulting in a Drug Safety Monitoring Board investigation and procedural modifications. Other serious adverse events related to the procedure included intraoperative pneumomediastinum (5.3%), COPD exacerbation (32.4%), and respiratory infection (27%). Bronchoscopic inspection of 26 stents at 6 months demonstrated a patency rate of 69%.

Broncus recently announced the results of a phase III double-blinded, randomized, sham-controlled trial (EASE) of the airway bypass procedure using the Exhale drug-eluting stent.[48] EASE was designed to demonstrate safety and efficacy of the procedure, but it failed to meet its composite primary end point of improving both FVC and mMRC dyspnea score when compared with sham controls. mMRC dyspnea score alone, however, did show significant improvement after the airway bypass procedure. Post hoc analysis of patients who met the composite primary end point showed that a reduction in RV of greater than or equal to 500 mL after treatment and at 1 month correlated with significant improvements in lung function and symptoms, whereas such improvements were not seen in those achieving lesser degrees of reduction in RV. At this date, peer review publication of the EASE results is pending.

Other LVR Techniques

Several other promising techniques to achieve lung volume reduction have recently been described in small numbers of patients. These techniques vary significantly in their approach but share the common feature of not being affected by the presence of collateral ventilation. In a pilot study, lung volume reduction coils (PneumRx, Inc, Mountain View, CA, USA) were bronchoscopically placed into the most diseased areas of lung bilaterally to achieve lung tissue compression.[49] Safety was the primary end point and efficacy outcomes were secondary end points in the 11 severe emphysema patients (8 homogeneous, 3 heterogeneous) that were studied. The 11 patients underwent 21 treatments with a total of 101 coils placed. A total of 33 adverse events were reported; none were severe, 64% were moderate, and 36% were mild. Adverse events possibly attributed to the procedure or device included dyspnea (10 events), cough (5 events), COPD exacerbations (3 events), and chest pain (1 event). Improvements in FEV_1, RV, TLC, SGRQ, and 6MWD were observed at 1 and 3 months following the first procedure. The greatest relative changes were observed in 6MWD, SGRQ, and mMRC in the patients with heterogeneous emphysema. Further testing of the device is ongoing.

The technique of bronchial thermal vapor ablation (BTVA; Uptake Medical Corp, Seattle, WA, USA), involves the bronchoscopic application of thermal energy to targeted areas of emphysema.[50] BTVA-induced injury triggers an inflammatory response in the airway and parenchyma, thereby producing lung volume reduction. BTVA uses a vapor generator and metal balloon vapor catheter, with target dosing at 3.0 to 7.5 cal/g according to a prior CT-based tissue-air algorithm. In a pilot study, 11 patients with heterogeneous emphysema, mean FEV_1 of 0.77 ± 0.17 L (32% predicted), and RV of 4.1 ± 0.9 L (219% predicted), underwent 9 right and 2 left upper lobe unilateral treatments (approximately 3 applications/lobe). Immediate mild opacification in the target areas was demonstrated by chest x-ray in all patients. All patients were discharged 24 to 48 hours after the procedure. Serious adverse events requiring hospitalization occurred in 5 patients; 2 patients had exacerbations of COPD and 3 patients had probable bacterial pneumonia, anxiety, and atrial tachycardia, respectively. Minor adverse events not requiring hospitalization included minor hemoptysis (n = 6) and inflammatory pneumonitis (n = 2). All patients had less dyspnea at 3 to 16 weeks after the procedure. Seven patients completed 1-month follow-up with a mean increase in FEV_1 of 9% ± 8% and decrease in RV of 7.4% ± 9.0%. However, at 6 months there was no difference compared with baseline in FVC, FEV_1, 6 MWD, and RV. In contrast, MRC dyspnea score (2.6 baseline to 2.1 at 6 months) and SGRQ (64.4 baseline to 49.1 at 6 months) both improved after BTVA. BTVA continues to undergo further investigation as a potential therapy for LVR at this time.

External placement of modified chest tubes into emphysematous regions produced increases in FEV_1 and 6MWD and reductions in RV, TLC, mMRC, and SGRQ in 3 patients.[51] These data support the concept that placing artificial spiracles into diseased emphysematous lung could enhance gas emptying, decrease end-expiratory lung volume, and potentially ameliorate the consequences of hyperinflation.

Finally, the presence of collateral ventilation is an important limitation to the success of endobronchial valve treatment.[52] A new system (Chartis; Pulmonx, Inc, Redwood City, CA, USA) is now available that consists of a console and balloon-tipped catheter that can be placed through the working channel of a bronchoscope to measure flow and pressures from isolated lung regions on a lobar to subsegmental level. During assessment, the balloon is inflated, the airway and lung region of interest are isolated, and airflow and pressure are measured. The absence of airflow during balloon occlusion signifies the lack of collateral ventilation and may help target appropriate emphysema patients and lung regions for endobronchial valve treatment. This device is currently being used in small pilot studies to optimize the selection of patients for endobronchial valve treatment.

SUMMARY

Hyperinflation is a major cause of morbidity and mortality in severe emphysema. LVRS offers a select group of patients with emphysema the opportunity for clinically meaningful improvements in exercise tolerance, lung function, quality of life, and in those with upper lobe predominant disease and low exercise, survival. A variety of novel, less invasive bronchoscopic techniques are currently undergoing study and show promise to effectively produce lung reduction in a broader group of patients with advanced emphysema. Additional well-designed prospective studies are needed to determine the optimum role of LVRS versus bronchoscopic LVR in the treatment of severe emphysema.[53]

REFERENCES

1. O'Donnell DE, Lam M, Webb KA. Measurement of symptoms, lung hyperinflation, and endurance during exercise in chronic obstructive pulmonary disease. Am J Respir Crit Care Med 1998;158(5 Pt 1):1557–65.
2. O'Donnell DE, Revill SM, Webb KA. Dynamic hyperinflation and exercise intolerance in chronic obstructive pulmonary disease. Am J Respir Crit Care Med 2001;164(5):770–7.
3. Jubran A, Tobin MJ. Pathophysiologic basis of acute respiratory distress in patients who fail a trial of weaning from mechanical ventilation. Am J Respir Crit Care Med 1997;155(3):906–15.
4. Casanova C, Cote C, de Torres JP, et al. Inspiratory-to-total lung capacity ratio predicts mortality in patients with chronic obstructive pulmonary disease. Am J Respir Crit Care Med 2005;171(6):591–7.
5. Barr RG, Bluemke DA, Ahmed FS, et al. Percent emphysema, airflow obstruction, and impaired left ventricular filling. N Engl J Med 2010;362(3):217–27.
6. Watz H, Waschki B, Meyer T, et al. Decreasing cardiac chamber sizes and associated heart

dysfunction in COPD: role of hyperinflation. Chest 2010;138(1):32–8.

7. Criner GJ. COPD and the heart: when less lung means more heart. Chest 2010;138(1):6–8.

8. Mineo D, Ambrogi V, Cufari ME, et al. Variations of inflammatory mediators and alpha1-antitrypsin levels after lung volume reduction surgery for emphysema. Am J Respir Crit Care Med 2010; 181(8):806–14.

9. Cooper JD, Trulock EP, Triantafillou AN, et al. Bilateral pneumectomy (volume reduction) for chronic obstructive pulmonary disease. J Thorac Cardiovasc Surg 1995;109(1):106–16 [discussion: 116–9].

10. McKenna RJ Jr, Brenner M, Gelb AF, et al. A randomized, prospective trial of stapled lung reduction versus laser bullectomy for diffuse emphysema. J Thorac Cardiovasc Surg 1996;111(2):317–21 [discussion: 322].

11. Bingisser R, Zollinger A, Hauser M, et al. Bilateral volume reduction surgery for diffuse pulmonary emphysema by video-assisted thoracoscopy. J Thorac Cardiovasc Surg 1996;112(4):875–82.

12. Cooper JD, Patterson GA, Sundaresan RS, et al. Results of 150 consecutive bilateral lung volume reduction procedures in patients with severe emphysema. J Thorac Cardiovasc Surg 1996; 112(5):1319–29 [discussion: 1329–30].

13. Miller JI Jr, Lee RB, Mansour KA. Lung volume reduction surgery: Lessons learned. Ann Thorac Surg 1996;61(5):1464–8 [discussion: 1468–9].

14. Daniel TM, Chan BB, Bhaskar V, et al. Lung volume reduction surgery. case selection, operative technique, and clinical results. Ann Surg 1996;223(5): 526–31 [discussion: 532–3].

15. Argenziano M, Moazami N, Thomashow B, et al. Extended indications for lung volume reduction surgery in advanced emphysema. Ann Thorac Surg 1996;62(6):1588–97.

16. Wisser W, Tschernko E, Senbaklavaci O, et al. Functional improvement after volume reduction: sternotomy versus videoendoscopic approach. Ann Thorac Surg 1997;63(3):822–7 [discussion: 827–8].

17. Health Care Financing Administration: Report to Congress. Lung volume reduction surgery and Medicare coverage policy: implications of recently published evidence. US Government: DHHS; 1998.

18. NETT Research Group. Rationale and design of the national emphysema treatment trial. A prospective randomized trial of lung volume reduction surgery. Chest 1999;116:1750.

19. Kolata G. Medicare says it will pay but patients say "No thanks". NY Times (Print) 2006.

20. Grady D. After early success, operations to remove damaged tissues have fallen sharply. NY Times (Print) 2007.

21. Toma TP, Hopkinson NS, Hillier J, et al. Bronchoscopic volume reduction with valve implants in patients with severe emphysema. Lancet 2003; 361(9361):931–3.

22. Watanabe Y, Matasuo K, Tamaoki A, et al. Bronchial occlusion with endobronchial Watanabe spigot. Journal of Bronchology 2003;10:264–7.

23. Sabanathan S, Richardson J, Pieri-Davies S. Bronchoscopic lung volume reduction. J Cardiovasc Surg (Torino) 2003;44(1):101–8.

24. Rendina EA, De Giacomo T, Venuta F, et al. Feasibility and safety of the airway bypass procedure for patients with emphysema. J Thorac Cardiovasc Surg 2003;125(6):1294–9.

25. Ingenito EP, Reilly JJ, Mentzer SJ, et al. Bronchoscopic volume reduction: a safe and effective alternative to surgical therapy for emphysema. Am J Respir Crit Care Med 2001;164(2):295–301.

26. Ingenito EP, Berger RL, Henderson AC, et al. Bronchoscopic lung volume reduction using tissue engineering principles. Am J Respir Crit Care Med 2003; 167(5):771–8.

27. Snell GI, Holsworth L, Borrill ZL, et al. The potential for bronchoscopic lung volume reduction using bronchial prostheses: a pilot study. Chest 2003; 124(3):1073–80.

28. Sciurba FC, Ernst A, Herth FJ, et al. A randomized study of endobronchial valves for advanced emphysema. N Engl J Med 2010;363(13):1233–44.

29. Sterman DH, Mehta AC, Wood DE, et al. A multicenter pilot study of a bronchial valve for the treatment of severe emphysema. Respiration 2010;79(3):222–33.

30. Fishman A, Martinez F, Naunheim K, et al. A randomized trial comparing lung-volume-reduction surgery with medical therapy for severe emphysema. N Engl J Med 2003;348(21): 2059–73.

31. Naunheim KS, Wood DE, Mohsenifar Z, et al. Long-term follow-up of patients receiving lung-volume-reduction surgery versus medical therapy for severe emphysema by the National Emphysema Treatment Trial Research Group. Ann Thorac Surg 2006;82(2): 431–43.

32. DeCamp MM, Blackstone EH, Naunheim KS, et al. Patient and surgical factors influencing air leak after lung volume reduction surgery: lessons learned from the National Emphysema Treatment Trial. Ann Thorac Surg 2006;82(1):197–206 [discussion: 206–7].

33. National Emphysema Treatment Trial Research Group. Safety and efficacy of median sternotomy versus video-assisted thoracic surgery for lung volume reduction surgery. J Thorac Cardiovasc Surg 2004;127:1350–60.

34. Ramsey SD, Berry K, Etzioni R, et al. Cost effectiveness of lung-volume-reduction surgery for patients with severe emphysema. N Engl J Med 2003; 348(21):2092–102.

35. Ramsey SD, Shroyer AL, Sullivan SD, et al. Updated evaluation of the cost-effectiveness of lung volume reduction surgery. Chest 2007;131(3):823–32.

36. National Emphysema Treatment Trial Research Group. Patients at high risk of death after lung-volume-reduction surgery. N Engl J Med 2001; 345(15):1075–83.

37. Naunheim KS, Wood DE, Krasna MJ, et al. Predictors of operative mortality and cardiopulmonary morbidity in the national emphysema treatment trial. J Thorac Cardiovasc Surg 2006;131(1):43–53.

38. Wan IY, Toma TP, Geddes DM, et al. Bronchoscopic lung volume reduction for end-stage emphysema: report on the first 98 patients. Chest 2006;129(3): 518–26.

39. Coxson HO, Nasute Fauerbach PV, Storness-Bliss C, et al. Computed tomography assessment of lung volume changes after bronchial valve treatment. Eur Respir J 2008;32(6):1443–50.

40. Criner GJ, Pinto-Plata V, Strange C, et al. Biologic lung volume reduction in advanced upper lobe emphysema: phase 2 results. Am J Respir Crit Care Med 2009;179(9):791–8.

41. Refaely Y, Dransfield M, Kramer MR, et al. Biologic lung volume reduction therapy for advanced homogeneous emphysema. Eur Respir J 2010 Jul;36(1):20–7.

42. Magnussen H, Kirsten A, Eberhardt R, et al. CT assessment of regional lung volume changes following endobronchial volume reduction therapy in emphysema patients using a synthetic adhesive hydrogel-foam. Am J Respir Crit Care Med 2010; 181:A5533.

43. Fessler HE. Collateral ventilation, the bane of bronchoscopic volume reduction. Am J Respir Crit Care Med 2005;171(5):423–4.

44. Choong CK, Haddad FJ, Gee EY, et al. Feasibility and safety of airway bypass stent placement and influence of topical mitomycin C on stent patency. J Thorac Cardiovasc Surg 2005;129(3):632–8.

45. Cardoso PF, Snell GI, Hopkins P, et al. Clinical application of airway bypass with paclitaxel-eluting stents: early results. J Thorac Cardiovasc Surg 2007;134(4):974–81.

46. Lausberg HF, Chino K, Patterson GA, et al. Bronchial fenestration improves expiratory flow in emphysematous human lungs. Ann Thorac Surg 2003;75(2): 393–7 [discussion: 398].

47. Choong CK, Phan L, Massetti P, et al. Prolongation of patency of airway bypass stents with use of drug-eluting stents. J Thorac Cardiovasc Surg 2006;131(1):60–4.

48. Broncus Technologies Inc. Broncus reports early EASE trial results for airway bypass with EXHALE drug-eluting stents. 2009. Available at: http://markets. hpcwire.com/taborcomm.hpcwire/?guid=1081574. Accessed October 22, 2010.

49. Herth FJ, Eberhard R, Gompelmann D, et al. Bronchoscopic lung volume reduction with a dedicated coil: a clinical pilot study. Ther Adv Respir Dis 2010;4(4):225–31.

50. Snell GI, Hopkins P, Westall G, et al. A feasibility and safety study of bronchoscopic thermal vapor ablation: a novel emphysema therapy. Ann Thorac Surg 2009;88(6):1993–8.

51. Saad R, Neto V, Botter M, et al. Therapeutic application of collateral ventilation with pulmonary drainage in the treatment of diffuse emphysema: report of the first three cases. J Bras Pneumol 2009;1(1):14–9.

52. Ernst A, Eberhardt R, Gompelmann D, et al. Low degree of collateral ventilation measurement in heterogeneous emphysema subject treated by endobronchial lung volume reduction predicts ELVR success. Am J Respir Crit Care Med 2010;181: A1571.

53. Criner GJ. Endoscopic interventions in severe emphysema. Am J Respir Crit Care Med 2009; 180:684.

Alternatives to Lung Transplantation: Treatment of Pulmonary Arterial Hypertension

Paul A. Corris, MBBS, FRCP

KEYWORDS

- Pulmonary arterial hypertension
- Chronic thromboembolic pulmonary hypertension
- Lung transplantation • Pulmonary endarterectomy
- Atrial septostomy

The Dana Point International Consensus Meeting in 2008 reclassified the clinical presentation of pulmonary hypertension into 5 categories. The first category comprises an intrinsic precapillary pulmonary arteriopathy called pulmonary arterial hypertension (PAH), including idiopathic PAH (IPAH) and familial/inherited pulmonary arterial hypertension, as well as pulmonary hypertension associated with connective tissue disease, congenital systemic-to-pulmonary shunts, portal hypertension, human immunodeficiency virus (HIV), and the use of anorexigens. The second category includes pulmonary hypertension as a consequence of left heart disease and increased left heart filling pressures. The third category is related to lung airway or parenchymal diseases with capillary destruction and hypoxic pulmonary vasoconstriction. The fourth category consists of chronic thromboembolic pulmonary hypertension (CTEPH) and is a consequence of pulmonary embolism. The fifth category is pulmonary hypertension of unclear or multifactorial etiologies associated with a mix of rare diseases.

For categories 2 and 3, treatment consists of improving the cardiac or pulmonary abnormalities by reducing left ventricular filling and afterload or by correcting hypoxemia. For categories 1 and 4, specific therapeutic approaches have been developed and are described here. In some patients, these targeted therapies may be very successful and may put off the need for transplantation indefinitely, while in other patients they will be insufficient to stabilize the disease and can only be considered as a bridge to transplantation. Overall, the proportion of lung transplantations performed for IPAH has decreased from about 12% in the 1990s to 2% in 2006.[1] The recent evolution toward a more aggressive approach driven by therapeutic goals derived from prognostic factors has led to consideration of transplantation earlier in disease course when it becomes clear that medical interventions are failing.

PAH

Prognostic Factors in PAH

In the preprostacyclin era, the median survival of untreated patients with IPAH was 2.8 years. However, patients with much better survival could be identified on the basis of favorable clinical indices. A low functional class (New York Heart Association [NYHA] 1 and 2) and better hemodynamics (right atrial pressure <10 mm Hg, cardiac index >2.5 L/min/m^2 and mixed venous oxygen

Institute of Cellular Medicine, Newcastle University and Newcastle upon Tyne Hospitals NHS Foundation Trust, NE77DN, UK
E-mail address: Paul.corris@ncl.ac.uk

Clin Chest Med 32 (2011) 399–410
doi:10.1016/j.ccm.2011.02.015
0272-5231/11/$ – see front matter © 2011 Published by Elsevier Inc.

saturation >63%) were first identified as important good prognostic factors.[2,3] Subsequently, other factors were described comprising:

- A relatively preserved exercise capacity: 6-minute walk distance greater than 332 m,[4] peak oxygen uptake greater than 10.4 mL/min/kg, and systolic blood pressure greater than 120 mm Hg[5]
- Preserved right ventricular contractile function: Tei index greater tan 0.8,[6] or tricuspid annular tricuspid annular plane systolic excursion greater than 18 mm[7]
- Less right ventricular strain: brain natriuretic peptide (BNP) lower than 150 pg/mL,[8] N terminal brain naturetic peptide (NTproBNP) lower than 1400 pg/mL,[9] or troponin C lower than 0.01 ng/mL.[10]

Similarly, factors have been identified that can predict outcome in patients treated with specific disease-targeted drugs. Sitbon and colleagues[11] showed that an NYHA class 1 or 2, a 6-minute walk distance greater than 380 m, or a 30% decrease in total pulmonary vascular resistance, obtained within 3 months of epoprostenol therapy, were associated with a good outcome (>80% survival at 3 years). This was confirmed by McLaughlin and colleagues,[12] showing a higher survival rate in patients in NYHA class 1 or 2 after 1 year of epoprostenol therapy. More recently, Provencher and colleagues[13] also showed that 6-minute walk distance and total pulmonary vascular resistance after 4 months of bosentan therapy were predictive for long-term survival. The use of these prognostic factors, both before and after the initiation of specific PAH therapy, can help to stratify patients according to their disease severity and to decide whether and when patients should be listed for lung transplantation.

Medical Treatment for PAH

This section describes the randomized controlled studies (RCTs) performed in PAH and summarized in **Table 1**.

Prostacyclin analogs

Prostacyclin or prostaglandin I_2 (PGI_2), first described in 1976, is still considered as the most potent pulmonary vasodilator. It is produced by endothelial cells, binds to specific membrane receptors of smooth muscles cells, and activates adenylate cyclase to increase intracellular cyclic adenosine monophosphate. Beside its vasodilator action, PGI2 also inhibits platelet aggregation and smooth muscle proliferation, both of which are abnormal in PAH.[14,15] Moreover, PGI_2 production has been shown to be insufficient in IPAH, providing a rationale for therapeutic use.[16]

Epoprostenol In 1987, Higenbottam and colleagues[17] reported the first chronic use of a prostacyclin analog, epoprostenol, in a patient with IPAH. Two RCTs, from Rubin and colleagues[18] in 1990 and Barst and colleagues[19] in 1996, confirmed that substantial improvements in symptoms, exercise tolerance, and pulmonary hemodynamics could be seen. The second study randomized 81 IPAH patients with NYHA functional class 3 and 4 to receive either continuous epoprostenol or conventional therapy. The mean epoprostenol dose at the end of the 12-week study was 9.2 ng/kg/min. The 6-minute walk distance, the primary end-point of the study, was significantly improved in epoprostenol-treated patients, while it deteriorated in patients under conventional therapy. Significant improvements were also seen in pulmonary hemodynamics, NYHA functional class, and quality of life. This pivotal study led to expanded use of epoprostenol, and, as a consequence of having an effective medical alternative, up to 70% of patients initially listed for lung transplantation were removed from the list as a result of improvement.[20,21] Epoprostenol has since been shown to improve hemodynamics and exercise capacity in patients with PAH related to scleroderma disease.[22] Uncontrolled studies also suggest improvement in patients with PAH related to congenital heart disease,[23,24] portal hypertension,[25] HIV infection,[26] and distal CTEPH.[24]

Because of its short half-life (3–5 minutes), epoprostenol has to be administered intravenously as a continuous infusion. This requires a tunneled central venous catheter and a portable infusion pump. The drug needs to be reconstituted daily and stored in refrigerated reservoirs connected to the portable pump. Patients and relatives need appropriate training by expert nurses to learn how to manage the system safely at home and how to solve the most frequent technical problems. The treatment is started at a dose of 2 ng/kg/min and progressively increased at a rate limited by side effects, including hypotension, flushing, headache, diarrhea, restlessness, jaw pain, leg pain, backache, abdominal discomfort, and nausea. Periodic dose increases are required to maintain efficacy because of tolerance to the drug. Adverse effects are ascites, probably related to increased permeability of the peritoneal membrane, hyperthyroidism, and thrombocytopenia. Complications related to the delivery system are pump malfunction, catheter obstruction and dislocations, local infection, and bacteremia. Excessive dosage can induce high cardiac

Table 1
Summary of randomized controlled trials in pulmonary arterial hypertension: efficacy results

Drug	Indication	NYHA	Borg	QoL	6MWD	PVR	NTproBNP	TTCW	Hospitalization	Progression
Epoprostenol	IPAH-CTD	✓	—	✓	✓	✓	—	Survival	—	—
Treprostinil	IPAH-CTD-CHD	✓	✓	NS	✓	✓	—	—	—	—
Iloprost	IPAH-CTD-CTEPH	✓	—	✓	✓	✓	—	—	—	—
Bosentan	IPAH-CTD	✓	✓	✓	✓	✓	—	—	✓	✓
Bosentan	CHD	✓	—	—	✓	✓	—	—	—	—
Bosentan	NYHA II	—	NS	✓	P = .08	✓	✓	✓	NS	✓
Bosentan	CTEPH	NS	NS	NS	NS	✓	✓	NS	NS	—
Sitaxentan	IPAH-CTD-CHD	✓	NS	✓	✓	✓	—	NS	NS	NS
Ambrisentan	IPAH-CTD-HIV	✓	✓	✓	✓	—	✓	✓	(↓)	(↓)
Sildenafil	IPAH-CTD-CHD	✓	NS	—	✓	✓	—	NS	(↓)	NS
Tadalafil	IPAH-CTD-HIV-CHD	NS	NS	✓	✓	✓	—	—	—	NS

Abbreviations: BNP, brain natriuretic peptide; Borg, Borg dyspnea score at the end of the 6-minute walk distance (6-MWD); CHD, PAH associated with congenital heart disease; CTD, pulmonary arterial hypertension (PAH) associated with connective tissue disease; CTEPH, chronic thromboembolic pulmonary hypertension; HIV, PAH associated with the human immunodeficiency virus; IPAH, idiopathic pulmonary arterial hypertension; NS, not significant; NTproBNP, N terminal brain natruretic peptide; NYHA, modified New York Heart Association functional class; PVR, pulmonary vascular resistance; QoL, quality of life; TTCW, time to clinical worsening.

output states, unnecessarily increasing cardiac work.[27]

Treprostinol Treprostinil is a chemically stable tricyclic benzidine analog of prostacyclin, stable at room temperature and with a longer half-life (30–80 minutes, depending on the administration route), suitable for intravenous and subcutaneous administrations. It was developed as a potential successor of epoprostenol. A large 12-week RCT enrolled 469 patients with NYHA class 2 through 4 IPAH, PAH related to congenital heart disease, and PAH related to connective tissue diseases.[28] As with epoprostenol, significant improvements in exercise capacity, functional class, and hemodynamics were reported. The effect on 6-minute walk distance was, however, much smaller than for epoprostenol, except for the patients receiving the highest doses. US Food and Drug Administration (FDA) approval was granted in 2002 because of substantial safety and convenience advantages over intravenous epoprostenol. Unfortunately, pain and redness at the infusion site are encountered by 85% of the patients when the drug is administered subcutaneously, and 8% of patients find the pain intolerable. This has clearly limited the use of the drug. Subcutaneous administration requires small subcutaneous catheters and micro-infusion pumps similar to those used to administer insulin to diabetic patients. The initial infusion rate is 1.25 ng/kg/min and gradually increases twice weekly by 1.25 ng/kg/min. Pain seems to be unrelated to the dose, is maximal 4 days after insertion, and decreases afterwards. Patients therefore maintain the catheter at the same place for 1 to several weeks. Patients on intravenous epoprostenol can be transitioned to subcutaneous treprostenil over 1 to 4 days, with no major adverse effects and without clinical deterioration.[29]

In 2004, the FDA also approved treprostinil for intravenous administration. Although this therapy shares with epoprostenol the risk of line infection and sepsis, it offers advantages of longer half-life and easier drug preparation. Three small uncontrolled studies, 1 after slow transition from intravenous epoprostenol,[30] 1 after rapid switch[31] and 1 for de novo treatment,[32] suggest similar efficacy for intravenous treprostinil and epoprostenol. However, the dosing of intravenous treprostinil is generally at least twice that of epoprostenol.

Inhaled treprostinil has been studied in a phase 3 trial, which showed significant but moderate improvements in exercise capacity.[33] An oral form of treprostinil is under investigation.

Iloprost Iloprost is another stable prostacyclin analog with an intermediate half-life (20–25 minutes) available for intravenous and inhaled administration. The inhalation route is attractive, because it delivers medication to ventilated lung areas exclusively, thereby limiting ventilation mismatch and hypoxemia. A 12-week RCT included 203 patients with NYHA class 3 and 4 IPAH, PAH related to connective tissue disease, and CTEPH.[34] The primary composite endpoint (improvement in NYHA class plus at least 10% improvement in the 6-minute walk distance plus no deterioration or death) was reached by 16.8% of the patients on iloprost treatment versus 4.9% on placebo. Fewer patients in the iloprost group died or deteriorated compared with the placebo group (4.9% vs 11.8%). Iloprost benefits also included hemodynamic, functional, and quality-of-life improvements. Adverse effects were increased cough, headache, flush, and jaw pain. The major limitation of this therapy is the short duration of effect requiring repetitive inhalations up to 9 times a day, each lasting 4 to 15 minuts, depending on the nebulizer type.[35]

Iloprost has also been studied as add-on therapy in patients treated with bosentan. Sixty-five patients were included in a 12-week RCT.[36] Significant improvements in functional class, hemodynamics, and time to clinical worsening were observed in the combination therapy group.

Endothelin receptor antagonists

Endothelin-1 (ET-1) is a potent vasoconstrictor and pro-proliferative substance. It is produced by endothelial cells and binds to two different receptors, ET_A and ET_B. Excessive production of endothelin in IPAH provides a rationale for receptor blockade. Selective ET_A and nonselective ET_A and ET_B receptor antagonists (ERA) have been developed.

Bosentan Bosentan, an orally active dual receptor antagonist, has been evaluated in two RCTs including NYHA-class 3 patients with IPAH and patients with PAH related to connective tissue disease. In the first study, significant improvements in exercise capacity, hemodynamics, and functional class were documented.[37] In the second one, bosentan (125 mg and 250 mg twice daily) significantly increased exercise capacity, delayed the time to clinical worsening, and improved Borg dyspnea score and functional class.[38] More recently, bosentan was shown to improve hemodynamics and time to clinical worsening but not 6-minute walk distance in NYHA class 2 patients with IPAH and PAH related to connective tissue disease.[39] Finally, in a RCT performed in patients with PAH related to congenital heart disease, bosentan significantly improved hemodynamics and 6-minute walk distance.[40]

Bosentan is well tolerated, except for a reversible, dose-related increase in liver enzymes in about 10% of the patients. This hepatotoxicity is attributed to inhibition of the canalicular bile salt export pump.[41] Significant drug interactions have been reported with cyclosporine, tacrolimus, gliburide, ketoconazole, itraconazole, and ritonavir. FDA approval was obtained in 2002.

Sitaxentan Sitaxetan is a highly selective ET_A receptor blocker. It has been evaluated in 2 large RCTs that included NYHA class 2 and 3 patients with IPAH and PAH related to connective tissue disease and to congenital heart disease. In the first trial, drug dosage was 100 mg and 300 mg once daily.[42] Sitaxentan significantly improved exercise capacity (6-minute walk distance but not peak oxygen consumption), functional class and pulmonary hemodynamics. In the second RCT, dosage was 50 and 100 mg for sitaxentan, and there was an additional open-label arm with bosentan.[43] Significant improvements in 6-minute walk distance and functional class were reported for the 100 mg and bosentan arms but not for the 50 mg arm. Notably, sitaxsentan has very recently been withdrawn by Pfizer from clinical use because of unpredictable acute hepatic failure.

Ambrisentan Ambrisentan is a modestly selective ET_A receptor blocker that has been studied in 2 large RCTs.[44] Significant improvements in 6-minute walk distance, functional class, Borg dyspnea score, quality of life, and time to clinical worsening were reported for all 3 dosages. No significant liver function abnormalities were reported. Peripheral edema was a common adverse effect, particularly in the 10 mg arm. FDA approval was obtained in 2007. No drug interactions have been reported to date.

Phosphodiesterase 5 inhibitors

Cyclic guanosine monophosphate (cGMP), the intracellular second messenger of nitric oxide (NO), is a potent vasodilator and inhibitor of smooth muscle cell proliferation. Inhibitors of cGMP phosphodiesterase (PDE) increase intracellular concentrations of cGMP, thereby enhancing the effects of endogenous NO. The cGMP-specific PDE5 is the predominant PDE isoenzyme in the pulmonary arteries.

Sildenafil Sildenafil is an orally active, selective PDE5 inhibitor with a half-life of 3 to 5 hours. One large RCT randomized NYHA class 2 to 4 patients with IPAH or PAH related to connective tissue disease and congenital heart disease to receive 20 mg, 40 mg, or 80 mg of sildenafil versus placebo three times daily for 12 weeks.[45]

Significant improvements in 6-minute walk distance and pulmonary hemodynamics were demonstrated, of similar magnitude for the 3 dose regimens. FDA approval was obtained in 2005. Because of the absence of a dose–response effect, only the 20 mg dosage was approved.

Adverse effects include headache, flushing, dizziness, dyspepsia, abnormal vision, back pain, myalgia, and epistaxis. A potentiation of the hypotensive effects of nitrates has been reported. Concomitant administration with bosentan causes a decrease in the plasma level of sildenafil and an increase in the level of bosentan; however, no dose adjustment has been recommended. Coadministration with ketoconazole, itraconazole, or ritonavir is discouraged.

Tadalafil Tadalafil is a newer, longer-acting PDE5 inhibitor. A recent 16-week RCT included patients with IPAH and PAH associated with connective tissue disease, congenital heart disease, and HIV who were randomized to placebo or tadalafil 2.5 mg, 10 mg, 20 mg, or 40 mg orally once daily.[46] Treatment was given as monotherapy, or, in 53% of patients, as add-on therapy to bosentan. Tadalafil 40 mg increased 6-minute walk distance and quality of life, delayed the time to clinical worsening, and improved hemodynamics. The most common treatment-related adverse event reported with tadalafil was headache.

Long-term survival data

With the exception of the original epoprostenol study,[19] all the previously mentioned 12- to 16-weeks RCTs were unable and not powered to show survival benefits. In a meta-analysis, Macchia and colleagues[47] could not demonstrate survival benefits for the PAH-specific therapies. However, in 2009, Galie and colleagues,[48] combining data from 21 studies involving 3140 patients, showed a 43% mortality reduction over 14.3 months, on average. Survival data have also been collected from long-term observational studies and compared against historical controls from a period when no therapy was available for PAH in the United States (**Table 2**).[2] These historical data were confirmed by more recent survival data from China, where these therapies are not widely available.[49]

Only a small number of IPAH patients with an acute vasodilator response to NO or epoprostenol demonstrate a beneficial response to calcium channel blockers (CCBs), but this characteristic is associated with a long-term survival advantage.[50] Recommended doses are up to 240 mg/d for nifedipine and 900 mg/d for diltiazem, but the effect of smaller doses has not been evaluated. It is

Table 2
Summary of large cohorts treated with epoprostenol, treprostinil, iloprost, and bosentan in comparison with conventional treatment

References	Drug	n	Type	NYHA	6MWD	OA	1-y	2-y	3-y	Comb[a]
D'Alonzo et al,[2] 1991	—	194	IPAH	—	—	20%	68	—	48	—
Christie et al,[1] 2008	LTx	710	IPAH	—	—	—	69	63	59	—
Barst, 1994	epo	18	IPAH	3.17	264 ± 160	100%	87	72	63	—
Sitbon et al,[11] 2002	epo	178	IPAH	—	240	—	85	70	63	—
McLaughlin et al,[12] 2002	epo	162	IPAH	—	—	—	88	76	63	—
Barst et al,[43] 2006	trepro	860	—	—	—	—	87	78	71	15%
Lang et al,[51] 2006	trepro	122	PAH/CTEPH	3.20 ± 0.04	305 ± 11	95%	89	—	71	18%
Opitz et al,[52] 2005	ilo inh	76	IPAH	—	—	47%	79	70	59	54%
Hoeper, 2008	ilo inh+iv	79	IPAH-CTD-CHD-PoPH	3.23	287 ± 112	—	86	73	59	—
McLaughlin et al,[55] 2005	bos	169	—	—	345 ± 87	88%	96	89	86	30%
Hoeper, 2005	bos	123	—	—	308 ± 133	—	93	83	80	43%
Provencher et al,[13] 2006	bos	103	IPAH	—	319 ± 105	99%	92	89	79	44%
Sandoval et al,[63] 1998	BDAS	14	IPAH	3.57 ± 0.6	107 ± 127	—	92	92	92	—
Rich et al,[50] 1992	CCB	17	IPAH (R)	2.39 ± 0.5	—	—	94	94	94	—
Sitbon, 2005	CCB	38	IPAH (LT R)	2.42	380 ± 112	—	97	97	97	—

Abbreviations: BDAS, baloon dilation atrial septostomy; bos, bosentan; CCB, calcium channel blockers; CHD, congenital heart disease; CTEPH, chronic thromboembolic pulmonary hypertension; epo, epoprostenol; ilo inh, inhaled iloprost; iv, intravenous; (I)PAH, (idiopathic) pulmonary arterial hypertension; LTx, lung transplant; PoPH, portopulmonary hypertension; trepro, treprostenil; 6-MWD, 6-min walking distance.

[a] Proportion of patients started with combination therapy during the course of the study.

recommended that treatment with CCBs only be considered for patients whose fall in mean pulmonary arterial pressure and pulmonary vascular resistance is dramatic and sustained.

Two single-center reports on the long-term follow up of patients with IPAH treated with epoprostenol showed an overall survival of 63% at 3 years and 55% at 5 years.[11,12] Treprostinil seems to have an effect on survival which is similar to that of epoprostenol.[51] This is clearly not the case for inhaled iloprost[52] nor for intravenous iloprost.[53] The improvement in prognosis observed with the oral agents (bosentan, sitaxentan and sildenafil) is clearly related to inclusion of less sick patients, and to the significant proportion of combined therapies in the most recent series. It is also quite remarkable that different series across different countries or continents provide similar survival data within each drug category.

A few observational studies have looked at the long-term outcome in specific PAH subgroups. In a subgroup of 66 patients with PAH related to connective tissue disease previously included in the two bosentan RCTs, Denton and colleagues[54] showed 1- and 2-year survival rates of 86% and 73%, respectively. These data, compared with the 96% and 89% survival reported for patients with IPAH by McLaughlin and colleagues,[55] emphasize again the poorer prognosis of patients with PAH related to connective tissue disease. However, in the recently published, open-label TRUST-study investigating the long-term effects of bosentan in PAH related to connective tissue disease, the authors reported 92% survival at 48 weeks with stabilized quality of life.[56] These results are in agreement with the significant improvement in survival reported by Williams and colleagues[57] in a cohort of 45 patients with PAH related to systemic sclerosis treated with bosentan as first-line therapy compared with a historical group of 47 patients from the prebosentan era. Similarly, Adriaenssens and colleagues[58] analyzed the effects of new therapies (mainly treprostinil and bosentan) in a cohort of patients with PAH related to congenital heart disease. The authors were able to show a prolonged time to clinical worsening (defined by death or inscription on the active list for transplantation) in patients receiving new therapies compared with patients on conservative therapy.

Patients with IPAH listed for lung transplantation have demonstrated a 50% reduction in mortality while on the list (33% vs 64%) when treated with iloprost or bosentan compared with non targeted therapy.[59] It is, however, important to emphasize the better survival of transplanted patients compared with those still waiting for transplantation and treated with iloprost or bosentan. Timely referral of these patients for transplantation centers should therefore be reinforced.

It also appears that a high proportion of patients who are dying from PAH nowadays receive monotherapy with oral agents.[60] This is suggested by the recent report of an American care provider on 821 patients initiated on bosentan between Oct. 1, 2004, and Dec. 31, 2004, and followed over 3 years. Overall survival at 3 years was only 64%. Of 190 patients who died, 169 were on bosentan monotherapy, and only 11% were escalated to prostanoid therapy before death. The vast majority of them had never been referred to an expert center.

In conclusion, it is important to realize that even if meta-analyses of RCTs are not able to demonstrate improved survival with new therapies for PAH, there is a large body of evidence for improved survival to be found in long-term observational studies. However, about 30% of the patients fail to respond even to epoprostenol therapy, and those who remain in NYHA class 3 and 4 have 3-year survival rates of about 30%.[11,12]

Atrial Septostomy for PAH

Rationale

Atrial septostomy has been used for a long time as a palliative procedure for certain congenital cardiac anomalies in children. Its use in patients with PAH is supported by the observation that IPAH patients with a patent foramen ovale live longer than those without intracardiac shunting.[61] Likewise, patients with Eisenmenger syndrome live longer and have heart failure less frequently than patients with IPAH.[62] Shunting decreases right ventricular afterload and increases left ventricular preload, inducing an increase in cardiac output. The drop in systemic arterial oxygen saturation induced by right–left shunting is compensated by increased cardiac output, systemic oxygen transport, and mixed venous oxygen saturation. There is also a decompression of the right ventricle and decreased symptoms of heart failure.

Techniques

The criteria to perform atrial septostomy are an NYHA class of 3 to 4, recurrent syncopal episodes, severe ascites, or clinical deterioration despite maximum medical treatment. The procedure is performed under sedation or light anesthesia, ideally under control of transesophageal echocardiography and careful hemodynamic monitoring titrated for a fall in arterial saturation of 5% to 10%. Once a hole is punctured using a Brockenbrough needle or a radiofrequency catheter, the fenestration can be made by different techniques: balloon dilation only, a self-expandable stent, a balloon-expandable stent with special technique to get a diabolo shape, or a fenestrated atrial septal defect occluder. In the first case, the hole is progressively dilated with increasingly larger balloons until an arterial saturation of 80% to 85% with FiO_2 21% is obtained.[63] A blade balloon can be used to get a better initial opening with tears, which subsequently can be enlarged.[64] Balloon dilatation is easy and relatively inexpensive. However, the disadvantages are multiple:

The final size of the connection is difficult to predict
Multiple sizes of balloons may be needed
Spontaneous closure of such a connection is usually observed over days to weeks.[65]

Redo-dilation after some weeks with a balloon is dangerous; the fenestration will have fibrous walls, which usually will resist dilation and can rupture with very big balloons, potentially resulting in a broad tear and excessive right to left shunt. By using a stent, it is possible to resize the hole at any time during the course of the disease. After release of the stent, the opening inside can be increased by balloon dilation. A diabolo shape has recently be used to improve stent stability.[66]

Results

In an early review of 62 cases, Rothman and colleagues[67] documented a mortality of 15%. Severe and refractory arterial hypoxemia, due to excessive communication, was the leading cause of death. This emphasizes the need for controlled fenestration. High right atrial pressure and pulmonary vascular resistance were associated with poor outcome, suggesting that septostomy should be performed earlier in the course of the disease. Improvement was reported in 70% of the patients, with resolution of ascites, edema, and syncopal episodes. Sandoval and colleagues[63] reported, in a series of 15 patients, that right atrial pressure decreased by about 5 mm Hg; cardiac index increased by more than 0.5 L/min/m^2, and the 6-minute walk distance was almost doubled. Kerstein and colleagues[64] noted further improvements in hemodynamics 7 to 27 months after septostomy. The complications were transient hypotension, femoral pseudo-aneurysm/arteriovenous fistula, and spontaneous closure in 20% of the cases. Overall, atrial septostomy seems to be a safe procedure in well selected PAH patients. In the modern era, mortality rates are in the range of 0% to 6% for balloon dilatation atrial septostomy[63,65] and for stent fenestration.[66]

Current therapeutic algorithms for PAH all position atrial septostomy as a late therapy and often consider it as a bridge to transplantation.[68,69] It is, however, crucial to have this procedure in mind from the diagnosis on, and certainly when medical treatment is not as satisfactory as it should be according to the already identified prognostic factors.

CTEPH

CTEPH is probably caused by single or recurrent embolization of thrombi that obstruct the pulmonary vascular bed. A history of symptomatic pulmonary embolism, however, is absent in up to 50% of patients who develop CTEPH. The reasons for incomplete resolution of the emboli are not fully understood. During the course of the disease, a distal vessel arteriopathy, caused by overperfusion in nonoccluded lung areas, sometimes becomes predominant. As the only potentially curable cause of pulmonary hypertension, CTEPH should be recognized so that appropriate interventions can be undertaken. The differential diagnosis between PAH and CTEPH is sometimes complicated, as central in situ thrombosis related to low flow can be seen in PAH. The presence of segmental perfusion defects on lung scan is a strong argument for CTEPH. Assessment of operability can be challenging, even when employing modern imaging procedures such as pulmonary angiography, computed tomography (CT) angiography or magnetic resonance tomography.

Pulmonary Endarterectomy

Procedure

Pulmonary endarterectomy (PEA) was introduced in 1958 but not commonly performed until 1985. Most of the procedures have been performed at the University of California at San Diego, but other centers worldwide are now performing the operation. Mortality of PEA has decreased from 22% originally to 4% to 8% in experienced centers.

The technique of bilateral PEA was originally described by Daily[70] and then further refined by Jamieson.[71] PEA is performed through a median sternotomy with cardiopulmonary bypass and periods of deep hypothermic (18°–20°C) circulatory arrest lasting 20 minutes. The superior vena cava is dissected free; the right pulmonary artery is incised, an endarterectomy plane is established and right endarterectomy is performed. The left pulmonary artery is then incised and left endarterectomy is performed. The atrial septum is inspected and a patent foramen ovale, if present, is closed. Recent modifications of the surgical approach include the use of intraoperative video-assisted angioscopy to enhance visibility in the distal pulmonary arteries[72] and selective antegrade cerebral perfusion with moderate rather than deep hypothermia.[73]

Although pulmonary hemodynamics improve immediately after surgery in most patients, the postoperative course can be complicated. In addition to the common complications of cardiac surgery, patients undergoing PEA can experience severe reperfusion edema and persistent pulmonary hypertension with hemodynamic instability.

Patient selection

Although PEA is the treatment of choice for CTEPH, not all patients are eligible for this surgery. Patients with very high pulmonary vascular resistance (>1200 dyne/s/cm^5) have a high perioperative mortality. The proportion of large vessel obstruction versus small vessel obliteration is a crucial determinant of the response to surgery. A discrepancy between angiographic obstruction and pulmonary hemodynamics should be handled with caution. Partitioning pulmonary vascular resistance by analyzing the pulmonary arterial pressure curve after inflation of the balloon of the Swan Ganz catheter gives information on the presence of small vessel disease and can help to predict postoperative pulmonary arterial pressure and outcome of PEA.[74] Comorbidities, such as morbid obesity, severe interstitial or obstructive pulmonary disease, chronic renal insufficiency, diabetes mellitus, inoperable coronary artery disease, hepatic dysfunction, and advanced age contribute to increased risk and should be considered. Age is not a contraindication to PEA if health status is otherwise good. If PEA is not an option or if an inadequate functional status is obtained after PEA, lung transplantation can be considered.

Long-term outcome

The untreated prognosis of advanced CTEPH is poor, with a 5-year survival of about 20%.[75–77] In contrast, 5-year survival following PEA is around 75%.[78] Most patients undergoing PEA also experience long-term improvements in functional class, exercise capacity and pulmonary hemodynamics.

Medical Treatment

In addition to the mechanical occlusion of a large part of the pulmonary circulation, remodeling of the nonoccluded vasculature—exposed to elevated pressure-related and flow-related physical forces—may contribute to a worsening of pulmonary hypertension. This observation has served as a rationale for the use of PAH-specific treatments in CTEPH.

Preoperative medical treatment

In patients with very high pulmonary vascular resistance and thereby a potentially high risk of perioperative mortality, pretreatment with epoprostenol[79] has been proposed. However, no RCT is available, and there is no clear consensus view other than that PEA should not be delayed by a trial of medical therapy. Any preoperative use of disease-modifying therapy should be within the context of an RCT.

Medical treatment for inoperable patients

Medical therapy is even more widely used for patients with inoperable disease or with persistent pulmonary hypertension after PEA. A recent 16-week large RCT showed significant decrease in pulmonary vascular resistance (24% from baseline) and in NTproBNP in CTEPH patients treated with bosentan, without change in the 6-minute walk distance.[80] A small RCT with sildenafil similarly showed significant improvement in pulmonary vascular resistance without effect on 6-minute walk distance,[81] but in an open-label trial including a larger number of patients, Reichenberger and colleagues[82] were able to show simultaneous improvements in hemodynamics and exercise capacity. A recent paper by Skoro-Sajer and colleagues[75] demonstrated a significant improvement in survival after 1 to 5 years of therapy with subcutaneous treprostinil compared with a matched historical control group. Five-year survival did not, however, reach the value obtained with PEA.

SUMMARY

Lung transplantation used to be the only hope for patients presenting with advanced PAH. The last 20 years has seen the development of disease-targeted drugs, directed toward different pathways of importance to the pathobiology of PAH. Favorable response to medical therapy frequently delays or obviates the need for transplantation. For refractory cases, atrial septostomy can provide significant palliation and serve as a bridge to transplant. For patients with CTEPH and proximal clot, PEA rather than transplantation is usually the surgical option of choice. The diagnosis, assessment, and management of PAH remain complex, underpinning the need to provide care for such patients via specialist centers.

REFERENCES

1. Christie JD, Edwards LB, Aurora P, et al. Registry of the International Society for Heart and Lung Transplantation: twenty-fifth official adult lung and heart/

lung transplantation report–2008. J Heart Lung Transplant 2008;27:957–69.

2. D'Alonzo GE, Barst RJ, Ayres SM, et al. Survival in patients with primary pulmonary hypertension. Results from a national prospective registry. Ann Intern Med 1991;115:343–9.

3. Fuster V, Steele PM, Edwards WD, et al. Primary pulmonary hypertension: natural history and importance of thrombosis. Circulation 1984;70:580–7.

4. Miyamoto S, Nagaya N, Satoh T, et al. Clinical correlates and prognostic significance of six-minute walk test in patients with primary pulmonary hypertension. Comparison with cardiopulmonary exercise testing. Am J Respir Crit Care Med 2000; 161:487–92.

5. Wensel R, Opitz CF, Anker SD, et al. Assessment of survival in patients with primary pulmonary hypertension: importance of cardiopulmonary exercise testing. Circulation 2002;106:319–24.

6. Yeo TC, Dujardin KS, Tei C, et al. Value of a Doppler-derived index combining systolic and diastolic time intervals in predicting outcome in primary pulmonary hypertension. Am J Cardiol 1998;81:1157–61.

7. Forfia PR, Fisher MR, Mathai SC, et al. Tricuspid annular displacement predicts survival in pulmonary hypertension. Am J Respir Crit Care Med 2006;174: 1034–41.

8. Nagaya N, Nishikimi T, Okano Y, et al. Plasma brain natriuretic peptide levels increase in proportion to the extent of right ventricular dysfunction in pulmonary hypertension. J Am Coll Cardiol 1998;31:202–8.

9. Fijalkowska A, Kurzyna M, Torbicki A, et al. Serum N-terminal brain natriuretic peptide as a prognostic parameter in patients with pulmonary hypertension. Chest 2006;129:1313–21.

10. Torbicki A, Kurzyna M, Kuca P, et al. Detectable serum cardiac troponin T as a marker of poor prognosis among patients with chronic precapillary pulmonary hypertension. Circulation 2003;108:844–8.

11. Sitbon O, Humbert M, Nunes H, et al. Long-term intravenous epoprostenol infusion in primary pulmonary hypertension: prognostic factors and survival. J Am Coll Cardiol 2002;40:780–8.

12. McLaughlin VV, Shillington A, Rich S. Survival in primary pulmonary hypertension: the impact of epoprostenol therapy. Circulation 2002;106:1477–82.

13. Provencher S, Sitbon O, Humbert M, et al. Long-term outcome with first-line bosentan therapy in idiopathic pulmonary arterial hypertension. Eur Heart J 2006;27:589–95.

14. Friedman R, Mears JG, Barst RJ. Continuous infusion of prostacyclin normalizes plasma markers of endothelial cell injury and platelet aggregation in primary pulmonary hypertension. Circulation 1997; 96:2782–4.

15. Mandegar M, Fung YC, Huang W, et al. Cellular and molecular mechanisms of pulmonary vascular remodeling: role in the development of pulmonary hypertension. Microvasc Res 2004;68:75–103.

16. Christman BW, McPherson CD, Newman JH, et al. An imbalance between the excretion of thromboxane and prostacyclin metabolites in pulmonary hypertension. N Engl J Med 1992;327:70–5.

17. Higenbottam T, Wheeldon D, Wells F, et al. Long-term treatment of primary pulmonary hypertension with continuous intravenous epoprostenol (prostacyclin). Lancet 1984;1:1046–7.

18. Rubin LJ, Mendoza J, Hood M, et al. Treatment of primary pulmonary hypertension with continuous intravenous prostacyclin (epoprostenol). Results of a randomized trial. Ann Intern Med 1990;112:485–91.

19. Barst RJ, Rubin LJ, Long WA, et al. A comparison of continuous intravenous epoprostenol (prostacyclin) with conventional therapy for primary pulmonary hypertension. The Primary Pulmonary Hypertension Study Group. N Engl J Med 1996;334:296–302.

20. Robbins IM, Christman BW, Newman JH, et al. A survey of diagnostic practices and the use of epoprostenol in patients with primary pulmonary hypertension. Chest 1998;114:1269–75.

21. Conte JV, Gaine SP, Orens JB, et al. The influence of continuous intravenous prostacyclin therapy for primary pulmonary hypertension on the timing and outcome of transplantation. J Heart Lung Transplant 1998;17:679–85.

22. Badesch DB, Tapson VF, McGoon MD, et al. Continuous intravenous epoprostenol for pulmonary hypertension due to the scleroderma spectrum of disease. A randomized, controlled trial. Ann Intern Med 2000;132:425–34.

23. Rosenzweig EB, Kerstein D, Barst RJ. Long-term prostacyclin for pulmonary hypertension with associated congenital heart defects. Circulation 1999; 99:1858–65.

24. Higenbottam T, Butt AY, McMahon A, et al. Long-term intravenous prostaglandin (epoprostenol or iloprost) for treatment of severe pulmonary hypertension. Heart 1998;80:151–5.

25. Kuo PC, Johnson LB, Plotkin JS, et al. Continuous intravenous infusion of epoprostenol for the treatment of portopulmonary hypertension. Transplantation 1997;63:604–6.

26. Aguilar RV, Farber HW. Epoprostenol (prostacyclin) therapy in HIV-associated pulmonary hypertension. Am J Respir Crit Care Med 2000;162:1846–50.

27. Rich S, McLaughlin VV. The effects of chronic prostacyclin therapy on cardiac output and symptoms in primary pulmonary hypertension. J Am Coll Cardiol 1999;34:1184–7.

28. Simonneau G, Barst RJ, Galie N, et al. Continuous subcutaneous infusion of treprostinil, a prostacyclin analogue, in patients with pulmonary arterial hypertension: a double-blind, randomized, placebo-controlled trial. Am J Respir Crit Care Med 2002;165:800–4.

29. Vachiery JL, Hill N, Zwicke D, et al. Transitioning from IV epoprostenol to subcutaneous treprostinil in pulmonary arterial hypertension. Chest 2002; 121:1561–5.

30. Gomberg-Maitland M, Tapson VF, Benza RL, et al. Transition from intravenous epoprostenol to intravenous treprostinil in pulmonary hypertension. Am J Respir Crit Care Med 2005;172:1586–9.

31. Sitbon O, Manes A, Jais X, et al. Rapid switch from intravenous epoprostenol to intravenous treprostinil in patients with pulmonary arterial hypertension. J Cardiovasc Pharmacol 2007;49:1–5.

32. Tapson VF, Gomberg-Maitland M, McLaughlin VV, et al. Safety and efficacy of IV treprostinil for pulmonary arterial hypertension: a prospective, multicenter, open-label, 12-week trial. Chest 2006;129: 683–8.

33. McLaughlin VV, Benza RL, Rubin LJ, et al. Addition of inhaled treprostinil to oral therapy for pulmonary arterial hypertension: a randomized controlled clinical trial. J Am Coll Cardiol 2010; 55:1915–22.

34. Olschewski H, Simonneau G, Galie N, et al. Inhaled iloprost for severe pulmonary hypertension. N Engl J Med 2002;347:322–9.

35. Gessler T, Schmehl T, Hoeper MM, et al. Ultrasonic versus jet nebulization of iloprost in severe pulmonary hypertension. Eur Respir J 2001;17:14–9.

36. McLaughlin VV, Oudiz RJ, Frost A, et al. Randomized study of adding inhaled iloprost to existing bosentan in pulmonary arterial hypertension. Am J Respir Crit Care Med 2006;174:1257–63.

37. Channick RN, Simonneau G, Sitbon O, et al. Effects of the dual endothelin-receptor antagonist bosentan in patients with pulmonary hypertension: a randomised placebo-controlled study. Lancet 2001;358: 1119–23.

38. Rubin LJ, Badesch DB, Barst RJ, et al. Bosentan therapy for pulmonary arterial hypertension. N Engl J Med 2002;346:896–903.

39. Galie N, Rubin L, Hoeper M, et al. Treatment of patients with mildly symptomatic pulmonary arterial hypertension with bosentan (EARLY study): a double-blind, randomised controlled trial. Lancet 2008;371:2093–100.

40. Galie N, Beghetti M, Gatzoulis MA, et al. Bosentan therapy in patients with Eisenmenger syndrome: a multicenter, double-blind, randomized, placebo-controlled study. Circulation 2006;114:48–54.

41. Fattinger K, Funk C, Pantze M, et al. The endothelin antagonist bosentan inhibits the canalicular bile salt export pump: a potential mechanism for hepatic adverse reactions. Clin Pharmacol Ther 2001;69: 223–31.

42. Barst RJ, Langleben D, Frost A, et al. Sitaxsentan therapy for pulmonary arterial hypertension. Am J Respir Crit Care Med 2004;169:441–7.

43. Barst RJ, Langleben D, Badesch D, et al. Treatment of pulmonary arterial hypertension with the selective endothelin-A receptor antagonist sitaxsentan. J Am Coll Cardiol 2006;16(47):2049–56.

44. Galiè N, Olschewski H, Oudiz RJ, et al. Ambrisentan for the treatment of pulmonary arterial hypertension: results of the ambrisentan in pulmonary arterial hypertension, randomized, double-blind, placebo-controlled, multicenter, efficacy (ARIES) study 1 and 2. Circulation 2008;117:3010–9.

45. Galie N, Ghofrani HA, Torbicki A, et al. Sildenafil citrate therapy for pulmonary arterial hypertension. N Engl J Med 2005;353:2148–57.

46. Barst RJ, Brundage BH, Ghofrani A, et al. Tadalafil improves exercise capacity, health-related quality of life and delays time to clinical worsening in patients with symptomatic pulmonary arterial hypertension. Chest 2008;134:s39003.

47. Macchia A, Marchioli R, Marfisi R, et al. A meta-analysis of trials of pulmonary hypertension: a clinical condition looking for drugs and research methodology. Am Heart J 2007;153:1037–47.

48. Galie N, Manes A, Negro L, et al. A meta-analysis of randomized controlled trials in pulmonary arterial hypertension. Eur Heart J 2009;30:394–403.

49. Jing ZC, Xu XQ, Han ZY, et al. Registry and survival study in chinese patients with idiopathic and familial pulmonary arterial hypertension. Chest 2007;132: 373–9.

50. Rich S, Kaufmann E, Levy PS. The effects of high doses of calcium channel blockers on survival in primary pulmonary hypertension. N Engl J Med 1992;327:76–81.

51. Lang I, Gomez-Sanchez M, Kneussl M, et al. Efficacy of long-term subcutaneous treprostinil sodium therapy in pulmonary hypertension. Chest 2006; 129:1636–43.

52. Opitz CF, Wensel R, Winkler J, et al. Clinical efficacy and survival with first-line inhaled iloprost therapy in patients with idiopathic pulmonary arterial hypertension. Eur Heart J 2005;26:1895–902.

53. Hoeper MM, Gall H, Seyfarth HJ, et al. Long-term outcome with intravenous iloprost in pulmonary arterial hypertension. Eur Respir J 2009;34(1):132–7.

54. Denton CP, Humbert M, Rubin L, et al. Bosentan treatment for pulmonary arterial hypertension related to connective tissue disease: a subgroup analysis of the pivotal clinical trials and their open-label extensions. Ann Rheum Dis 2006;65:1336–40.

55. McLaughlin VV, Sitbon O, Badesch DB, et al. Survival with first-line bosentan in patients with primary pulmonary hypertension. Eur Respir J 2005;25:244–9.

56. Keogh AM, McNeil KD, Wlodarczyk J, et al. Quality of life in pulmonary arterial hypertension: improvement and maintenance with bosentan. J Heart Lung Transplant 2007;26:181–7.

57. Williams MH, Das C, Handler CE, et al. Systemic sclerosis associated pulmonary hypertension: improved survival in the current era. Heart 2006;92:926–32.

58. Adriaenssens T, Delcroix M, Van Deyk K, et al. Advanced therapy may delay the need for transplantation in patients with the Eisenmenger syndrome. Eur Heart J 2006;27:1472–7.

59. Dandel M, Lehmkuhl HB, Mulahasanovic S, et al. Survival of patients with idiopathic pulmonary arterial hypertension after listing for transplantation: impact of iloprost and bosentan treatment. J Heart Lung Transplant 2007;26:898–906.

60. Tankersley MA, D'Albini LD, Ozanich AN, et al. A 36-month survival analysis of patients beginning oral PAH monotherapy: an indication for escalation of therapy? Houston (TX): PHA; 2008.

61. Glanville AR, Burke CM, Theodore J, et al. Primary pulmonary hypertension. Length of survival in patients referred for heart–lung transplantation. Chest 1987;91:675–81.

62. Hopkins WE, Ochoa LL, Richardson GW, et al. Comparison of the hemodynamics and survival of adults with severe primary pulmonary hypertension or Eisenmenger syndrome. J Heart Lung Transplant 1996;15:100–5.

63. Sandoval J, Gaspar J, Pulido T, et al. Graded balloon dilation atrial septostomy in severe primary pulmonary hypertension. A therapeutic alternative for patients nonresponsive to vasodilator treatment. J Am Coll Cardiol 1998;32:297–304.

64. Kerstein D, Levy PS, Hsu DT, et al. Blade balloon atrial septostomy in patients with severe primary pulmonary hypertension. Circulation 1995;91: 2028–35.

65. Kurzyna M, Dabrowski M, Bielecki D, et al. Atrial septostomy in treatment of end-stage right heart failure in patients with pulmonary hypertension. Chest 2007;131:977–83.

66. Troost E, Delcroix M, Gewillig M, et al. A modified technique of stent fenestration of the interatrial septum improves patients with pulmonary hypertension. Catheter Cardiovasc Interv 2009;73:173–9.

67. Rothman A, Sklansky MS, Lucas VW, et al. Atrial septostomy as a bridge to lung transplantation in patients with severe pulmonary hypertension. Am J Cardiol 1999;84:682–6.

68. Badesch DB, Abman SH, Simonneau G, et al. Medical therapy for pulmonary arterial hypertension: updated ACCP evidence-based clinical practice guidelines. Chest 2007;131:1917–28.

69. Galie N, Torbicki A, Barst R, et al. Guidelines on diagnosis and treatment of pulmonary arterial hypertension. The task force on diagnosis and treatment of pulmonary arterial hypertension of the European Society of Cardiology. Eur Heart J 2004;25:2243–78.

70. Daily PO, Dembitsky WP, Iversen S. Technique of pulmonary thromboendarterectomy for chronic pulmonary embolism. J Card Surg 1989;4:10–24.

71. Jamieson SW, Auger WR, Fedullo PF, et al. Experience and results with 150 pulmonary thromboendarterectomy operations over a 29-month period. J Thorac Cardiovasc Surg 1993;106:116–26.

72. Dartevelle P, Fadel E, Chapelier A, et al. Angioscopic video-assisted pulmonary endarterectomy for postembolic pulmonary hypertension. Eur J Cardiothorac Surg 1999;16:38–43.

73. Thomson B, Tsui SS, Dunning J, et al. Pulmonary endarterectomy is possible and effective without the use of complete circulatory arrest—the UK experience in over 150 patients. Eur J Cardiothorac Surg 2008;33:157–63.

74. Kim NH, Fesler P, Channick RN, et al. Preoperative partitioning of pulmonary vascular resistance correlates with early outcome after thromboendarterectomy for chronic thromboembolic pulmonary hypertension. Circulation 2004;109:18–22.

75. Skoro-Sajer N, Bonderman D, Wiesbauer F, et al. Treprostinil for severe inoperable chronic thromboembolic pulmonary hypertension. J Thromb Haemost 2007;5:483–9.

76. Riedel M, Stanek V, Widimsky J, et al. Long-term follow-up of patients with pulmonary thromboembolism. Late prognosis and evolution of hemodynamic and respiratory data. Chest 1982;81:151–8.

77. Lewczuk J, Piszko P, Jagas J, et al. Prognostic factors in medically treated patients with chronic pulmonary embolism. Chest 2001;119:818–23.

78. Archibald CJ, Auger WR, Fedullo PF, et al. Long-term outcome after pulmonary thromboendarterectomy. Am J Respir Crit Care Med 1999;160: 523–8.

79. Bresser P, Fedullo PF, Auger WR, et al. Continuous intravenous epoprostenol for chronic thromboembolic pulmonary hypertension. Eur Respir J 2004; 23:595–600.

80. Jais X, D'Armini AM, Jansa P, et al. Bosentan for treatment of inoperable chronic thromboembolic pulmonary hypertension: BENEFiT (Bosentan Effects in iNopErable Forms of chronIc Thromboembolic pulmonary hypertension), a randomized, placebo-controlled trial. J Am Coll Cardiol 2008;52: 2127–34.

81. Suntharalingam J, Treacy CM, Doughty NJ, et al. Long-term use of sildenafil in inoperable chronic thromboembolic pulmonary hypertension. Chest 2008;134:229–36.

82. Reichenberger F, Voswinckel R, Enke B, et al. Long-term treatment with sildenafil in chronic thromboembolic pulmonary hypertension. Eur Respir J 2007;30: 922–7.

Index

Note: Page numbers of article titles are in **boldface** type.

Clin Chest Med 32 (2011) 411–416
doi:10.1016/S0272-5231(11)00039-6
0272-5231/11/$ – see front matter © 2011 Elsevier Inc. All rights reserved

Printed and bound by CPI Group (UK) Ltd, Croydon, CR0 4YY

03/10/2024

01040359-0001